Mental Health in Historical Perspective

Series Editors
Catharine Coleborne
School of Humanities and Social Science
University of Newcastle
Callaghan, NSW, Australia

Matthew Smith
History of Psychiatry
University of Strathclyde
Glasgow, UK

Covering all historical periods and geographical contexts, the series explores how mental illness has been understood, experienced, diagnosed, treated and contested. It will publish works that engage actively with contemporary debates related to mental health and, as such, will be of interest not only to historians, but also mental health professionals, patients and policy makers. With its focus on mental health, rather than just psychiatry, the series will endeavour to provide more patient-centred histories. Although this has long been an aim of health historians, it has not been realised, and this series aims to change that.

The scope of the series is kept as broad as possible to attract good quality proposals about all aspects of the history of mental health from all periods. The series emphasises interdisciplinary approaches to the field of study, and encourages short titles, longer works, collections, and titles which stretch the boundaries of academic publishing in new ways.

More information about this series at
http://www.springer.com/series/14806

Alice Mauger

The Cost of Insanity in Nineteenth-Century Ireland

Public, Voluntary and Private Asylum Care

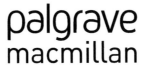

palgrave
macmillan

Alice Mauger
Centre for the History of Medicine in
  Ireland, School of History
University College Dublin
Dublin, Ireland

Mental Health in Historical Perspective
ISBN 978-3-319-65243-6   ISBN 978-3-319-65244-3   (eBook)
https://doi.org/10.1007/978-3-319-65244-3

Library of Congress Control Number: 2017949204

Cover credit: © book cover art Joana Kruse/Alamy Stock Photo

Printed on acid-free paper

This Palgrave Macmillan imprint is published by Springer Nature
The registered company is Springer International Publishing AG
The registered company address is: Gewerbestrasse 11, 6330 Cham, Switzerland

In Memory of my Mother, Mary

Acknowledgements

This book is the product of the immense levels of support and encouragement given to me over the last few years, not just in University College Dublin, where I studied, but in archives, other universities and at home. Dr. Catherine Cox was a constant source of guidance, providing me with the essential and thought-provoking feedback, comments and criticism she is uniquely qualified to make. I would also particularly like to thank Dr. Lindsey Earner-Byrne, for her kindness, thoroughness and professional insights into all my academic pursuits and her continued interest and support. In addition, I am indebted to my colleagues who have worked at the School of History and Archives and the Centre for the History of Medicine in Ireland at University College Dublin for their stimulating academic conversations, helpful advice and friendship. These include Drs. Anne Mac Lellan, David Durnin, Fiachra Byrne, Richard McElligott, Sarah York, Niamh NicGhabhann, Sean Lucey, Philomena Gorey, Clara Cullen, Claire Poinsot, Ian Miller and Keith Smith, and my former colleagues at William Fry, including Maria Butler and Deirdre McGuinness. I am also indebted to everyone who has provided feedback, comments and questions at the various places I presented my work. I am especially grateful to the Wellcome Trust, who kindly funded both my master's and doctoral studies and made it possible for me to spend periods of time in different parts of Ireland conducting research and to share it with colleagues abroad. Thanks also to the editorial team at Palgrave MacMillan, especially Molly Beck and the anonymous reviewer for their generous and insightful feedback on drafts of this manuscript.

The archival research, which forms the basis of this book, would not have been possible without the confidence vested in me by those who granted me access to the nineteenth-century records of nine Irish psychiatric hospitals. I am extremely grateful to these individuals and collectives, who include Emma Balmaine, Sile McManus, Stewarts' Ethics Committee and the HSE. I would especially like to thank Dr. Denis Eustace, who not only took the time to meet with me and grant me access to his treasure trove of historic records but also provided me with his keen insight and unparalleled knowledge of Hampstead and Highfield Houses. His tour of the demesne, encompassing its unspoiled nineteenth-century pleasure grounds, really brought to life for me the history I was writing.

Archival research would have proven rather isolating and daunting were it not for the kindness, patience and immeasurable assistance of the archivists, librarians and records keepers at the various places I worked. They include Brian Donnelly and Gregory O'Connor at the National Archives of Ireland, Gráinne Doran at the Wexford County Council Archive Service, Irene Franklin at Clare County Council, Richard Bennett at Grangegorman Museum, Glynn and Shirley Douglas and all the gang at the Friend's Historical Library in Rathfarnham, Joan Rappel and Sean Priestly at Stewarts, Kate McCallion at St John of God Hospital and Harriet Wheelock at the Royal College of Physicians of Ireland. Their inspiring suggestions and interest in my research made archival visits an enjoyable and productive pursuit and were a testament to their dedication in furthering the study of Irish history. Many went beyond their call of duty, providing me with transport to and from archives and even lunch! I would also like to thank the staff at the National Archives of Ireland, the National Archives (Kew), the National Library of Ireland and the Public Records Office Northern Ireland.

I want to thank all my close friends and my family, especially Ralph Mauger, Jack and Emma Carroll, and Catherine, Philip and Sophie Mitchell. Their endurance and encouragement have been unwavering and I am forever indebted to them. I would not be where I am today without the guidance, love and support of my mother, Mary, who always believed in me. Finally, thanks to Richard for his unceasing patience, direction and moral support, and for being my best friend.

Alice Mauger

CONTENTS

Abbreviations

CCA	Clare Country Archives
CSORP	Chief Secretary's Office Registered Papers
FHL	Friend's Historical Library, Rathfarnham, Dublin
GM	Grangegorman Museum
NAI	National Archives of Ireland
PRONI	Public Records Office of Northern Ireland
SJOGH	St. John of God Hospital
WCC	Wexford County Council

LIST OF FIGURES

LIST OF TABLES

CHAPTER 1

Introduction

Recent decades have witnessed growing fascination with the development of Irish mental healthcare.[1] Scholars have delved into nineteenth-century records to uncover astonishingly colourful and detailed accounts of institutionalisation. Their studies have recaptured the very fabric of asylum life: the sort of people committed, their behaviour, the treatments they received and their experiences and views of incarceration. The emerging pictures tend to be punctuated by staff violence, filth, overcrowding and a mounting pessimism about medicine's ability to cure 'insanity'. In spite of this undeniable progress in reclaiming the history of Ireland's mentally ill and their caregivers, scholarship has focused overwhelmingly on the poor.

This tendency arguably reflects a historical reality. Those admitted to asylums, but not as paupers, were relatively few. Yet by shifting our focus away from the poor and assessing the assortment of care options for other social groups, we can gain vivid insights into how families from a variety of social backgrounds coped with mental illness. A far cry from Charlotte Brontë's 'madwoman in the attic', more than one of Ireland's asylums was kept exclusively for respectable ladies. As this book will reveal, the sense of class identity and social status shared by families, along with their collective spending power, had overwhelming consequences for patients' care and treatment. The high importance rural Irish families placed on property—especially land—lends to this study a particularly interesting dimension. This book interrogates the popular notion that relatives were routinely locked away to be deprived of land

© The Author(s) 2018
A. Mauger, *The Cost of Insanity in Nineteenth-Century Ireland*, Mental Health in Historical Perspective,
https://doi.org/10.1007/978-3-319-65244-3_1

or inheritance and queries how often "land grabbing" Irish families really abused the asylum system for personal economic gain.

Focusing on Britain, wide-ranging and sophisticated studies have grappled with non-pauper patients' institutionalisation, diagnosis, experience and treatment.[2] But save for Elizabeth Malcolm's study of Dublin's Swift's Hospital, their Irish counterparts have been awarded little more than a supporting role.[3] This may be rooted in an expectation that the Irish experience differed little from Britain's. Ireland and Britain, after all, had forceful political and cultural ties. As Mark Finnane noted in his highly regarded exploration of Ireland's public asylum system, 'the Irish government was, of course, the English government in Ireland'.[4] Moreover, some historians have convincingly suggested that post-Famine Ireland was mid-Victorian, at least where the absorption of Victorian attitudes towards living standards, devotional routine and the decline of the Irish language were concerned.[5] Nonetheless, to assume that Ireland is unworthy of separate investigation would be to ignore key disparities between Ireland and Britain. These include Ireland's overwhelmingly rural character, greater poverty levels and prominent religious and political divisions, which permeated the welfare landscape and resulted in Catholic and Protestant controlled hospitals. This book builds on existing surveys of Ireland's lunatic asylums by arguing that a myriad of political, religious, economic and socio-cultural factors came to define public, voluntary and private provision, creating a uniquely Irish institutional framework. It also considers the type of people institutionalised, their expectations of asylum life and the roles played by families, communities and doctors in their care and treatment.

Case Studies

To address these questions, nine asylums were selected as case studies. These were the three private asylums, Hampstead House, Highfield House and St John of God's; two voluntary asylums, Bloomfield Retreat and Stewarts Institution; and the four district asylums at Belfast, Ennis, Enniscorthy and Dublin (Richmond). Together these hospitals housed patients from urban and rural settings in the north, south, east and west of the country. Of the nine asylums, six were in Dublin, reflecting the geographical concentration of private and voluntary care in Ireland's capital.

Nineteenth-century Ireland, subject to a quasi-colonial administration in Dublin Castle (1801–1922), famine, massive land-agitation, emigration and, at the end of the century, an enduring economic depression (c. 1879–1895), lends a stimulating backdrop. From 1801 until the Great Famine (c. 1845–1850), the rising middle classes began to gain a footing in both urban and rural Ireland. When Irish peers and the richest gentry steadily withdrew from Dublin after the union (1801), this vacuum was filled by the rising professional classes, especially lawyers and physicians.[6] From the eighteenth century, Dublin had become a key player in medical education and by the mid-nineteenth century had numerous teaching hospitals and medical schools as well as being home to the Irish medical colleges.[7] In this era, the focus of power had shifted from the Protestant ascendancy towards Catholics, who gradually came to control local politics and, to a lesser degree, Dublin's businesses and professions.[8] In relation to occupational profile, late nineteenth-century Dublin was much closer to London than any other English or Irish provincial city.[9] Several industries also registered steady progress in Dublin, including flour milling, brewing and textiles.[10] Of course, like other cities in the United Kingdom, there also existed extreme poverty and Dublin's poorest inhabitants fell victim to contagious diseases, poor sanitation, tenement accommodation and overcrowding.[11]

But Dublin remained both geographically and demographically isolated from the rest of Ireland. While the north-east of Ireland and particularly Belfast continued to industrialise and areas such as Cork in the south of Ireland urbanised, a staggering residual population inhabited the 'very backward', 'little urbanised or industrialised' and 'over-populated' landscape of rural Ireland.[12] In rural communities, there were immense inequalities in income and holding size prior to the Famine.[13] While the effects of the Famine on Ireland's population are well known, there is a lesser-told tale underlying the more common chronicles of death, disease and economic downturn. Although some landlords suffered from declining net incomes and land values, others held fast to their position and even as late as the 1880s, almost half of Ireland comprised estates of 5000 acres or more owned by only 700 landlords.[14] While this was taking place, a middling class of farmer, not poles apart from his British equivalent, began to strengthen his position in rural Ireland.[15] The smaller tenants and cottiers who suffered during the Famine paved the way for a more successful commercial farmer. In post-Famine Ireland, the growing non-renewal of long leases meant an increasing consolidation of farmland, which in turn engendered a rural landscape not dissimilar in appearance to Britain.[16] In the words of R.V. Comerford, 'the newly progressing—if not universally prosperous—multitudes of rural society were ready for a lifestyle more obviously "respectable" than that of their parents'.[17]

Post-Famine rural Ireland saw greater social diversity than previous eras, with the increased visibility of a growing middle class. The extension of railways and introduction of bank branches to rural towns attracted people with reasonably paid jobs, while growing numbers of specialised retail shops 'gave an air of progress, even modest affluence, to the streets'. Those who prospered included managers, shopkeepers, bankers, professional men, administrators and the upper levels of skilled artisans.[18] Landless labourers, unskilled or semi-skilled industrial workers and the unemployed, however, were more precariously positioned and for many, emigration offered the most hopeful future.[19] Thus, after the Famine, the landscape inhabited by Irish asylums had undergone dramatic changes. This trend continued following the Land Wars of the late nineteenth century, which brought about a decline in landlords' incomes and a gradual emergence of land ownership among peasants.[20] From 1879, Ireland experienced an agricultural depression that affected most areas of the economy.[21] These shifts, along with the cultural and political upheaval of the nineteenth century, had complex ramifications for the institutions and actors at the centre of this story.

Within this setting, Irish asylum care flourished. In 1817, the state authorised the creation of public asylums intended exclusively for the 'lunatic poor' and these institutions, which became known as district asylums, quickly expanded beyond all expectations.[22] By 1830, four district asylums housed some 300 patients; by 1900, twenty-two accommodated almost 16,000.[23] Importantly, these asylums preceded their English and Welsh equivalents, predating the Poor Law and falling instead under the direct control of central government. This fashioned the criteria for those eligible for relief. While the substantial accommodation in workhouse lunatic wards from the 1840s was restricted to the destitute, the only requirement for entering a district asylum was a certificate of poverty, which stated that neither the patient nor their family or 'friends' could afford accommodation in a private asylum. As a result, most of the patients committed to district asylums were considered poor but not destitute.[24]

By the 1840s, national and local lunacy administrators came under increasing pressure due to overcrowding and high admissions rates to district asylums. The continuing expansion of this system on a scale seemingly far higher than elsewhere in the United Kingdom provoked debates and anxieties about Irish susceptibility to mental illness.[25] Against this backdrop, care options for the non-pauper insane began to increase. In 1870, new rules allowing paying patients into district asylums were introduced. Private asylums catered for a much smaller pool of potential patients. In 1830, seven private asylums housed 117 patients and by 1900, only 306 patients resided in thirteen such institutions.[26] While parishes in England and Wales often boarded-out paupers in private asylums,[27] the Irish Poor Law was never allowed to adopt this practice, partly because the public system had been established earlier there. This, combined with the expense of private asylum care, was the principal reason why Irish private asylums remained comparatively small, catering instead for primarily wealthier clients.[28]

Meanwhile, four separate charitable asylums were founded from the bequests and donations of various philanthropic groups interested in lunacy. These voluntary institutions, often termed 'mixed' because they admitted both charity and private patients, were considered distinct from private asylums because their managing bodies did not profit from patient fees. Instead, any surplus funds were diverted towards the care of less wealthy patients or improvements to the accommodation provided. Although these voluntary hospitals eventually housed more patients than the private asylums, they remained small compared with the district system. In 1830, two voluntary asylums accommodated 154 patients; by 1900, there were four catering for 403 patients.[29]

Together, the records of the nine selected institutions are the foundations for this book's exploration of public, voluntary and private asylum care. The three private asylums, Hampstead House, its sister asylum, Highfield House, and the Hospital of St John of God, were in Dublin City's suburbs. Hampstead was founded in 1825, when Drs. John Eustace, Isaac Ryall and Richard Grattan formed a partnership to manage it. Ryall purchased the property on the north side of Dublin, which included Hampstead House, and co-leased the house and an acre of land to Grattan and Eustace.[30] Ryall left the partnership the following year and a new contract was drawn up between Eustace and Grattan for the joint ownership of Hampstead. A further twenty-three acres were leased in 1836, and in 1862, all of Hampstead's female patients were removed to the nearby Highfield House, which occupied the same demesne. Both Hampstead and Highfield remained small. Within five years of opening, Hampstead had only thirteen patients; by 1900, Hampstead had twelve male patients and Highfield had eighteen female patients.[31] Based in the south Dublin suburb of Stillorgan, St John of God's had its origins in the arrival of members of the Hospitaller Order of St John of God from France in 1877. Members of this order, which had a tradition of caring for the mentally ill, established and gave their name to the private asylum in 1885.[32] St John of God's was run by these religious brothers and admitted only men. In contrast to Hampstead and Highfield, it quickly became one of the largest private asylums in Ireland. Within five years of opening, twenty-nine patients resided at St John of God's and by 1900, there were seventy-six.[33]

The two voluntary asylums selected for study are the Bloomfield Retreat and Stewarts Institution, also located in Dublin's suburbs. Members of the Society of Friends founded the Bloomfield Retreat in Donnybrook in 1812. Society members supported this asylum through donations and subscriptions and were also allowed to nominate charity patients, while a committee composed of Society members managed the asylum.[34] This managing committee modelled Bloomfield on the principles developed at the York Retreat in England, where the Tuke family had famously advocated moral therapy (see Chaps. 5, 6 and 7).[35] Like the York Retreat, Bloomfield was small by national standards. Within five years of opening, Bloomfield had only eleven patients and by 1900, there were thirty-three.[36]

The other voluntary asylum chosen was originally called the Lucan Spa but was renamed Stewarts Institution in the 1870s after its proprietor, Dr. Henry Hutchinson Stewart, a medical doctor and philanthropist with an especial interest in the welfare of the insane.[37] Following the introduction of the Poor Law in 1838, he became a governor of the Hardwicke Hospital, which housed chronic pauper lunatics. This hospital had formed part of the House of Industry in North Brunswick Street, Dublin, which was remodelled as the North Union Workhouse. No further patients were admitted to the Hardwicke and by 1856, its remaining chronic patients had been transferred to a former military barracks at Islandbridge, Dublin.[38] The following year, Stewart purchased the former Spa Hotel in Lucan and transferred the 102 Islandbridge patients under his charge to these premises.[39] Vacancies arose as these mainly elderly patients died and Stewart began to admit paying patients of an 'intermediate class' at a 'moderate rate' of payment. By 1867, there were thirty-seven paying patients along with the sixty-two remaining Islandbridge patients.[40] Despite his best efforts, demand for accommodation persistently outstripped supply and in the same year, Stewart wrote that he had 'constantly been obliged to refuse patients for want of room'.[41]

Around this time, Stewart became interested in the plight of 'idiot' children and this had lasting consequences for his asylum. In 1865, Dr. George Kidd, the editor of the *Dublin Quarterly Journal of Medical Science* (1863–1868) published an appeal in that journal for the establishment of an institution for 'idiotic' children.[42] Kidd, who would later become an obstetric surgeon (1868–1875), assistant master (1875–1876) and finally master (1876–1883) at the Coombe Lying-In Hospital in Dublin, was sensitive to the needs of 'idiot' children and visited asylums in Scotland and England in 1865.[43] The following year, Kidd and Stewart formed part of a committee to establish a special institution for the education of 'idiot' children and the two men co-founded a children's institution.[44] A property adjacent to the Lucan Spa asylum was acquired and admitted the first twelve children in 1869. The committee took charge of both the asylum and the children's institution and Stewart agreed to divert the asylum's profits to the latter.[45] While the children's branch catered for both charity and private patients, the asylum reserved its accommodation for paying patients.[46] In the early 1870s, the committee purchased a new site in nearby Palmerstown and building work commenced. Once completed, patients from both the children's institution and the Lucan Spa asylum were transferred to this new facility, which was, at this point, named the Stewarts Institution.[47] Stewarts was principally devoted to caring for 'idiot' children but in the late 1890s, the accommodation for private patients was greatly enlarged. By 1900, there were sixty-two private patients and ninety-six 'imbecile' patients.[48] With the exception of St John of God's, both the private and voluntary asylums in this study had a Protestant ethos and, accordingly, accommodated mainly patients who were Church of Ireland (see Chaps. 2 and 4).

The last Dublin-based asylum was the Richmond district asylum (est. 1815), known in more recent years as Grangegorman. While Richmond served the bordering counties of Wicklow and Louth, its primary catchment area was Dublin City and County and most of the paying patients admitted came from Dublin. The other three district asylums selected were in Belfast (est. 1829), Ennis (est. 1868) and Enniscorthy (est. 1868). Belfast, an industrial city located in the north of Ireland, had, by the end of the nineteenth century, overtaken Dublin to become Ireland's largest city and had the country's largest port. Internationally renowned for its strong shipbuilding industry, including Harland and Wolff, Belfast was also host to expanding textiles industries in the later part of the century and had a higher proportion of skilled workers, higher female participation rates and higher incomes than Dublin.[49] The religious profile of Belfast's population was at odds with other cities in Ireland, with a comparatively high proportion of members of the Church of Ireland and Presbyterians, and this is mirrored among the asylum's paying patients.[50] Ennis, a small town in the rural west of Ireland, experienced a short-lived retail boom in the immediate aftermath of the Famine. Although the railway was extended to Ennis from the neighbouring city of Limerick in 1859, both the town and its surrounding parishes settled into a slow decline from the 1860s, with little opportunity for any significant commercial or industrial development or the expansion of local trades.[51] Enniscorthy, a town in the more prosperous County Wexford in the rural south-east of Ireland, had strong trade compared with towns like Ennis. Wexford was also traditionally one of the wealthier farming areas in Ireland and boasted many large estates as well as smaller holdings.[52] These four district asylums differed in size. Richmond and Belfast were mammoth institutions, accommodating some 2200 (forty-nine paying) patients and 1300 (six paying) patients respectively in 1900. By comparison, Enniscorthy and Ennis were moderately sized, housing approximately 450 (twenty-four paying) patients and 380 (twelve paying) patients in the same year.[53]

While the proportion of paying patients in the four district asylums was small, their numbers equalled those in many of the smaller private and voluntary asylums in this era, revealing that district asylums had become an important form of care for non-paupers. Meanwhile, accommodation for paying patients had greatly increased within the private and voluntary sectors from 270 patients in 1830 to 700 in 1900.[54] This expansion is particularly significant given that the general Irish population had halved between 1845 and 1900. While the immediate consequences of the Famine brought about a dramatic population decline in Ireland through both death and emigration, further depopulation occurred after 1850 when famine conditions had all but disappeared.[55]

CONTEXT

In contrast to the plethora of research on the history of Irish psychiatry, sparse scholarly attention has been devoted to paying patients. Finnane's survey fails to acknowledge the existence of paying patients in the district system. Catherine Cox has briefly outlined the legalisation of paying patients' admission into district asylums and contended that the resulting revenue generated was negligible, yet her discussion of patients in the Enniscorthy and Carlow asylums does not distinguish between paying and pauper patients.[56] Although several scholars have examined the social profile of district asylum patients,[57] few have focused on patients in other asylums.[58] Malcolm's commissioned history of St Patrick's (Swift's) Hospital is the only academic study of a non-public asylum in Ireland. While much of Malcolm's work concerns administrative and financial aspects of the hospital's history, she also examines patients' social profile in the 1870s and 1880s. This analysis, however, falls short of distinguishing between paying and charitable patients.[59] Oonagh Walsh has completed an article-length investigation of the implications of patients' gender on their admission, treatment and discharge in both district and private asylums in nineteenth-century Ireland. Yet her study relies solely on the reports of the lunacy inspectors for her analysis of private patients.[60] My own previous research on the social role of Irish private asylums also focuses primarily on these reports.[61]

This book expands on current scholarship to provide a more rounded and focused study of paying patients in nineteenth-century Ireland. It considers the role of public, voluntary and private asylums and assesses the social profile of paying patients in these sectors. Given the existence of substantial surveys of the pauper insane, much of the research underpinning this book focuses on non-paupers, while comparisons are drawn with existing findings on pauper patient groups. It therefore adds complexity to our understanding of the impact of factors such as class, social status, spending power, religion and gender on patterns of committal, care and treatment in Ireland.

Throughout, comparisons are drawn between Ireland and Britain. Scholarship on British asylums and paying patients has focused mainly on urban and industrial settings.[62] One notable exception is the work of Joseph Melling and Bill Forsythe, which explores public and private mental healthcare in Devon in the largely rural south-west of England.[63] The emphasis on the urban and industrial has its origins in Andrew

Scull's revisionist argument that the institutionalisation of the insane was evidence of bourgeois elites' concerns to regulate insanity within the labouring masses. For Scull, the expansion of the English county asylum system was a consequence of the 'commercialisation of existence', as those who were unable to function in a capitalist market economy were no longer tolerated and essentially 'dumped' in these institutions.[64]

Subsequent counter- and post-revisionist scholarship has revised Scull's model, re-assessing the role of the family in the committal and discharge process and recognising the existence of family bonds.[65] Scholars, including David Wright and, in the Irish context, Finnane, have stressed the importance of the role of the family in identifying mental illness and in committing relatives to asylums.[66] However, Cox has shown that there were limits to the degree of autonomy families enjoyed and that they were 'obliged to negotiate with other actors, including police, magistrates and dispensary doctors, and to operate within specific legal frameworks'.[67] Various studies have also highlighted how predominantly rural Ireland offers a context in which industrially focused models can be challenged.[68] As Scull has acknowledged, his model cannot so readily be applied to rural contexts, arguing, for example, that Wales' 'economic backwardness' meant more traditional modes of care persisted because rural families were less likely to 'dump' inconvenient relatives into asylums.[69] This book engages with these debates, in demonstrating that the families of paying patients negotiated fees with asylum authorities and often had the luxury of selection between the three sectors of asylum care. In doing so, it reveals that families did not simply pay to 'dump' relatives in institutions but, rather, their decision to commit a relative was complicated by property and business interests and the welfare of the entire family unit.

RECORDS

This study investigates a range of sources from government records to medical literature and asylum records. Government sources are indispensable for situating Irish lunacy provision within the wider context of state affairs. At national level, the Irish prison inspectors and, from 1845, the lunacy inspectors were central figures in lunacy administration. These inspectors, based in Dublin Castle, were required to visit all 'receptacles for the insane' and reported annually on their observations. During the nineteenth century, the government also initiated several commissions of inquiry into lunacy provision, the reports of which contain evidence from protagonists including the lunacy inspectors, asylum managing bodies and resident physicians.[70] During these inquiries, interest groups debated, contested and explored the various methods of providing for Ireland's non-pauper insane.

Drawing on admissions registers, casebooks, minute books and annual reports for the nine selected asylums, two databases of paying patients' social profile were compiled for the periods 1826–1867 and 1868–1900. Analysis of this material establishes the sectors of Irish society found in different types of asylums (see Chap. 4). As outlined in Appendix A, for the district asylums, paying patients were identified using admissions registers, minute books and financial accounts and then, through nominal linkage, in the casebooks. By using all available records to identify paying patients, those who were admitted as paupers but were later charged maintenance are captured in the study. Where patients were admitted as paying patients but later maintained at the expense of the asylum, this is noted in discussions of their case histories. The decision was made to include all patients who were charged at one point or another during their stay to highlight the fluidity between paying and pauper patients in the district asylum system.

Chapters 5, 6 and 7 draw heavily on asylum doctors' case notes on patients. Analysis of this source is still a relatively new practice in the history of psychiatry and scholars have adopted differing stances on its credibility.[71] Aside from its time-consuming nature, problems with censorship are rife. While case notes often contain direct statements from patients, friends and relatives, historians including Jonathan Andrews have cautioned that these sources are mediated through the reporting physician, therefore reflecting medical preoccupations and biases.[72] Yet, as Andrews has acknowledged, case notes 'may provide the surest basis we have' for understanding the changing nature of the experience of the insane in asylums since 1800.[73] Certainly, as Hilary Marland has suggested, lay commentary in case notes should not be ignored.[74] In the Irish context, Cox has found that patients, relatives and friends often provided medical and social histories of patients which, while lacking contextual information, can be useful, particularly where they appear in quotations in case notes.[75]

In addition, many scholars have begun to seek out the patient's view in such diverse materials as their letters, accounts by their family and friends, their art and poetry, their diaries and memoirs and even fictional literature on patient experiences.[76] This has largely been in response to Roy Porter's call to arms, in 1985, for a 'patient-orientated history'. Despite the enthusiasm of the 1980s, however, much work remains to be done. Some thirty years after Porter's call, Flurin Condrau observed that the history of the patient's experience was still undeveloped.[77] Patients' letters provide unrivalled insight into their experiences of asylum life. However, where letters have survived, they are often those withheld by the asylum authorities, which might be expected to contain complaints about the asylum, casting it in a disproportionately negative light. Yet, as Allan Beveridge has shown, frequent similarities in patients' responses to the Morningside Asylum in Scotland demand that their 'claims are considered seriously'.[78] In the course of researching this book, several hundred letters were found, mostly appended to case notes.

SOCIAL CLASS IN IRELAND

Defining class boundaries in nineteenth-century Ireland is a difficult, even impenetrable, task, and poses challenges for most historians. The label 'middle classes'—rather than 'middle class'—is often adopted when discussing any individual or group who could not be described as working class or aristocratic.[79] Such appellations are unhelpful in an Irish context and Irish historians have favoured a Weberian understanding of class, which more heavily relies on notions of social status.[80] This book does not purport to resolve these challenges. Instead, by analysing various social groups, it meditates on the influence of social class and status on responses to mental illness. In this regard, it engages simultaneously with the hitherto unrelated discourses of social class and psychiatry in nineteenth-century Ireland.

Ireland's class boundaries were not rigidly defined. Ireland's lack of urbanisation and industrialisation did not allow for clear-cut economic stratification. Instead, the rural Irish placed a high importance on land, which was inextricably bound up in both social status and class-specific gender constructions.[81] Among the rural Irish, inheritance was a determining factor for living standards. After the Famine, families abandoned the practice of subdividing their land between all heirs and this adoption of impartible inheritance fostered succession disputes, family tensions and class and gender conflicts.[82] Despite the immense importance the rural Irish placed on land, Maura Cronin has suggested that appropriate or 'respectable' behaviour, rather than economic position, defined class boundaries in Ireland.[83] In consequence, there is little sense of the emergence of a working-class identity in rural Irish contexts. Instead, divisions were often in terms of the amount of land owned, if it was owned at all. Designations such as 'small farmer', broadly speaking those with at least five acres of land, 'grazier', those occupying at least one holding of 150–200 acres, and 'large farmer' are thus commonly found.[84]

This book draws on these existing approaches in its definition of class boundaries. Within the realm of asylum provision, it distinguishes between the 'pauper' insane, or those considered unable to contribute towards their maintenance, and the 'non-pauper' insane, those who were considered capable of contributing. It is important to note that the labels of pauper and non-pauper do not accurately reflect patients' social or economic condition, nor does the term pauper in this context imply destitution.[85] Rather, they best represent contemporary characterisations of asylum populations.

More nuanced class boundaries are identified among diverse groups of asylum patients—those committed to district, voluntary and private asylums as paying patients. While it is difficult to accurately assess the social origins of asylum patients solely based on their occupational profile, a more complete picture begins to emerge when a comprehensive survey of patients' occupational status, maintenance fees and, where possible, landholdings is undertaken (see Chap. 4). The importance placed on social class in nineteenth-century Ireland is further measured against the perceptions, expectations and experiences of the patients themselves (see Chaps. 5 and 6). In addition, the responses of families, communities and doctors to non-pauper insanity reveal the forms of behaviour and lifestyle deemed appropriate for distinct social groups.

OUTLINE OF CHAPTERS

This book comprises seven chapters, each focusing on the complex interplay between various actors involved in providing for the non-pauper insane. Chapter 2 outlines the political development of non-pauper lunacy provision in nineteenth-century Ireland. Focusing on Ireland's lunacy inspectors, the national press and the emerging psychiatric community, it is concerned with the debates aired at national level on how best to accommodate different social groups. It concludes that in the absence of a single effective model, the result was a patchwork of public, voluntary and private accommodation, each the outcome of a set of shared convictions as to how, why and by whom the non-pauper insane should be treated.

Chapter 3 considers the realities of providing care at local level. Concentrating on the managing bodies and resident physicians of the nine selected asylums, it traces their experiences of administrating non-pauper lunacy. It also considers the interactions between families, communities and these administrative figures when negotiating patients' maintenance fees. Revisiting the conclusion of Chap. 2, this chapter contends that the piecemeal and fragmented approach to non-pauper lunacy provision resulted in an institutional marketplace. As will be argued, patients and their relatives often had the luxury of selection, which created competition between the voluntary and private sectors. Families choosing between these sectors based their decisions not only on price and location, but on the religious ethos of institutions and the standard of accommodation provided. An analysis of the duration of stay and outcome for patients committed to these asylums suggests that more expensive asylums offered a greater chance of cure, or at least relief from the symptoms of insanity, than did the district asylums.

Centring on patients in the nine case studies, Chap. 4 delineates the socio-economic background of paying patients committed to public, voluntary and private asylums in the periods 1826–1867 and 1868–1900. It reveals that many paying patients in district asylums occupied a precarious social position just above the rank of pauper. Charitable and especially private asylum patients, meanwhile, were usually drawn from comparably comfortable circumstances. Exploration of patients' social profile is supplemented by analysis of their maintenance fees and property holdings, shedding further light on the spending power of discrete social groups. The existence of an institutional marketplace is further depicted through evidence of the socio-economic overlap of patients in the three types of asylums.

Focusing primarily on the period from 1868 to 1900, Chap. 5 considers the extent to which the social class, gender and occupational profile of paying patients influenced medical and lay identification of the causes of their insanity. It argues that asylum doctors in Ireland often constructed gender- as well as class-specific aetiologies for their non-pauper patients: primarily work for men and domesticity for women. Contrary to Britain, 'alcohol' was often attributed as a cause of illness, particularly among private asylum patients, reflecting cultural disparities in attitudes towards alcohol consumption on the two islands.

As Chap. 6 examines, the emphasis on work went beyond the medical identification of causes and symptoms of non-pauper insanity to encompass therapy. A significant tenet of moral therapy, which remained the dominant form of treatment in nineteenth-century Irish asylums, was work therapy. However, patients' social origins impacted on this component of their treatment as, not unlike the British context, those caring for patients from more privileged backgrounds struggled to offer what was considered class-appropriate employment.[86] Instead, doctors at the voluntary and private asylums prescribed more varied and extensive programmes of recreation consistent with patients' accustomed pastimes outside the asylum.

Chapter 7 centres specifically on the experiences and impressions of paying patients in the selected asylums, exploring their care and treatment primarily in the 1890s. It suggests that social status and class identity heavily influenced expectations of care. In district asylums, paying patients were particularly anxious to affirm their social standing to distance themselves from the pauper patients with whom they were forced to share lodgings. This led to the kind of class, religious and political tensions between patients largely absent in the voluntary and private asylums. Asylum doctors' expectations of paying patients were equally informed by class and status. Yet, staff's attempts to maintain a sense of social decorum in even the most expensive asylums were often frustrated by patients' violence and 'inappropriate' behaviour.

Overall, this book argues that the failure of the nineteenth-century Irish state to provide accommodation for the non-pauper insane when setting up the district asylum system gained public, state and medical recognition, both at national and local level. Fresh and revised legislation and increased centralisation sought to address the challenges of accommodating this social cohort, while the lunacy inspectors, the medical community and the press raised the question of who should be legally, financially and morally accountable. No single solution was reached; instead, the state, philanthropists and private asylum proprietors came to share responsibility. This enabled many families to select between rival sectors of asylum provision. Meanwhile, the emerging psychiatric profession, sometimes sharing a sense of social equality with their paying patients, constructed class- and gender-based readings of their disorders, fashioning treatments and accommodation accordingly. The patients, acutely conscious of their own status and the threat incarceration posed to their social standing, entertained certain expectations of what their care should entail. Ultimately, however, mental illness apparently overtook class identity and often patients themselves threatened to disrupt the social decorum of the institutions in which they resided.

NOTES

1. For example, Finnane (1981), Robins (1986), Malcolm (1989, 1999, 2003), Reynolds (1992), Walsh (2001, 2004), Cox (2012), Kelly (2016).
2. Most notably Parry-Jones (1972), Digby (1985), MacKenzie (1992), Marland (2004), Andrews and Digby (2004), Melling and Forsythe (2006).
3. Malcolm (1989).
4. Finnane (1981, p. 14).
5. Comerford (1989, pp. 372–373, 387, 391). See also Lane (2010b).
6. MacDonagh (1989, p. 193).
7. Jones and Malcolm (1999, p. 1).
8. Daly (1984, p. 1).
9. Ibid., p. 4.
10. Ó Gráda (1989a, p. 146), Ó Gráda (1989b, p. 113).
11. Prunty (1998, p. 1).
12. Guinnane (1997, pp. 55–56), Ó Gráda (1989b, pp. 110, 119), Comerford (1989, p. 373).
13. Ó Gráda (1989b, pp. 117, 114).
14. Ó Gráda (1999, p. 127), Hoppen (1998, p. 574), Vaughan (1994, p. 6).
15. Ó Gráda (1989b, p. 114).
16. Daly (1986, p. 27).
17. Comerford (1989, p. 387).
18. Gribbon (1989, pp. 334–335).
19. Ibid., p. 335.
20. Daly (1984, p. 12).
21. See Ó Gráda (1994, pp. 236–254).
22. 57 Geo. III, c. 106, see Finnane (1981, pp. 18–52).
23. Ninth Report of the Inspectors General on the General State of the Prisons of Ireland [172], H.C. 1830–1831, iv, p. 269; Fiftieth Report of the Inspectors of Lunatics (Ireland) [CD 760], H.C. 1901, xxviii, p. 487.
24. Cox (2012, p. 172). See also Finnane (1981, pp. 29–30).
25. Cox (2012, p. 34). See also Finnane (1981).
26. Ninth Report of the Inspectors General on the General State of the Prisons of Ireland, H.C. 1830–1831; Fiftieth Report of the Inspectors of Lunatics (Ireland), H.C. 1901.
27. Parry-Jones (1972, p. 7), Melling and Forsythe (2006, pp. 31–32).

28. Cox (2012, p. 2), Mauger (2012).
29. Ninth Report of the Inspectors General on the General State of the Prisons of Ireland, H.C. 1830–1831; Fiftieth Report of the Inspectors of Lunatics (Ireland), H.C. 1901.
30. O'Hare (1998, pp. 1–2).
31. Admissions Registers, 1826–1900 (Highfield Hospital Group, Hampstead and Highfield Records); Fiftieth Report of the Inspectors of Lunatics (Ireland), H.C. 1901.
32. O'Donnell (1991, pp. 18–49).
33. Admissions Registers, 1885–1900 (SJOGH, Patient Records); Fiftieth Report of the Inspectors of Lunatics (Ireland), H.C. 1901.
34. *Annual Report of the State of the Retreat* (Dublin 1811, p. 23).
35. For the York Retreat see Digby (1983, pp. 52–72).
36. Admissions Registers, 1812–1900 (FHL, Bloomfield Records); Fiftieth Report of the Inspectors of Lunatics (Ireland), H.C. 1901.
37. For more on Henry Hutchinson Stewart see (Breathnach 1998, pp. 27–33).
38. O'Brien and Lunney (2002).
39. Report on District, Local and Private Lunatic Asylums in Ireland [3894], H.C. 1867, xviii, 453, p. 40.
40. Eighteenth Report on the District, Criminal, and Private Lunatic Asylums in Ireland [4181], H.C. 1868–1869, xxvii, 419, p. 36.
41. Report on District, Local and Private Lunatic Asylums in Ireland, H.C. 1867, p. 40.
42. O'Brien and Lunney (2002), Andrews (2002).
43. Ibid.
44. Ibid.
45. O'Brien and Lunney (2002). Stewart also donated £5000 to the children's institution.
46. Eighteenth Report on the District, Criminal, and Private Lunatic Asylums in Ireland, H.C. 1868–1869, p. 36.
47. Twenty-First Report on the District, Criminal, and Private Lunatic Asylums in Ireland [C 647], H.C. 1872, xxvii, 323, p. 33.
48. Fiftieth Report of the Inspectors of Lunatics (Ireland), H.C. 1901.
49. Daly (1984, pp. 2, 11, 39, 317–318). For more on industry in the North of Ireland and particularly Belfast see Gribbon (1989, pp. 298–309).
50. Vaughan and Fitzpatrick (1978, pp. 88–89).
51. Ó Murchadha (1998, pp. 232–233, 243–244).
52. Bell and Watson (2009, p. 18).
53. Admissions and Receptions Registers, 1841–1900 (PRONI, Purdysburn Hospital, HOS/28/1/3); Admissions-Refusals, 1868–1900 (CCA, Our Lady's Hospital, OL3/1.3); Admissions Registers, 1868–1900 (WCC, St

Senan's Hospital, Enniscorthy); Admissions Registers, 1870–1900 (GM, Richmond District Lunatic Asylum); *Fiftieth Report of the Inspectors of Lunatics (Ireland)*, H.C. 1901. The number of paying patients resident is an estimate based on those identified in the admissions registers.
54. Fiftieth Report of the Inspectors of Lunatics (Ireland), H.C. 1901.
55. Guinnane (1997, p. 3).
56. Cox (2012).
57. Malcolm (1999), Walsh (2004), Cox (2012). See also Finnane (1981).
58. Fiachra Byrne's examination of the representations of twentieth-century Irish mental hospitals and patients for the period includes a survey of St Patrick's hospital. See Byrne (2011).
59. Malcolm (1989).
60. Walsh (2004).
61. Mauger (2012).
62. Especially Parry-Jones (1972), Wright (1997, pp. 137–155), Smith (1999), Suzuki (2006), Houston (2001, pp. 19–44).
63. Melling and Forsythe (2006), Melling (2004, pp. 177–221), Melling et al. (2001, pp. 153–180), Forsythe, Melling and Adair (1999, pp. 68–92).
64. Scull (1993, pp. 3, 10–11, 26–29, 32–34, 45–46, 62–63, 105–107, 352).
65. See, for example Walsh (2001, p. 145), Cox (2012, pp. xviii, 108–109, 148–149), Wright (1998, pp. 93–112), Michael (2003), Cherry (2003), Wright (1997), Suzuki (1991, 1992, 2001, 2006).
66. For example, Wright (1998), Finnane (1981, pp. 175–220, 1985, pp. 134-48), Walton (1979–1980, pp. 1–22).
67. Cox (2012, p. 241).
68. See, for example, Cox (2012), Malcolm (1999).
69. Scull (1982, p. 247).
70. Report of the Commissioners of Inquiry into the State of the Lunatic Asylums and Other Institutions for the Custody and Treatment of the Insane in Ireland, Part II [2436], H.C. 1857–1858, xxvii (henceforth cited as Report into the State of Lunatic Asylums); Poor Law Union and Lunacy Inquiry Commission (Ireland) Report [C 2239], H.C. 1878–1879, xxxi (henceforth cited as Trench Commission Report); First and Second Reports of the Committee appointed by the Lord Lieutenant of Ireland on Lunacy Administration (Ireland) [C 6434], H.C. 1890–1891, xxxvi (henceforth cited as Report of Committee on Lunacy Administration).
71. See, for example, Cox (2012, pp. 195–196), Marland (2004, pp. 99–105), Andrews (1998, pp. 255–281), Condrau (2007, pp. 525–540).
72. Andrews (1998), Melling and Forsythe (2006, p. 200).
73. Andrews (1998, p. 281).

74. Marland (2004, p. 101).
75. Cox (2012, pp. 195–196).
76. See for example, Cox (2012, pp. 195–239), Andrews (1998), Beveridge (1998, pp. 431–469), Ingram (1998), Lane (2002, pp. 205–248), Marland (2004), Porter (1987).
77. Porter (1985, p. 181), Condrau (2007, p. 526).
78. Beveridge (1998, p. 461).
79. Lane (2010a, pp. 1–2).
80. Ibid., p. 2.
81. Cronin (2010, pp. 107–129).
82. Ó Gráda (1993).
83. Cronin (2010).
84. Jones (1995, pp. ix, 1).
85. As Cox has pointed out, 'the language of pauperism pervaded prison and lunacy inspectors' reports' wherein district asylums were referred to as institutions for the reception of 'pauper' insanity. Cox (2012, p. 170).
86. For discussion of this issue in a colonial context see Ernst (1996, pp. 357–382).

REFERENCES

Andrews, Helen. 'George Hugh Kidd.' In *Dictionary of Irish Biography*, edited by James McGuire and James Quinn. Cambridge: Cambridge University Press, 2002.

Andrews, Jonathan. 'Case Notes, Case Histories and the Patient's Experience of Insanity at Gartnaval Royal Asylum, Glasgow, in the Nineteenth Century.' *Social History of Medicine* 11, no. 2 (1998): 255–281.

Andrews, Jonathan and Anne Digby (eds.). *Sex and Seclusion, Class and Custody: Perspectives on Gender and Class in the History of British Psychiatry.* Amsterdam and New York: Rodopi, 2004.

Bell, Jonathan and Mervyn Watson. *A History of Irish Farming 1750–1950.* Dublin: Four Courts Press, 2009.

Beveridge, Allan. 'Life in the Asylum: Patient's Letters from Morningside, 1873–1908.' *History of Psychiatry* 9 (1998): 431–469.

Breathnach, C.S. 'Henry Hutchinson Stewart (1798–1879): From Page to Philanthropist.' *History of Psychiatry* 9 (1998): 27–33.

Byrne, Fiachra. 'Madness and Mental Illness in Ireland: Discourses, People and Practices, 1900 to c. 1960.' PhD diss., University College Dublin, 2011.

Cherry, Steven. *Mental Healthcare in Modern England: The Norfolk Lunatic Asylum/St Andrew's Hospital circa 1810–1998.* Suffolk: The Boydell Press, 2003.

Comerford, R.V. 'Ireland 1850–1870: Post-Famine and Mid-Victorian.' In *A New History of Ireland V: Ireland under the Union, I, 1801–1870*, edited by W.E. Vaughan, 371–385. Oxford: Oxford University Press, 1989.

Condrau, Flurin. 'The Patient's View meets the Clinical Gaze.' *Social History of Medicine* 20, no. 3 (Dec 2007): 525–540.

Cox, Catherine. *Negotiating Insanity in the Southeast of Ireland 1830–1900.* Manchester: Manchester University Press, 2012.

Cronin, Maura. '"You'd be Disgraced!": Middle-Class Women and Respectability in Post-Famine Ireland.' In *Politics, Society and Middle Class in Modern Ireland*, edited by Fintan Lane, 107–129. Basingstoke: Palgrave MacMillan, 2010.

Daly, Mary E. *Dublin, The Deposed Capital: A Social and Economic History, 1860–1914.* Cork: Cork University Press, 1984.

Daly, Mary E. *The Famine in Ireland.* Dublin: Dundalgan Press, 1986.

Digby, Anne. 'Moral Treatment at the Retreat 1796–1846.' In *The Anatomy of Madness: Essays in The History of Psychiatry Vol. II: Institutions and Society*, edited by W.F. Bynum, Roy Porter and Michael Shepherd, 52–72. London and New York: Tavistock, 1983.

Digby, Anne. *Madness, Morality and Medicine: A Study of the York Retreat, 1796–1914.* Cambridge: Cambridge University Press, 1985.

Ernst, Waltraud. 'European Madness and Gender in Nineteenth-Century British India.' *Social History of Medicine* 9 (1996): 357–382.

Finnane, Mark. *Insanity and the Insane in Post-Famine Ireland.* London: Croom Helm, 1981.

Finnane, Mark. 'Asylums, Families and the State.' *History Workshop Journal* 20, no. 1 (1985): 134–148.

Forsythe, Bill, Joseph Melling and Richard Adair. 'Politics of Lunacy: Central State Regulation and the Devon Pauper Lunatic Asylum, 1845–1914.' In *Insanity, Institutions and Society, 1800–1914*, edited by Joseph Melling and Bill Forsythe, 68–92. London and New York: Routledge, 1999.

Gribbon, H.D. 'Economic and Social History, 1850–1921.' In *A New History of Ireland VI: Ireland Under Union, 1870–1921*, edited by W.E. Vaughan, 260–356. Oxford: Oxford University Press, 1989.

Guinnane, Timothy. *The Vanishing Irish: Households, Migration, and the Rural Economy in Ireland, 1850–1914.* Princeton: Princeton University Press, 1997.

Hoppen, K. Theodore. *The Mid-Victorian Generation, 1846–1886.* Oxford: Oxford University Press, 1998.

Houston, Robert A. '"Not Simply Boarding": Care of the Mentally Incapacitated in Scotland during the long Eighteenth Century.' In *Outside the Walls of the Asylum: The History of Care in the Community, 1750–2000*, edited by Peter Bartlett and David Wright, 19–44. London: Athlone Press, 2001.

Ingram, Allan. *Patterns of Madness in the Eighteenth Century: A Reader.* Liverpool: Liverpool University Press, 1998.

Jones, David Seth. *Graziers, Land Reform, and Political Conflict in Ireland.* Washington D.C.: Catholic University of America Press, 1995.

Jones, Greta and Elizabeth Malcolm. 'Introduction: An Anatomy of Irish Medical History.' In *Medicine, Disease and the State in Ireland, 1650–1940,* edited by Elizabeth Malcolm and Greta Jones, 1–17. Cork: Cork University Press, 1999.

Kelly, Brendan. *Hearing Voices: The History of Psychiatry in Ireland.* Newbridge: Irish Academic Press, 2016.

Lane, Fintan. Introduction to *Politics, Society and Middle Class in Modern Ireland,* edited by Fintan Lane, 1–6. Basingstoke: Palgrave Macmillan, 2010a.

Lane, Fintan (ed.). *Politics, Society and the Middle Class in Modern Ireland.* Basingstoke: Palgrave Macmillan, 2010b.

Lane, Joan. '"The Doctor Scolds Me": The Diaries and Correspondence of Patients in Eighteenth-Century England.' In *Patients and Practitioners: Lay Perceptions of Medicine in Pre-Industrial Society,* edited by Roy Porter, 205–248. Cambridge: Cambridge University Press, 2002.

MacDonagh, Oliver. 'Ideas and Institutions, 1830–1845.' In *A New History of Ireland V: Ireland under the Union, I, 1801–1870,* edited by W.E. Vaughan, 193–217. Oxford: Oxford University Press, 1989.

MacKenzie, Charlotte. *Psychiatry for the Rich: A History of the Private Madhouse at Ticehurst in Sussex, 1792–1917.* London: Routledge, 1992.

Malcolm, Elizabeth. *Swift's Hospital: A History of St. Patrick's Hospital, Dublin, 1746–1989.* Dublin: Gill and Macmillan, 1989.

Malcolm, Elizabeth. 'The House of Strident Shadows: The Asylum, the Family and Emigration in Post-Famine Rural Ireland.' In *Medicine, Disease and the State in Ireland 1650–1940,* edited by Elizabeth Malcolm and Greta Jones, 177–195, Cork: Cork University Press, 1999.

Malcolm, Elizabeth. '"Ireland's Crowded Madhouses": The Institutional Confinement of the Insane in Nineteenth- and Twentieth-Century Ireland.' In *The Confinement of the Insane: International Perspectives, 1800–1965,* edited by Roy Porter and David Wright, 315–333. Cambridge: Cambridge University Press, 2003.

Marland, Hilary. *Dangerous Motherhood: Insanity and Childbirth in Victorian Britain.* Basingstoke: Palgrave Macmillan, 2004.

Mauger, Alice. '"Confinement of the Higher Orders": The Social Role of Private Lunatic Asylums in Ireland, c. 1820–1860.' *Journal of the History of Medicine and Allied Sciences* 67, no. 2 (2012): 281–317.

Melling, Joseph. 'Sex and Sensibility in Cultural History: The English Governess and the Lunatic Asylum, 1845–1914.' In *Sex and Seclusion, Class and Custody: Perspectives on Gender and Class in the History of British Psychiatry,* edited by Jonathan Andrews and Anne Digby, 177–221. Amsterdam and New York: Rodopi, 2004.

Melling, Joseph and Bill Forsythe. *The Politics of Madness: The State, Insanity and Society in England, 1845–14*. London and New York: Routledge, 2006.

Melling, Joseph, Bill Forsythe and Richard Adair. 'Families, Communities and the Legal Regulation of Lunacy in Victorian England: Assessments of Crime, Violence and Welfare in Admissions to the Devon Asylum, 1845–1914.' In *Outside the Walls of the Asylum: The History of Care in the Community, 1750–2000*, edited by Peter Bartlett and David Wright, 153–180. London: Athlone Press, 2001.

Michael, Pamela. *Care and Treatment of the Mentally Ill in North Wales 1800–2000*. Cardiff: University of Wales Press, 2003.

Ó Gráda, Cormac. 'Industry and Communications, 1801–45.' In *A New History of Ireland V: Ireland under the Union, I, 1801–70*, edited by W. E. Vaughan, 137–157. Oxford: Oxford University Press, 1989a.

Ó Gráda, Cormac. 'Poverty, Population, and Agriculture, 1801–1845.' In *A New History of Ireland V: Ireland under the Union, I, 1801–70*, edited by W.E. Vaughan, 108–136. Oxford: Oxford University Press, 1989b.

Ó Gráda, Cormac. *Ireland before and after the Famine: Exploration in Economic History, 1800–1925*. Manchester: Manchester University Press, 1993.

Ó Gráda, Cormac. *Ireland: A New Economic History, 1780–1939*. Oxford: Oxford University Press, 1994.

Ó Gráda, Cormac. *Black '47 and Beyond: The Great Irish Famine in History, Economy, and Memory*. Princeton: Princeton University Press, 1999.

Ó Murchadha, Ciarán. *Sable Wings over the Land: Ennis County Clare and its Wider Community during the Great Famine*. Ennis: CLASP Press, 1998.

O'Brien, Andrew and Linde Lunney. 'Henry Hutchinson Stewart.' In *Dictionary of Irish Biography*, edited by James McGuire and James Quinn. Cambridge: Cambridge University Press, 2002.

O'Donnell, Brian. *John of God: Father of the Poor*. Burwood, Australia: Oceania Province, 1991.

O'Hare, Pauline. *In the Care of Friends*. Dublin: Highfield Healthcare, 1998.

Parry-Jones, William Ll. *The Trade in Lunacy: A Study of Private Madhouses in England in the Eighteenth and Nineteenth Centuries*. London: Routledge & Kegan Paul, 1972.

Porter, Roy. 'The Patient's View: Doing Medical History from Below.' *History and Society*, 14 (1985): 175–198.

Porter, Roy. *A Social History of Madness: Stories of the Insane*. London: Weidenfeld and Nicolson, 1987.

Prunty, Jacinta. *Dublin Slums, 1800–1925: A Study in Urban Geography, 1800–1925*. Dublin and Portland: Irish Academic Press, 1998.

Reynolds, Joseph. *Grangegorman: Psychiatric Care in Dublin Since 1815*. Dublin: Institute of Public Administration, 1992.

Robins, Joseph. *Fools and Mad: A History of the Insane in Ireland.* Dublin: Institute of Public Administration, 1986.

Scull, Andrew. *Museums of Madness: The Social Organisation of Insanity in Nineteenth-Century England.* Harmondsworth: Penguin, 1982.

Scull, Andrew. *The Most Solitary of Afflictions: Madness and Society in Britain, 1700–1900.* New Haven: Yale University Press, 1993.

Smith, Leonard D. *Cure, Comfort and Safe Custody: Public Lunatic Asylums in Early Nineteenth-Century England.* London and New York: Leicester University Press, 1999.

Suzuki, Akihito. 'Lunacy in Seventeenth- and Eighteenth-Century England: Analysis of Quarter Sessions Records.' Parts I and II. *History of Psychiatry* 2 (1991): 437–456; 3 (1992): 29–44.

Suzuki, Akihito. 'Enclosing and Disclosing Lunatics within the Family Walls: Domestic Psychiatric Regime and the Public Sphere in Early Nineteenth-Century England.' In *Outside the Walls of the Asylum: The History of Care in the Community, 1750–2000,* edited by Peter Bartlett and David Wright, 115–132. London: Athlone Press, 2001.

Suzuki, Akihito. *Madness at Home: The Psychiatrist, the Patient and the Family in England, 1820–1860.* Berkeley and Los Angeles: University of California Press, 2006.

Vaughan, W.E. *Landlords and Tenants in Mid-Victorian Ireland.* New York: Oxford University Press, 1994.

Vaughan, W.E. and A.J. Fitzpatrick (eds.). *Irish Historical Statistics: Population, 1821–1971.* Dublin: Royal Irish Academy, 1978.

Walsh, Oonagh. 'Lunatic and Criminal Alliances in Nineteenth-Century Ireland.' In *Outside the Walls of the Asylum: The History of Care in the Community 1750–2000,* edited by Peter Bartlett and David Wright, 132–152. London: Athlone Press, 2001.

Walsh, Oonagh. 'Gender and Insanity in Nineteenth-Century Ireland.' In *Sex and Seclusion, Class and Custody: Perspectives on Gender and Class in the History of British Psychiatry,* edited by Jonathan Andrews and Anne Digby, 69–93. Amsterdam and New York: Rodopi, 2004.

Walton, John. 'Lunacy in the Industrial Revolution: A Study of Asylum Admission in Lancashire, 1848–1850.' *Journal of Social History* 13, no. 1 (1979–1980): 1–22.

Wright, David. 'Getting out of the Asylum: Understanding the Confinement of the Insane in the Nineteenth Century.' *Social History of Medicine* 10, no. 1 (1997): 137–155.

Wright, David. 'Family Strategies and the Institutional Confinement of "Idiot" Children in Victorian England.' *Journal of Family History,* 23, no. 2 (April, 1998): 190–208.

PART I

Governing Insanity

CHAPTER 2

The Non-Pauper Insane: Private, Voluntary and State Concerns

One would think that our legislators imagined insanity to spring only from the pride of wealth or the misery of poverty. They have never thought of making provision for the lunatic of the great class which lies between.[1]

This observation, which appeared in an *Irish Times* editorial in 1860, summed up widespread public concerns that Irish asylums were failing to cater for a specific group: those who could not afford private care but were not considered destitute. Accommodation of this kind had been available in England since the eighteenth century, where the private, public and voluntary sectors gradually coalesced to form a 'mixed economy of care'.[2] The *Irish Times* editors' incredulous tone is unsurprising, given that the government had shown enormous energy when intervening in other areas of Irish lunacy provision.[3] At national level, the issue gained increasing importance, attracting the attention of government officials as well as igniting interest among the medical community, philanthropists and the national press. The overwhelming question was how, where and to what extent to provide for the 'great class which lies between'.

This question had resonated during the 1850s, most notably during a commission of inquiry held between 1857 and 1858. This commission was established to inquire into the state of lunacy laws, lunatic asylums and other institutions for the 'custody and treatment of the insane' in Ireland. While not intended exclusively as an inquiry into fee-paying asylum care, its proceedings sparked journalistic interest in that issue, receiving coverage in the leading national newspaper of the day, the *Freeman's*

© The Author(s) 2018
A. Mauger, *The Cost of Insanity in Nineteenth-Century Ireland*, Mental Health in Historical Perspective,
https://doi.org/10.1007/978-3-319-65244-3_2

Journal.[4] Meanwhile, official reports on Irish asylums repeatedly voiced government and medical concerns. From 1823 until the formation of the medical lunacy inspectorate in 1845, the prison inspectors were required to visit and submit reports on all receptacles for the insane in Ireland. In their reports, the prison inspectors provided rather sketchy outlines of each 'place of profit', focusing most of their attention on the burgeoning district system. The first medical lunacy inspectors, Dr. Francis White (1846–1857) and Dr. John Nugent (1847–1890) drew clear distinctions between private and district asylums and delineated 'mixed' or voluntary asylums as a category in their own right. White, Nugent and their successors, Dr. George William Hatchell (1857–1889), Dr. George Plunkett O'Farrell (1890–1907) and Dr. E. Maziere Courtenay (1890–c. 1911) reported annually on Irish asylums. Their reports did not follow a specified format and the statistical data included varied from year to year. The inconsistent nature of these data poses difficulties when attempting to trace trends at specific intervals and, for this reason, statistical information examined in this chapter is often selective.

This chapter surveys national concerns about the admission of paying patients to private, voluntary and district asylums. It reviews proposals to establish separate accommodation for paying patients, negative coverage of private asylums by the press and lunacy inspectors, the growing social importance of Ireland's four voluntary asylums and the implications of the eventual reception of paying patients in district asylums. Ultimately, it argues, in the absence of a single effective solution to the problem of maintaining 'the great class which lies between', district, voluntary and private asylums came to provide distinct forms of care.

'CONFINEMENT OF THE HIGHER ORDERS'

In Ireland, private asylums played a relatively small role for much of the nineteenth century. In comparison with England and Wales, they were slow to develop. The origins of the earliest private asylums remain obscure, as were the grounds on which they were established.[5] Prior to 1800, Cittadella in County Cork (est. 1799) was the only private asylum in Ireland. During the 1810s and 1820s, a number of small-scale establishments sprang up, mainly located in Dublin. The remainder of the century saw greater expansion, with the establishment of a further twenty-eight private asylums between 1840 to 1900. Unremarkable for a period of economic prosperity, thirteen of these asylums had appeared during the 1860s and 1870s. Yet, the depression which began in 1879 and continued until the mid-1890s witnessed only a small decline in patient numbers, while the number of private asylums reached a peak of twenty in 1890. Nonetheless, some institutions, such as Rose Bush House in Dublin and the private asylum at Moate in Westmeath, remained open for less than a year. Others, such as Rathgar House and No. 174 Rathgar Road in Dublin, received only three patients each. As will be discussed, this period of depression also saw the closure of institutions which had been in operation for quite some time.

These modest beginnings were probably the reason that, excluding annual inspection, private asylums evaded government reform until 1842.[6] Early nineteenth-century legislators instead fixed their gaze on the burgeoning district system. The Private Asylums (Ireland) Act of 1842 significantly extended central government's regulatory control over private asylums and sat well with contemporary political objectives towards centralisation, at a time when the state was rapidly reforming areas such as education, economic development, police, prisons and public health.[7] As such, it may be viewed as just one element of the wider governmental reform sweeping through Ireland. Yet, the Act was the most important piece of legislation targeting non-pauper lunacy provision during the nineteenth century and in many respects brought Irish legislation in line with England and Wales, at least temporarily.

The 1842 Act aimed to increase protection for private patients. It introduced licensing measures, in place in England and Wales since 1774, and a rigorous tightening up of regulations.[8] New measures included more frequent and unannounced inspections, while paying patients now required medical certification by two doctors.[9] The latter signalled official recognition of public hysteria over the perceived vulnerability of private patients to wrongful or over-lengthy confinement; pauper patients required only one medical certificate. Finnane suggests this disparity resulted from the assumption that 'no advantage, other than a social one, would accrue to the partners in the committal of a poor person'. By contrast, legislators considered private patients to be at risk of wrongful confinement for the pecuniary advantage of their relatives.[10] In England and Wales, similar protective procedures for private patients had been in place since 1828.[11]

Although these regulatory measures might have inspired the public's confidence, the reality was different. By 1860, the editors of the *Irish Times* had launched a tirade against private asylums, labelling them a 'crying evil', 'moral pest-houses' and appealing that these 'engines of ill so monstrous are swept from our land'. The editors went further, expressing disbelief that 'any person would be so hardhearted as, knowing the nature of these dens, to consign an afflicted relative or friend to such misery and woe'.[12] The three key areas under criticism had been summarised in an article the previous year. Firstly, the editors were especially sceptical about the agendas of private asylum proprietors, pointing out that it was in their best financial interests to retain patients rather than cure them. Secondly, they heavily criticised the families of patients for failing to care for them in the home. In doing so, they revealed that their issue lay more with confinement itself, rather than any unpleasant conditions identified in the private asylums:

> To read the prospectus of some Private Asylums, we would fancy them to be each a little paradise. Employment is provided, and amusement. There are games, balls, private theatricals, and concerts. In fact, all are to be treated as 'members of a family.' Why, then, does not the family to which a lunatic belongs provide all this solace which we are so ready to pay for? Why must we cloak our selfishness under the guise of affectionate relationship? Why must we bury each insane member of our kindred, as we do our dead, out of our sight, and comfort ourselves with the complacent notion that we pay largely to provide a haven for him?

Finally, the editors turned their attention to the cure rates which had been published in the inspectors' report for the year ending April 1859. Having provided some rather inconsistent calculations, the editors concluded 'it would appear, then, that the District Asylums offer, at least, as great a chance of cure as the most pretentious of Private Licensed Houses'.[13] Comparing the figures provided by the inspectors confirms that the proportion of cures to admissions for district asylums was higher (49.3% for year-end March 1859) than for those admitted to private asylums (40% for year-end December 1859). As Chap. 3 will outline, while cure rates for patients admitted to St John of God's, Hampstead and Highfield tended to be higher than those to the voluntary and district asylums studied, the proportion of those discharged relieved was higher than for pauper patients admitted to the district system.[14] As will be discussed, the high rate of those discharged prior to being 'cured' can be interpreted as evidence against the over-lengthy confinement of private asylums' patients for financial gain.

The editors' criticisms echoed those expressed in Britain since the eighteenth century, where humanitarian reformers challenged private asylum care as 'cruel in nature and inadequate in scale'.[15] In fact, the *Irish Times* reprinted reports of the English Commissioners in Lunacy as evidence of the abuses in the private asylum system.[16] In contrast, the Irish lunacy inspectors' commentary on private asylums was so positive in this era that Hampstead House published extracts of their 1861 report as a classified advertisement for that institution.[17] In his comprehensive study of English and Welsh private asylums, William Ll. Parry-Jones attributes the longstanding public prejudices against private asylums to an over-hasty acceptance of sensationalist disclosures.[18] Likewise, in spite of sporadic condemnations by the press, there is no evidence of abuses in Irish private asylums before the 1860s.[19]

By the late 1860s, the lunacy inspectors' views on private asylums had become more mixed. In 1867, they claimed that many private asylums, including Farnham House, Hampstead House and Lisle House in Dublin and the Midland Retreat in Queen's County (now County Laois) were 'admirably conducted and the patients in them treated with great care and attention, their personal wants, comforts and cleanliness being sedulously attended to'. However, the inspectors described other, unnamed, private asylums as 'less satisfactory' and reported they had administered 'very severe rebukes for culpable neglect in several instances'. In one case, having visited an unnamed Dublin private asylum in very cold weather and late in the evening, the inspectors found 'a want of fire and lights and an apparent disregard of order, cleanliness and comfort'.[20] The inspectors did not identify these asylums in their reports, excerpts of which appeared in national and local newspapers throughout the nineteenth century. Had they exposed them, they might have dissuaded potential clientele from committing their relatives to these institutions. Although the 1842 Act had not vested the inspectors with the power to revoke licences, it stipulated they could recommend a withdrawal of a licence to the Lord Chancellor of Ireland,[21] who, along with the Lord Lieutenant,[22] had this authority.[23] Yet Nugent and Hatchell did not exercise this authority. In their 1867 report, they wrote, 'were it not for the difficulty ... of providing other accommodation ... we would long since have recommended the withholding of licenses and closing the establishments'.[24] The importance of this statement should not be overlooked. In the absence of any other provision, the inspectors claimed they had little alternative but to tolerate, if not partially obscure, the poor conditions prevailing in some of Ireland's private asylums.

After 1867, little official attention was directed at private asylum conditions until the late 1880s, when the inspectors appeared to approve of the majority which were, they claimed, 'for the most part creditably conducted' and 'suitable abodes for patients in the better classes of society'. By this time, some private asylum proprietors were offering accommodation on a graded scale: while they still charged extremely high fees for most patients, they now provided inferior accommodation for others at much lower fees (see Chap. 3). As will be discussed, the inspectors took issue with these reduced rates of board but continued to display a fatalistic attitude towards conditions of care.[25] Their approach to private asylums in this era reflects their declining authority and vitality towards the end of their careers. After 1870, the inspectors were apparently unable to go beyond the routine administrative function of their office and, by the 1880s, both inspectors were 'old, even invalid and had little energy to carry out their duties efficiently'.[26] In this period, Nugent, who was reputed to have had a particularly difficult personality, came into conflict with asylum governors and central government, while the less controversial Hatchell was often too ill to carry out his duties.[27] In his final report, Nugent had apparently resigned himself to the state of private asylums in Ireland, arguing it was his duty only to see that proprietors carried out the provisions of the legislation.[28]

In 1890, a new Lunacy Act was introduced in England, which prohibited the granting of any further private asylum licences and barred existing ones from expanding their accommodation.[29] This development followed continuing pressure for reform, which included proposals to abolish the entire private system. As Parry-Jones reasons, this pressure was closely associated with concerns for the middle-class insane and criticism centred on the principle of profit underpinning the system.[30] Meanwhile, in Ireland, the Lord Lieutenant appointed three commissioners to investigate current lunacy laws. These commissioners were Arthur Mitchell, a Scottish lunacy commissioner, R.W.A. Holmes, the Treasury Remembrancer for Ireland, and F.X.F. MacCabe, a medical inspector with the local government board.[31] The commissioners drew attention to the English Lunacy Act but did not recommend corresponding restrictions for Ireland:

Private Asylums receiving patients in affluent circumstances will soon die, if they have not the confidence of the public and if they are not reported on favourably … All classes of private patients are on the whole, in our opinion, best situated in asylums which are not carried on for the profit of proprietors. There are Private Asylums, however, in which the insane are treated with much skill and liberality and as Ireland does not possess great accommodation for private patients, either rich or not rich, in endowed and chartered institutions, we do not think it desirable to recommend prohibitive provisions like those of the new English Lunacy Law (1890) to be introduced into fresh Lunacy legislation for Ireland.

However, the commissioners condemned the maintenance of private patients at low rates, arguing it was 'difficult to obtain a profit ... without a stinting of necessary comforts and advantages'.[32]

The commission coincided with the appointment, in 1890, of two new lunacy inspectors, O'Farrell and Courtenay, who replaced Nugent and Hatchell. Although the new inspectors showed little imagination in administration or policy, they brought a new energy and were less complacent about poor asylum conditions.[33] This latter appraisal also applies to the inspectors' attitude towards private asylums. From the outset, the new inspectors expressed discontent with private asylums, stating that with few exceptions they were 'not entirely satisfactory'. Like the 1890–1891 inquiry commissioners, the inspectors were strongly opposed to private asylums receiving patients at low rates, especially those containing only a few patients.[34] In 1891, they successfully recommended the withdrawal of a licence from Cittadella in Cork. The closure of Cittadella was a landmark event. The asylum was established and initially managed by the renowned mad-doctor and moral therapy enthusiast, Dr. William Saunders Hallaran, who published the first Irish textbook on psychiatry and had been influential in implementing moral therapy in district asylums.[35] When its licence was revoked, Cittadella had been in operation for over ninety years. It is plausible the inspectors were making an example of Cittadella, sending a message to other private asylum proprietors that the inspectorate would not tolerate poor conditions of care.

Notably, the inspectors claimed to be protecting private patients whom they feared were not being given the 'comforts' and 'even luxuries' allegedly on offer in other countries.[36] A few years later, they argued that private patients kept at low rates 'cannot afford those comforts which are now considered necessary for the treatment of the insane'.[37] The inspectors feared proprietors lacked sufficient capital to operate in accordance with 'modern ideas' which could be seen abroad, though they did not specify what these ideas actually were.[38] In spite of their remonstrance, the inspectors echoed the resolution of the 1890–1891 commissioners, concluding that 'high-class licensed houses will always be preferred by the wealthy and if not found to provide excellent treatment, they will very soon die out from want of patients'.[39] Clearly, the inspectors now felt 'wealthy' families had the luxury of selection and in turn protection.

The closure of Cittadella signalled the inspectors' consolidation of their regulatory powers. Following this, they systematically identified poor conditions in private asylums, threatening to advocate the withdrawal of licences on several occasions. In addition to reporting on the general state of private asylums as a group, the inspectors began to append individual reports on each asylum. This represented a divergence from the old inspectors' practice of obscuring the identity of asylums they found fault with, and proprietors were visibly unnerved. For instance, in their 1895 report on Course Lodge in County Armagh, the inspectors stated:

> We trust at the next renewal of the licence, the magistrates will consider the reports which my colleague and I have made during the past two years on this establishment and we would suggest if they see fit to renew the licence, that they obtain an undertaking in writing and forward a copy of same to our office, that the proprietor will in future receive only quiet and harmless cases.[40]

The following year, they reported that the Armagh Retreat had failed to record in the asylum books that a female patient had set fire to her clothes and sustained burns. They criticised this 'serious disregard of an important duty' and threatened that if they uncovered evidence of any similar neglect in the future they would recommend the asylum's licence be withdrawn.[41] Even in cases where this was not threatened, the inspectors' simple expression of disapproval of a heating system or bed sheets met with rapid improvements. For example, in 1895, the inspectors were pleased to report that Belmont Park had taken steps 'to supply each bed with an under-blanket, as suggested in last report'.[42]

The influence of the new inspectors is further implied by the closure of several private asylums in the late nineteenth century. Of the ten that were established during the 1880s and 1890s, only two remained open in 1900, along with eleven pre-existing establishments. These were Belmont Park in Waterford and the House of St John of God (St John of God's) in Dublin. Their survival speaks volumes about the changing face of Irish private asylum care. Contrary to their criticism of other private asylums, the inspectors commended both Belmont and St John of God's for charging lower fees than other private asylums. Their praise was because both charged exclusively low fees, which they now felt safeguarded against inequalities between different classes of patients.[43] This meant these asylums catered for a social group distinct from other private asylums and suggests that patients in these institutions did not have the same luxury of selection. In 1895, the inspectors acknowledged that in reality these hospitals met the needs of comparatively few patients (fewer than 100 between them in that year).[44] However, in their last report, which included patient numbers for the year ending 1917, the lunacy inspectors recorded that Belmont and St John of God's had expanded to accommodate almost one-fifth of all private asylum patients.[45] Despite the inspectors' unfaltering approval of these institutions, there were limitations. Each received only male patients and was run by a religious community: the Brothers of Charity managed Belmont and, as discussed earlier, the Hospitaller Order of St John of God managed and gave their name to that asylum. Both St John of God's and Belmont therefore maintained a strong Catholic ethos and catered primarily for men of that religion.

Reporting in 1898, the lunacy inspectors did not seem troubled by the closure of eight private asylums since their appointment. Instead, they appeared self-congratulatory in their claim that the asylums which had closed were the very ones receiving patients at low rates of board and 'must of necessity be open to suspicion'.[46] Accordingly, in 1900, they reported:

a decided improvement has taken place in the accommodation provided in many of these houses and that there is a manifest desire on the part of most of the proprietors, to render the surrounding of their establishments in keeping with modern requirements for the care and treatment of private patients.[47]

Just ten years after their appointment, the inspectors alleged to have consolidated their influence over private asylums. They put forward, as evidence, a lack of abuses within the remaining thirteen private asylums. As the subsequent sections reveal, this development occurred in tandem with the expansion of alternative forms of non-pauper accommodation.

'THE GREAT CLASS WHICH LIES BETWEEN'

During the nineteenth century, there were several proposals for alternatives to private asylums. Official, lay and medical men frequently supported, debated and contested these various solutions. Beginning in the 1850s, official commentators, including the lunacy inspectors, advocated increased philanthropic activity, while the national press appealed for state-supported relief for the 'great class which lies between'. These public appeals may have been rooted in a realisation that public benevolence was failing to provide accommodation, but they were couched in criticism of private asylums.

The editors of the *Irish Times* demanded the replacement of private asylums with state-funded establishments catering for all social classes above paupers.[48] Thomas Bakewell, the proprietor of Staffordshire private asylum (1808–1835) had imagined a similar system for England as early as 1814. He recommended that the state should be the 'guardian of every lunatic' and oversee an alternative system of curative hospitals. Yet Bakewell's plans never came to fruition. Smith attributes this failure to the authorities' reluctance to raise the necessary funds, arguing that this vision was 'well beyond the level of intervention the politicians could contemplate'.[49] While state intervention in Irish lunacy provision was well established by the 1850s,[50] dedicated facilities for paying patients seemed to lie outside the realm of government aid.

Contrary to the *Irish Times'* support for state involvement, some members of the Irish medical community strictly opposed it. For example, in the 1850s, Dr. James Foulis Duncan, who was visiting physician to several Dublin private asylums, including the expensive Farnham House, highlighted the potential shortcomings of a state-funded system, both in a dedicated treatise and in a letter to the *Irish Times*.[51] Duncan, who clearly had a stake in private asylums, maintained that 'government asylums' would not prove an attractive alternative to the public. Presumably mindful of contemporary concerns about wrongful or over-lengthy confinement in private asylums, he also claimed it was in their proprietors' financial interests to effect a 'large number of cures ... in a short time'. Duncan went on to warn that if government asylums were established, they would come to monopolise asylum care:

Admitting that the Government were even to do this, the question remains to be asked, will they create several asylums of each grade and by doing so, leave the parties requiring accommodation the power of selecting between rival institutions, so as to have in some measure the option of disposing their invalid relative where they may think most for his advantage? Or will they, by creating one only of each kind, virtually establish a monopoly which they must necessarily be satisfied with?[52]

Looking beyond his vested interest in private asylums, Duncan's views underscored some of the key criticisms of state intervention in non-pauper lunacy administration. Ironically, at the time Duncan was writing, private asylums had virtually established a monopoly on non-pauper lunacy provision in the absence of alternative care options.

By the 1860s, the lunacy inspectors were also agitating for the setting up of what they termed 'intermediate asylums' for non-paupers. Contrary to public demands, the inspectors recommended these asylums should be charitable, deeming provision for this social group 'a question of local importance' and therefore falling outside state responsibility.[53] This mirrored the recommendations of the 1857–1858 commissioners, which concluded:

we should gladly see the existing [private] establishments of that class in Ireland give place to institutions of a self-supporting character and where this most helpless class would be cared for and maintained without reference to the profits to be derived from their infirmity. It is not to be expected that individuals will invest their capital, the source of support for themselves and their families, without looking for as large an income in return as it can fairly be made to produce, or that they will devote their time, labour and skills as professional men, to the care of the insane, from purely philanthropic motives.

In the face of this rather pessimistic assessment, the commissioners appealed to philanthropists:

Such an asylum ... would be an incalculable boon to society and we cannot but hope that in a city so remarkable for the charity of its inhabitants as Dublin the tide of benevolence may one day turn in this direction.[54]

Nineteenth-century Dublin certainly boasted an abundance of philanthropic initiatives in other areas of health and welfare provision.[55] These initiatives took place against a backdrop of state provision that philanthropists often viewed as inadequate.[56] Ratepayers resented their lack of authority over decisions about district asylums, particularly those incurring additional local taxation,[57] and it is likely many would-be philanthropists were similarly loath to contribute towards voluntary asylums. By the late 1860s in Ireland, appeals for further voluntary provision for the non-pauper insane had ceased. As the subsequent section discusses, this resulted in part from the arrival of two new voluntary asylums in the previous decade.

'A HIGHLY USEFUL AND BENEVOLENT FOUNDATION'

In the 1850s, St Vincent's and Stewarts joined Ireland's two existing voluntary asylums, St Patrick's (est. 1757) and Bloomfield (est. 1812). Their arrival symbolised the recognition by two distinct philanthropic groups of the need for dedicated facilities for members of their own class or faith. These four establishments differed from private asylums in a number of ways. While the lunacy inspectors described certain private institutions such as St John of God's and Belmont as charitable, they singled out the four Dublin-based 'mixed' or voluntary asylums for sharing one attribute: they were not kept for profit. This had important implications for attitudes towards the voluntary sector. Amidst public anxieties over the potential wrongful or over-lengthy confinement of private patients by profiteering proprietors, the profits generated from voluntary asylum patients' fees were diverted to maintain charity patients or to make improvements to the accommodation and care provided.[58] This practice, coupled with the lower fees they charged, resulted in voluntary asylums becoming the most widely used institutions for the non-pauper insane.

Each of the four voluntary asylums had strong religious affiliations, which in turn decided the sectors of society they served. St Patrick's, the first institution for the insane in Ireland, was founded in 1757 from the bequest of Irish writer and dean of St Patrick's Cathedral, Jonathan Swift. In her study of the hospital, Malcolm has shown that between 1841 and 1850, three-quarters of patients at St Patrick's were Church of Ireland, while between 1874 and 1883 they accounted for 81%.[59] As already discussed, the second voluntary asylum, the Bloomfield Retreat, was set up by members of the Society of Friends in 1812 to provide relief for members of that persuasion. By its very design, Bloomfield was therefore intended principally for a minority group; by 1901, Quakers made up less than 2% of the population of both Dublin and Ireland.[60] Until

1821, only Quakers were admitted. However, the managing committee quickly realised that there was an insufficient number of Quaker patients to fill the available beds and began to advertise vacancies for non-Quakers.[61] This followed suit with the York Retreat in England, which also began admitting non-Quaker patients at this point.[62] The admission of patients from other denominations increased and, by 1858, only half of Bloomfield's patients were members of the Society—a discernible shift from the institution's initial sectarian ethos.[63]

Founded almost half a century after Bloomfield in 1857, St Vincent's asylum was superintended by an order of nuns called the Sisters of Charity and received only female patients.[64] According to the lunacy inspectors, in 1857, Elizabeth Magan, sister of Francis, a barrister and high-ranking member of the United Irishmen, bequeathed 'many thousand pounds' to be used for 'some charitable purpose' in Dublin. Following Elizabeth's death, the relatives who inherited her property settled on establishing St Vincent's 'for the benefit of persons mentally affected belonging to the middle classes'. On opening, it could accommodate up to thirty patients and by 1870 it was reportedly 'full to capacity' at eighty-seven. The asylum subsequently expanded and by 1900 had more than tripled to accommodate 105 patients. Despite its Catholic ethos, and unlike the initial practice at Bloomfield, St Vincent's did not restrict entrance to members of one religious persuasion.[65] Nonetheless, in 1896, approximately 70% of patients attended Catholic mass, which was said three times on Sundays and religious holidays, suggesting most patients were Catholic.[66]

Although, Stewart's motivations for founding his institution were primarily medical and philanthropic, the asylum also had a religious character. Stewart came from a strictly Church of Ireland background. His father, the Reverend Abraham Augustus Stewart, had been the rector of Donabate and chaplain to the Lord Lieutenant of Ireland and this influenced the religious character at Stewarts.[67] The children's institution, while open to patients of all religions, was conducted on what the inspectors termed 'Protestant principles', and religious instruction formed the basis of patients' training. This practice did not extend to the lunatic asylum, however, which boasted two paid chaplaincies, one Protestant and one Roman Catholic.[68] Yet, as Chap. 4 outlines, patients admitted to Bloomfield and Stewarts were primarily Church of Ireland or Quaker.

The innately denominational ethos of voluntary asylums is unsurprising. As Maria Luddy has reasoned, 'philanthropic provision in nineteenth-century Ireland was denominational provision'.[69] In fact, Irish charities, and particularly those of a Protestant leaning, were often the subject of public mistrust and allegations of proselytising behaviour.[70] These anxieties were deeply rooted in Irish Catholic grievances surrounding the Famine period, when evangelical missionaries used hunger as an instrument to win converts to the Protestant faith by providing soup in designated kitchens.[71] Mindful of these apprehensions, many charities limited their assistance to members of their own denomination.[72] Another way of guarding against such charges was to provide religious ministrations to patients of all denominations. Yet this did little to sway cautious family members who were undoubtedly cognisant of the religious character of institutions. As will be seen, members of one creed were unlikely to select asylums that primarily received patients of another.

In addition to catering chiefly for members of one religion, voluntary asylum care was aimed at those who could not afford expensive private asylum accommodation, often following a descent down the social scale. Dr. Thomas Fitzpatrick, who would later become the first medical officer at St Vincent's, told the 1857–1858 commissioners that St Vincent's was intended for the 'middle classes'. Highlighting the delicacy of these individuals' status, he stated that those:

> belonging to the educated portion of the middle classes and depending on the continued exercise of their talent and industry, fall at once, when affected with even temporary mental disorder, from comfort to ruin and whose families are hopelessly dragged down with them to poverty and want ... the class between the rich and the poor suffer without resources and often long unknown, till the prolonged pains and grief of concealed poverty beset and torture them; and no relief presents itself until they have wholly fallen into the ranks of paupers.[73]

Fitzpatrick's evidence reflected contemporary unease about the fragility of social status. Even beyond those seeking asylum care, individuals who encountered a sudden change of fortune met with sympathy both from Irish Poor Law guardians and charitable organisations.[74] For example, the applications of middle-class women to charitable organisations tended to be subject to different criteria from those from the working classes, with social class often determining the type of aid given.[75] These practices were the result of philanthropists' anxieties about the delicate nature of their own financial security and status in society. Writing about the Association for the Relief of Ladies in Distress through Non-Payment of Rent in Ireland, Luddy has found that the comparable social backgrounds of the committee and the charity's recipients, combined with the realisation a similar fate could befall them, spurred the committee to action. She also asserts 'the possibility that such "ladies" could be forced to enter a workhouse was greeted with horror'.[76] Likewise, members of the public agitating for asylum provision for the middle classes were evidently concerned with the relief of their own social class. In 1874, a contributor using the pseudonym 'middle class' wrote to the *Irish Times* highlighting the want of increased asylum provision for the middle classes, which he argued would be a 'real boon to the community'.[77]

The managing bodies of voluntary asylums seemed anxious to cater for those who could not afford private asylum care. However, as Chap. 3 reveals, they often struggled to strike a balance between remaining charitable and financially solvent. As Ireland's system of district asylums expanded, St Patrick's patient base had become what Malcolm terms the 'middling classes' or those maintained at moderate sums. While this hospital's board of governors preferred even non-paying patients to be from the 'better classes' who had 'fallen on hard times', it was constantly compelled to adjust maintenance fees to simultaneously house the poor and attract wealthier patients. Tellingly, in 1845, most boarders were maintained at £30 or £40, yet by 1889, free patients were no longer admitted and the minimum fee was raised to £65 per annum.[78]

At Bloomfield, the managing committee was chiefly concerned with providing inexpensive care to members of the Society of Friends. Contributions of £100 from a Society meeting or £25 from an individual Friend entitled the donor to nominate one 'poor patient' maintained at the lowest terms (minimum £13 p.a.). Private patients, meanwhile, were charged a minimum of £26 per annum or more, 'according to circumstances'.[79] While Quaker patients were often received at these low rates and some free of charge, by the 1850s those of other religious persuasions were paying at least £78 per year. Bloomfield's superintendent, John Moss, attempted to account for this disparity, stating:

those who are belonging to the Society of Friends have an especial claim to be admitted at the lowest rate … because the Society in the first place subscribed the money for the purchasing of the ground and for the building and soforth [sic] and also additional sums in order that the additional expenses may in a great measure be defrayed.[80]

Although fees for Quakers competed well with private asylums, Bloomfield did not deliver affordable accommodation for those of other denominations. This was also the practice at the York Retreat, where by 1910, the lowest terms for Quaker patients were twelve shillings (approx. £30 p.a.), while non-Quaker patients were charged as much as seven guineas per week (approx. £380 p.a.).[81]

The two newer voluntary asylums offered more competitive rates. St Vincent's, which also admitted free and paying patients, charged on average £21 per year.[82] The inspectors predicted early on that the institution would 'prove a very useful addition to the private lunatic establishments of this country' and praised the self-supporting nature of the establishment, from which the religious community would derive 'no emoluments whatever from their self-imposed duties'.[83] Throughout the century, the inspectors continued to commend the institution's work. As has been discussed, Stewarts also offered 'moderate rates'. A letter to the editor of the *Irish Times* in 1874 stated that the hospital charged patients £36 per annum.[84] Ireland's four voluntary asylums therefore offered varying rates at different points in their history. By the late nineteenth century, St Patrick's board of governors no longer admitted free patients, while Stewarts and St Vincent's apparently adhered more rigidly to their initial philosophy. Bloomfield, meanwhile, continued to charge non-Quakers fees on a par with private care.

A final defining feature of the four voluntary asylums was their exemption from the 1842 licensing legislation. Fitzpatrick explained the reasoning behind this practice in his evidence at the 1857–1858 commission, in his assertion that St Vincent's should be exempt because the expense of obtaining a licence:

takes away from the accumulation of funds intended for benevolent purposes. The object of such an institution is to increase or extend its benefits, in case there is any surplus arising from its receipts.[85]

In consequence, any revenue accumulated by voluntary asylums was exempt from tax.

Other sections of the 1842 Act did apply: the lunacy inspectors inspected all institutions, including voluntary asylums, and paying patients required certification by two medical men.[86] Although voluntary asylums were subject to inspection, the exemption from licensing limited the lunacy inspectors' regulatory powers over them. In contrast to the anxieties of private asylum proprietors, outlined above, the managing bodies of voluntary asylums could choose to ignore the inspectors' advice. For instance, in 1897, the new inspectors complained about St Patrick's:

> It does not appear that any of the suggestions made in our annual reports have received attention from the managing committee, but it is nevertheless our duty to go on from year to year calling attention to the very obvious requirements of the hospital.[87]

Failure to make these unspecified improvements may have resulted from a lack of financial resources. As Malcolm has argued, the government often demanded modernisation but offered no financial aid.[88] But by the turn of the century, the inspectors praised St Patrick's, recording that 'a great deal of work' had been carried out.[89] In the meantime, the inspectors continued to applaud other voluntary asylums, suggesting they tended to offer a high standard of accommodation.

Following the establishment of St Vincent's and Stewarts, and Bloomfield's expansion, increasing numbers of patients came to reside in voluntary asylums. Numbers in private asylums, meanwhile, declined, presumably because the more competitive voluntary asylums proved attractive to their potential clients (see Fig. 2.1). This indicates the existence of a market for voluntarism prior to the 1870s and reflects contemporary demand for accommodation for the 'middling classes'. From 1870, there were consistently more patients in voluntary asylums than in private institutions.

Examined individually, a striking feature is the proportional decline in patients at St Patrick's (see Fig. 2.2). This can be attributed to mounting financial difficulties experienced by the institution.[90] In consequence of the board's decision to raise patient fees, St Patrick's failed to compete with the other voluntary asylums. Despite the burgeoning popularity of

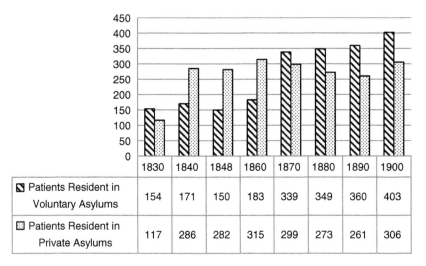

	1830	1840	1848	1860	1870	1880	1890	1900
▨ Patients Resident in Voluntary Asylums	154	171	150	183	339	349	360	403
▨ Patients Resident in Private Asylums	117	286	282	315	299	273	261	306

Fig. 2.1 Patient numbers in voluntary and private asylums in Ireland, 1830 to 1900. Compiled from *Reports of the Inspectors General on the General State of the Prisons of Ireland, 1831, 1841; Reports on District, Local and Private Lunatic Asylums in Ireland, 1849, 1861, 1871, 1881, 1890–1891, 1901*

voluntarism, no additional philanthropic initiative was launched following the establishment of Stewarts.

'Asylums for the Lunatic Poor'?

While it not is entirely surprising that the state was unwilling to finance separate accommodation for paying patients, it is striking that there was apparently no contemplation of a joint venture between state and charity. In England, following the introduction of the 1808 Lunacy Act, four such joint asylums were created, funded by both charitable bodies and the county and catering for pauper, charity and private patients.[91] Instead, from the early nineteenth century, officials in Ireland paid increasing homage to the feasibility of housing paying patients in the public asylums, a practice introduced to England in 1815. There, fees for paying patients in the county asylums were competitive with the private sector, enabling wider access.[92]

In Ireland, families had been appealing for district asylums to admit paying patients since at least the 1830s. In 1835, the 'friends' of a female

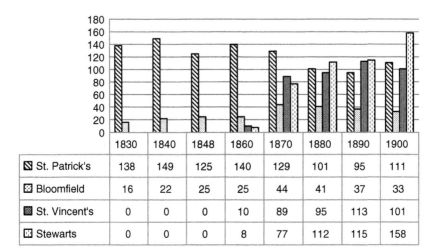

	1830	1840	1848	1860	1870	1880	1890	1900
St. Patrick's	138	149	125	140	129	101	95	111
Bloomfield	16	22	25	25	44	41	37	33
St. Vincent's	0	0	0	10	89	95	113	101
Stewarts	0	0	0	8	77	112	115	158

Fig. 2.2   Patient numbers in St Patrick's, Bloomfield, St Vincent's and Stewarts, 1830–1900. Compiled from *Reports of the Inspectors General on the General State of the Prisons of Ireland, 1831, 1841; Reports on District, Local and Private Lunatic Asylums in Ireland, 1849, 1861, 1871, 1881, 1890–1891, 1901*

lunatic applied to John Hitchcock, the manager of the Clonmel asylum, stating their willingness to pay for her care if he agreed to admit her. Hitchcock wrote to the Chief Secretary of Ireland for guidance.[93] In his letter, Hitchcock recognised that district asylums were legally required to provide relief for the 'lunatic poor', whose qualifying affidavit for admission must state 'they are paupers and have no friend, who will, or can be obliged to support them in a private lunatic establishment'. On the other hand, Hitchcock was willing to acknowledge:

> there are in this and other asylums a few, whose friends are many degrees above those belonging to the quite destitute poor – and though they might not be able to provide for them in a private asylum, yet might be brought, were it made a rule, to contribute at least, as much, as would indemnify the County for their maintenance.

Among this class, Hitchcock included people of reduced circumstances or limited incomes and large families, such as small farmers and second-rate shopkeepers.[94]

Clonmel was not the only asylum to receive applications of this sort. From the 1840s, the Richmond, Carlow and Maryborough district asylums had all begun to admit paying patients. Meanwhile, other asylums, including Belfast, refused to admit them until the practice was legally sanctioned. These earliest paying patients were maintained out of their own income or pension, the income from a farm or through contributions from their relatives.[95] By 1857, eleven district asylums housed fifty-three paying patients, who represented just over 1% of the total resident population.[96] The lunacy inspectors' attitude towards the practice was inconsistent at this point. As Cox has argued, they simply attempted 'to excuse and justify it', while at the same time stressing their disapproval.[97]

The uncertainty shared by asylum board members and the inspectors can be attributed to several factors, including the Irish medical community's concerns that a payment system was open to both abuse and tax-payer resentment.[98] In 1845, the newly appointed lunacy inspectors reported that the question of district asylums accepting paying patients warranted 'immediate and most serious attention on the part of the Government'. Apparently supporting this proposal, the inspectors maintained that local boards now favoured the measure and equivalent provisions were already in place in England and Scotland owing to the 'mixed character' of institutions there.[99] While the inspectors were aware that mixing paying and pauper patients might create class distinctions between them to the disadvantage of pauper patients, they claimed it was the right of middle-and lower-class farmers 'to participate in the benefits of institutions, towards the erection and support of which they are assessed'.[100] This cohort comprised the local ratepayers for whom district asylums had become a heavy financial burden.[101] Again, in 1852, the inspectors urged the propriety of admitting 'agriculturists and people in trade' who, under the present law, were 'in great measure debarred relief when labouring under insanity'. They advised against giving preferential treatment to paying patients and proposed that patients should be charged at the 'common annual expense for maintenance', stressing that this low rate should 'go simply to the support of the lunatic, without any derivable profit to a third party'.[102]

In 1856, attempts were made to legalise the admission of paying patients formally. The inspectors' influence was clear in a bill introduced 'to explain and amend the acts relating to lunatic asylums in Ireland'.[103] This bill was primarily concerned with devolving future authority for appointments to the Irish executive.[104] It also proposed a clause to legalise the admission of paying patients.[105] However, when the bill was passed later that year, this clause had been omitted, most likely neglected due to controversies over asylum staff appointments.[106] The following year, the question of legalising the admission of paying patients gained momentum during the 1857–1858 commission of inquiry, comprising Sir Thomas Nicholas Redington, Robert Andrews, Robert Wilfred Skeffington Lutwidge, James Wilkes and Dominic John Corrigan. The fact that these men were prominent members of their professions probably intensified the publicity surrounding the commission. Corrigan was a renowned member of the Irish medical community, the first Catholic president of the Royal College of Physicians of Ireland, had a private practice in Dublin and held numerous public appointments, often in relation to poor relief. Redington was an Irish administrator, a politician and a civil servant and held various posts including becoming the first Catholic Under-Secretary of State for Ireland (1846–1852) and Secretary to the Board of Control (1852–1856).[107] Wilkes, previously medical superintendent at the Staffordshire county asylum in England (1841–1855) was also a commissioner of lunacy in England. Finally, Skeffington Lutwidge served as a legal member of the lunacy commission in England from 1855 until his death in 1873. Together, these commissioners interviewed the lunacy inspectors, resident physicians, visiting physicians, governors and chaplains at asylums throughout Ireland on various aspects of lunacy administration and legislation. The commission was a crucial forum and the extensive discussions of sanctioning the reception of paying patients in district asylums reveal the importance attached to this issue by mid-century. Their responses were as diverse as they were plentiful.

Several resident physicians, visiting physicians and board members were in favour of admitting paying patients, although they remained uncertain of the legalities.[108] When queried, White claimed 'the law is so vague ... that in some asylums they refuse them'. He went on to recount the case of the Maryborough asylum board, which had applied to the inspectors for permission to admit a paying patient earlier that year. White had approved of the plan but then the board produced a document from 'some years past' which clearly showed that the law officers of the time had found 'that the law would not permit it'.[109] This was not the only discrepancy in the interpretation of the law regarding paying patients. For example, except for two pensioners, the Londonderry asylum did not cater for paying patients. Sir Robert Alexander Ferguson

M.P., a member of the asylum boards at both Omagh and Londonderry, spoke about the irregularity within the system:

> our idea in Derry has been that we had not a right to admit paying patients unless there was a superabundance of room; if there was room for more than the pauper patients that then we might admit the paying patients. That has been our understanding of the law both in Derry and in Omagh. At Omagh, having the room for them, we admitted them.[110]

In contrast, one governor of the Waterford asylum informed the commission 'I was always of the opinion it was not possible to do it under the existing law till Dr. White explained on the last Board day that it may be done'.[111]

Yet more confusion engulfed the question of whether families who could afford to pay only part of a patient's maintenance could do so. Board members and medical superintendents were particularly outspoken in this debate, touching as it did on their anxieties about the tax base for asylums. Although the Treasury initially covered construction costs for district asylums, ratepayers were required to repay these advances, meaning that the county rates ultimately funded the system. The counties were also expected to repay the total maintenance charges for patients, which the Treasury advanced.[112] Thus, when it came to patients whose maintenance came only partially from private sources, the question of who would make up the difference was fraught with tension.

Several boards opposed the reception of these part-paying patients altogether, insisting that neither the state nor the local ratepayer should be obliged to subsidise them. Adopting a more moderate stance, Reverend Henry Montgomery, a member of the Belfast board, urged that only those able to pay £5 or £10 per year should be allowed to, asking 'what are you doing with public rates but supporting the poor?'[113] Despite Montgomery's comments, at this point the Belfast board was still refusing to accept paying patients altogether.

Meanwhile, Samuel Haughton, a governor of the Carlow asylum, stated that his fellow board members were worried about the additional administrative pressure that admitting part-paying patients would create. Haughton feared it would be impossible to apportion payment according to patients' means, claiming that subsidising this group out of the local rates 'would be going from bad to worse, because they have not the machinery in the asylum to ascertain the truth with regard to the localities from which the persons came'. While Carlow had actually been admitting part-paying patients since at least 1854,[114] Haughton was correct in his forewarning. As Chap. 3 discusses, calculating means-appropriate fees became a time-consuming process for boards later in the nineteenth century.[115]

The medical community also held conflicting views about part-paying patients. The resident physician at Clonmel, Dr. James Flynn, argued that counties should not be compelled to support them. Mullingar's visiting physician, Dr. Joseph Ferguson, meanwhile, stated that lunatics were 'an interesting class', who, if 'allowed to go at large', produced multiple considerations for the state including crime, poverty and the extension of disease. In light of this, Ferguson maintained that the 'state ought to contribute any deficiency there might be, rather than throw it on the cess payers', contending it was up to the state to ensure the insane were institutionalised.[116] This appeal was probably rooted in Ferguson's recognition of the state's role in providing for pauper lunatics. As Finnane has contended, insanity at this time was commonly viewed as providential and accordingly was characterised as a national rather than a local problem.[117] Some asylum doctors in Ireland clearly subscribed to this view, which accounts for their demands for state recognition of the 'blameless' nature of the ailment. As will be discussed, the eventual outcome of these debates was to divide the outstanding maintenance for part-paying patients between the Treasury and the local rates, using the 'four shillings' rule.

Another concern about the reception of paying patients was whether they should receive superior food, clothing and accommodation. In theory, some argued, those who paid should be entitled to higher standards. However, proposals to provide better conditions for paying patients prompted anxieties both nationally and at local level. Many commentators feared that jealousies would arise between the pauper and paying patients. Nugent urged that both groups should be given identical accommodation and care, although he did not consider 'an injurious effect' would result from accommodating paying and non-paying patients together as 'the gradation is so imperceptible in social life'.[118] The Dean of Waterford asylum, Reverend Edward Newenham Hoare, adopted a contradictory stance, envisioning the number of 'difficulties' that might arise where paying patients' friends expected them to receive 'a mode of treatment as to dietary and other comforts better than what was ordinarily given to the pauper inmates'.[119]

Approaches to care for paying patients already in the asylums fluctuated widely. Most resident physicians favoured providing higher standards of accommodation. At Sligo, some paying patients were given 'every comfort they were accustomed to', along with a 'distinct attendant', and were housed in a separate ward. Fees were means-based and, in one or two cases, patients paid approximately £1 per week (£52 p.a.) before being removed to a private asylum. Notably, the asylum's resident physician, Dr. John McMunn, was against continuing to care for these patients:

> persons of that class require others of their own class to associate with them, in order to make them comfortable. It is most annoying to them to associate with persons of a lower class, which association, I think, materially retards their recovery. I think a pauper asylum totally unsuited to persons of a different class.

Sligo also received paying patients for as little as £10 per annum. Based on his experiences, McMunn prescribed a superior mode of care for paying patients, recommending that the 'rate-payers must pay the additional expense' incurred. He asserted that patients should be treated in a manner 'as near as possible to what they were accustomed to'. Thus, he stated, while pauper patients would receive their 'ordinary breakfast' of porridge, 'if a patient was accustomed to tea at home for breakfast, I would give him tea'. When one commissioner mockingly enquired whether McMunn might extend this 'to allow a man a carriage to drive in because he had been accustomed to one', McMunn disagreed. He did not share the concerns of several of his fellow resident physicians about the potential for jealousy between patients.[120]

Other asylum physicians and managers took pains to justify their preferential treatment of paying patients. Like McMunn, they framed their actions in terms of their moral obligation to accommodate patients in accordance with their previous living standards. For example, while the Ballinasloe asylum's manager, John B. M'Kiernan, placed non-violent paying patients in a 'better class' in the house, 'amongst the quiet and orderly', he attributed this to:

> a moral point of view, as regards their moral treatment, thinking they have been accustomed to more comforts than they would have in this asylum

as pauper patients and the want of which they would feel worse than the others.[121]

In relation to food, paying patients at Omagh were allowed 'nothing further than, perhaps, meat on Friday ... the day on which all the others get bread and milk'. They were also allowed to dress in their own clothes.[122] Omagh's resident physician, Francis John West, assured the commissioners he had seen no instance of jealousy between patients and that there had been no inconvenience. At Killarney, paying patients invariably received a 'better class of food'. Martin Shine Lawler, resident physician and governor at the asylum, said he felt obliged to these patients, citing the following example:

> there may be a paying patient who filled the rank of a gentleman; and who will not eat oatmeal gruel for breakfast and I am obliged to give him a more luxurious diet or better class of food.

Lawler conceded this had caused resentment, though he stated this was 'amongst persons who have been in a better position of life themselves, not amongst the humbler or poorer classes'.[123]

Only a minority of the resident physicians interviewed were against giving paying patients better treatment. Flynn warned of the confusion it would cause, resulting in 'interference with officers and servants corrupted and attempting to give patients advantages'.[124] Limerick's resident physician, Dr. Robert Fitzgerald, maintained that he should not be expected to provide a higher scale of diet for paying patients. At Limerick, paying patients' friends were generally responsible for their clothing and frequently provided some food items.[125] What emerged from the 1857–1858 inquiry was the uncertainty surrounding how best to accommodate this group, once admitted. It is plausible the asylum authorities felt a degree of sympathy for paying patients and were thus inclined to treat them preferentially. However, factors such as cost of accommodation and a sense of obligation towards the pauper patients also influenced these decisions.

On completing their inquiry, the commissioners found that the legislation did not 'appear to have contemplated the reception of paying patients', stating that the terms:

which indicated that Asylums were to be erected for the 'lunatic poor,' are not to be and, indeed, have not been, considered as limiting them to the 'destitute poor,' or those whom, by that technical definition, the law recognises as qualified to be relieved out of the poor rates.

They recommended that the admission of paying patients should be 'distinctly recognised' to protect the ratepayers from 'undue taxation' and the lunatic poor from 'unfair encroachment upon the accommodation intended more especially for them'. The commissioners also advised that managers should make no distinction between paying and pauper patients, unless, with the knowledge of the physician, their friends supplied extras. Finally, they suggested that paying patients should be entitled to wear their own clothes in the asylum, though they encouraged the extension of this privilege to all patients.[126]

Despite its emphasis on paying patients and the resulting publicity, the commissioners' report did not generate any new legislation either sanctioning or regulating their admission. On 12 June 1860, an editorial in the *Irish Times* criticised the inquiry's outcome. This editorial cited Flynn's interpretation of the inquiry:

the volumes of evidence are taken; a report in the face of the weight of evidence is made. Then the Commissioners differ and publish separate reports; counter reports in vindication are got up and published; the public is divided; statesmen who know nothing of Ireland are puzzled; and, at last, all legislation is 'abandoned'.

Here, Flynn referred to the letters of dissent written by various individuals, including Corrigan and the Governor of Belfast, to the Chief Secretary.[127] In 1859, Nugent also wrote to the Chief Secretary reviewing the findings of the commissioners' report and reiterating his support for the admission of paying patients.[128] The *Irish Times* editorial also related Flynn's recommendations for district asylums:

every county should have its own Asylum, with at least 200 beds, of which 30 should be allocated to paying patients, at £20 or £30 each per annum. These, with one chronic hospital for each province, would accommodate 8000 lunatics of the humbler and middle classes.[129]

This proposal garnered support from the press. The editors were advocates and the following day, a local paper, the *Nenagh Guardian*, characterised Flynn as the 'able physician' who offered 'some excellent suggestions'.[130]

Despite the commission's failure to engender new legislation, public interest in the paying patient question persisted. In 1864, the *Freeman's Journal* reprinted an editorial from another local paper, the *Clonmel Chronicle*, in which the editors argued:

> For rich and for poor – the millionaire, the tradesman, the mechanic and the pauper – for all classes and grades, there ought to be accommodation according to the means which can be afforded by the relatives of the patients, in public asylums.

They acknowledged that Flynn had been pressing this issue since the 1840s and complained that 'twenty years have since passed away and nothing has been done as yet'.[131] It is plausible that the foundation of St Vincent's and Stewarts and expansion of Bloomfield in the intervening decades had somewhat pacified appeals for state provision, alleviating the pressure on the state to provide for this group.

THE PRIVY COUNCIL CLAUSE

Whether or not public pressure played a role, in 1870 a clause was added to the Privy Council's rules for asylums authorising the admission of paying and part-paying patients to district asylums.[132] These rules contained limiting measures which largely echoed the commissioners' findings. As Cox has outlined, it prohibited access for paying patients in cases where pauper admissions were pending. Unlike entry as a pauper, paying patient applications required a certificate signed by a magistrate and a clergyman, verifying the applicant's unwillingness or inability to pay for private asylum care. While resident medical superintendents were tasked with submitting applications to the asylum board, the inspectors had the final say, as no paying patients could be admitted without their prior approval. Patient fees could not exceed the average cost of maintaining a pauper patient and could be no less than one-quarter of that amount. In real terms, this was between approximately £6 and £24 per annum, making it the least expensive asylum accommodation in Ireland, and protecting district asylums from allegations of profiting from paying patients.[133]

In response to some asylum doctors' preferential treatment of paying patients, they would now be subject to the same rules and regulations as pauper patients 'in regard to their treatment, care and maintenance'.[134]

Those rules were greeted with exceptional optimism. Once the Privy Council regulated the admission of paying patients, the inspectors seemed to become more comfortable with the practice.[135] They predicted that the rules would be 'of the greatest benefit to a number of persons hitherto without the advantages of asylum treatment' and reported that they met with 'very general approbation' from the various asylum boards.[136] The report of the 1878–1879 Trench commission inquiring into Poor Law unions and lunacy went so far as to project that 'twenty-five per cent of the beds in district asylums would be occupied by paying patients, if admissible'.[137] Yet, uptake remained limited and, after 1870, both the actual and proportionate numbers of paying patients dropped off (see Table 2.1). These figures are low compared with voluntary and private asylums. As seen earlier, between 1860 and 1880, the number of patients in voluntary asylums rose from 183 to 349, while those in private asylums had dropped from 349 to 261. While the increase in voluntary asylum patients resulted largely from the establishment of St Vincent's and Stewarts in the 1850s, it also reflects the relatively small uptake of district asylum provision for paying patients. Numbers admittedly fell far short of the 25% anticipated by the Trench commissioners. From 1877, the inspectors recorded the number of paying patients admitted as opposed to numbers resident. As Table 2.2 indicates, only a small proportion of admissions to district asylums were paying patients. From 1890 onwards, the newly elected lunacy inspectors ceased recording the number of paying patients in district asylums altogether.

Rather sheepishly, the lunacy inspectors repeatedly attempted to account for the persistently low numbers of paying patients admitted to district asylums. Among their explanations was the limiting nature of the Privy Council rules. As Cox has rightly contended, the inspectors failed to consider the difficulties paying patients might face in attempting to secure admission. Overcrowding, coupled with the fact that pauper admissions were given preference, meant admission was a slow process that proved unpopular with families.[138] When the Trench commissioners questioned Nugent about the inconvenient mode of admitting paying patients, he volunteered no solutions and essentially evaded discussion

Table 2.1 Number of paying patients resident in district asylums and the proportion of paying patients to total patients resident in district asylums, 1857–1889

Year	Number of paying patients resident	(%) Paying patients to total resident
1857	53	1.1
1860	84	2.0
1865	71	1.5
1870	122	1.8
1875	91	1.2

Compiled from *Reports on District, Local and Private Lunatic Asylums in Ireland, 1857, 1861, 1866, 1871, 1876*

Table 2.2 Number of paying patients admitted to district asylums and the proportion of paying patient admissions to total admissions to district asylums, 1880–1890

Year	Number of paying patients admitted	(%) Paying patients to total admitted
1880	65	2.8
1885	57	2.0
1889	53	1.8

Compiled from *Reports on District, Local and Private Lunatic Asylums in Ireland, 1881, 1886, 1890*

of the problem by reciting the relevant sections of the Privy Council rules.[139]

In contrast to Nugent's apathy, various medical superintendents lambasted the 'difficulty and delay' the Privy Council rules occasioned. Dr. John Charles Robertson, medical superintendent at Monaghan, complained in 1878:

In the first instance the forms when perfected are submitted to the Board of Governors, who meet but once a month and the admission approved by them, then the form has to be forwarded to the Inspector's office for their approval and when returned to the Resident Medical Superintendent, approved, he can then notify the patient's friends, that the lunatic can be admitted.

Robertson recognised that these patients might be admitted provisionally, pending approval, but warned 'there is some trouble in making the friends fill up the forms agreeing to pay the sum stipulated'. Dr. William Daxon, medical superintendent at Ennis, also criticised this mode of admission, adding that on a medical superintendent's refusal to admit a paying patient, 'the friends commit the patients as a dangerous lunatic and the institution loses the benefit of the money'.[140]

Difficulties obtaining fees after patients had been admitted were reportedly widespread.[141] Richmond's medical superintendent, Dr. Joseph Lalor, suggested that the Privy Council clause should be abolished, drawing the Trench commissioners' attention instead to the 1875 Lunatic Asylums (Ireland) Act. This Act allowed resident medical superintendents to apply to a court of summary jurisdiction to seize assets to the value of the fees owed, in cases where patients had means beyond those needed to support their family.[142] If a patient had no assets, any person responsible for their support outside the asylum became liable for their maintenance once incarcerated.[143] Lalor claimed these powers were sufficient to 'meet the cases of persons able to pay in whole or in part the cost of support' but were 'not carried out or very little carried out'. When he had, some years earlier, sent the Richmond board of governors a list of patients whose friends were believed to have means, the board 'had two or three cases put into the hands of their solicitor, but there was some difficulty in the way and it was not acted on'.[144] According to Lalor, there had been between thirty and forty patients of this class at Richmond.[145]

Nonetheless, the proportion of district asylum patients 'supposed to have means' who did not contribute was reportedly low. According to the lunacy inspectors, they accounted for less than 1% of resident patients, both before and after the new Privy Council rules and the passing of the 1875 Act (see Table 2.3). In real terms, these patients numbered no more than forty in any one year.

Still at pains to explain the small number of paying patients, by the 1880s the lunacy inspectors declared that 'the truth is there are no intermediate grades in Ireland sufficient for the purpose [of contributing towards their maintenance]'. At this point, the inspectors had almost completely reversed their former opinions on paying patients. They now suggested that the farming classes, the very people for whom they had previously urged the measure, should be immune to maintenance charges, because they had already contributed towards the rates.[146] This factor likely deterred many families from applying to pay for care because they felt they had already contributed to the system. However, it is also

Table 2.3 Proportion of paying patients and patients supposed to have means but do not pay to total resident population of district asylums in Ireland, 1865–1875

	(%) Paying patients	(%) Patients supposed to have means but do not pay
1865	1.5	0.6
1870	1.8	0.5
1875	1.2	0.5
1880	Unknown[a]	0.3
1885	Unknown	0.3
1890	Unknown	0.4

[a]From 1880, the inspectors recorded the number of paying patients admitted to district asylums. Comparison between those resident from 1880–1890 is thus not possible. Compiled from *Reports on District, Local and Private Lunatic Asylums in Ireland, 1866, 1871, 1876, 1881, 1886, 1890*

conceivable that these claims were rooted in the decreasing prosperity of Ireland during this period as the economic depression worsened. In 1890, the new inspectors recognised that 'the poverty existing in Ireland will to a certain degree explain why the number supported, wholly or in part, by family contributions is so small'.[147]

The lunacy inspectors also blamed asylum boards. In 1874, a state grant of four shillings per head per week was introduced towards the maintenance of lunatics in public asylums in Britain and Ireland.[148] This rule was important for paying patients. If the cost of maintenance in a district asylum was £22, patients paying approximately £11 12 *s* or less would be eligible for a Treasury grant. For patients charged more than this amount, the remainder came out of the local rates. The lunacy inspectors criticised the boards, whom they accused of 'best consulting the interests of the rate-payers by not putting pressure upon the relatives to contribute more than a certain amount' in order to qualify for the Treasury grant.[149] However, this was apparently a temporary problem. By the late 1890s, the inspectors were 'glad to report' that the boards displayed 'greater energy' in obtaining fees.[150]

Paying for district asylum care also proved unpopular because standards of accommodation and treatment could not surpass those offered to pauper patients.[151] Evidence given during the Trench commission suggests that families were reluctant to pay for the same level of care the pauper patients received free of charge. The disgrace of pauperising a family member was probably seen as payment enough.[152] As Richmond's medical superintendent, Lalor, told the commission:

> My experience is that people say, 'If I pay will my friends get better treatment?' and under the Privy Council rules they are not allowed to get better treatment and when they find this they let the thing go, as they say there is no advantage from paying.

Lalor also noted 'a great objection amongst people to let it be known that their friends are in an asylum', although he conceded that in some cases 'there is the proper pride not to have a person supported as a pauper who is not so'.[153] Nugent portrayed Irish families in similar terms: 'they say that "if we go into a public asylum, why go in with the disgrace, while we are paying;" so they go in and don't pay.' When asked whether separate accommodation for non-paupers would 'meet a want largely felt', Nugent replied: 'I think it would in England, but it is not congenial to the feelings of the Irish', demonstrating the continued failure to gain official support for this proposal.[154] As a means of compromise, Ennis' medical superintendent, Daxon, suggested that paying patients should be allowed to pay higher sums, 'as many of this class require better diet than the ordinary run of patients and their friends would much prefer to pay liberally for any extras that might be given to them'.[155] By the late 1890s, the lunacy inspectors concurred, arguing it was unfortunate that paying patients 'have to associate with persons below them in social position and education'.[156] They proposed that the local authorities should be empowered to supply separate lodgings for paying patients.[157] Still, by the turn of the century no drastic alterations took place and the Privy Council rules remained the principal guidelines for the reception of this group.

CONCLUSIONS

While Ireland was unusual for the early degree of state intervention in lunacy, provision for paying patients was slow to emerge. Because the private sector depended on profit, private care remained an expensive commodity out of reach for most of society, particularly during periods of economic hardship. Sporadic sensationalist press coverage of alleged abuses must also have deterred potential clientele. While by the end of the century, Belmont Park in Waterford and St John of God's in Dublin charged much lower than average fees, gaining favour with the lunacy inspectors, their scale and Catholic ethos left a large gap for others seeking affordable asylum care.

It was thus left to philanthropists and the state to grapple with how best to accommodate those between pauper and privileged. Contrasting discourses gave rise to two distinct solutions: the voluntary creation of mixed asylums catering for paying and charity patients, and sanctioning the admission of paying patients in district asylums. It was not until the founding of St Vincent's and Stewarts in the 1850s that voluntary provision became significant. These asylums offered moderate rates and even free accommodation to what they termed the 'middle classes' and the 'respectable poor'. Their managing bodies were sensitive to social distinctions between the various classes of patients and accommodation reflected the amounts charged. The state was more concerned with the protection of the poor, whom the district asylum system was initially created for, and the ratepayers who financed it. This resulted in the clumsily constructed Privy Council clause, which placed severe limitations on admissions and care for paying patients. Because of the varied agendas of these interest groups, non-pauper asylum care remained a patchwork of state, voluntary and private institutions, charging very different rates and offering vastly different standards of accommodation.

NOTES

1. 'Editorial Article 2,' *Irish Times*, 12 June 1860.
2. Smith (1999a, p. 12).
3. MacDonagh (1989, p. 206).
4. 'Lunatic Asylums' Commission,' *Freeman's Journal*, 24 Oct. 1857.
5. For a discussion of the grounds on which Hampstead House, Highfield House and St John of God's were established, see Chap. 3.
6. 5 & 6 Vic., c. 123.
7. MacDonagh (1989, p. 206).
8. 14 Geo. III, c. 49.
9. 5 & 6 Vic., c. 123, s. 14, 15, 18, 20, 28, 30.
10. Finnane (1981, p. 92).
11. Parry-Jones (1972, p. 17).
12. 'Editorial Article 1,' *Irish Times*, 29 Feb. 1860.
13. 'Editorial Article 1,' *Irish Times*, 12 Dec. 1859.
14. Ninth Report of the Inspectors General on the General State of the Prisons of Ireland, H.C. 1830–1831.

15. Bartlett (1999, p. 48).
16. For example, 'Article 1,' *Irish Times*, 6 Oct. 1859.
17. 'Classified Ad 24,' *Irish Times*, 8 March 1861.
18. Parry-Jones (1972, p. 282).
19. Mauger (2012).
20. Report on District, Local and Private Lunatic Asylums in Ireland, H.C. 1867, pp. 38–39.
21. The Lord Chancellor was the highest judicial officer in Ireland.
22. The Lord Lieutenant was the British monarch's official representative and head of the Irish executive.
23. 5 & 6 Vic., c. 123, s. 13.
24. Report on District, Local and Private Lunatic Asylums in Ireland, H.C. 1867, p. 39.
25. Thirty-Seventh Report on the District, Criminal, and Private Lunatic Asylums in Ireland [C 5459], H.C. 1888, lii, 595, p. 33.
26. Finnane (1981, p. 63).
27. Cox (2012, p. 48).
28. Thirty-Eighth Report on the District, Criminal, and Private Lunatic Asylums in Ireland [C 5796], H.C. 1889, xxxvii, 641, p. 19.
29. 53 Vic., c. 5.
30. Parry-Jones (1972, p. 26).
31. Finnane (1981, p. 67).
32. Report of Committee on Lunacy Administration, p. 27.
33. Finnane (1981, p. 63), Cox (2012, p. 51).
34. Thirty-Ninth Report on the District, Criminal, and Private Lunatic Asylums in Ireland [C 6148], H.C. 1890, xxxv, 609, p. 4.
35. Cox (2012, p. 2), Kelly (2008, pp. 79–84), Kelly (2016, pp. 25–28).
36. Fortieth Report of the Inspectors of Lunatics (Ireland) [C 6503], H.C. 1890–1891, xxxvi, 521, p. 15.
37. Report into the State of Lunatic Asylums, Part II, p154. Forty-Third Report of the Inspectors of Lunatics (Ireland) [C 7466], H.C. 1894, xliii, 401, p. 23.
38. Forty-Second Report of the Inspectors of Lunatics (Ireland) [C 7125], H.C. 1893–1894, xlvi, 369, p. 15.
39. Forty-Sixth Report of the Inspectors of Lunatics (Ireland) [C 8639], H.C. 1897, xxxviii, 527, p. 39.
40. Forty-Fourth Report of the Inspectors of Lunatics (Ireland) [C 7804], H.C. 1895, liv, 435, p. 172.
41. Forty-Fifth Report of the Inspectors of Lunatics (Ireland) [C 8251], H.C. 1896, xxxix, Part II, 1, pp. 171–172.
42. Forty-Fourth Report of the Inspectors of Lunatics (Ireland), H.C. 1895, p. 181.

43. Fortieth Report of the Inspectors of Lunatics (Ireland), H.C. 1890–1891, p. 190; Report into the State of Lunatic Asylums, Part II, p. 154. Forty-Third Report of the Inspectors of Lunatics (Ireland), H.C. 1894, pp. 170–171.
44. Forty-Fourth Report of the Inspectors of Lunatics (Ireland), H.C. 1895, p. 22.
45. Sixty-Seventh Report of the Inspectors of Lunatics (Ireland) [CMD 32], H.C. 1919, xxv, 305, p. 39.
46. Forty-Seventh Report of the Inspectors of Lunatics (Ireland) [C 8969], H.C. 1898, xliii, 491, p. 30.
47. Forty-Ninth Report of the Inspectors of Lunatics (Ireland) [CD 312], H.C. 1900, xxxvii, 513, p. xl.
48. 'Article 1,' *Irish Times*, 14 Dec. 14 1859.
49. Smith (1994, pp. 191, 210, 212–213).
50. See Cox (2012), Finnane (1981).
51. Dr. James Foulis Duncan is not to be confused with his father, Dr. James Duncan, the proprietor of Farnham House Private Asylum. For more on James Foulis Duncan, see Kelly (2016, pp. 55–59).
52. Duncan (1853, pp. 257–258, 260–261).
53. Fourteenth Report on the District, Criminal, and Private Lunatic Asylums in Ireland [3556], H.C. 1865, xxi, 103, p. 13.
54. Report into the State of Lunatic Asylums, Part I, p. 32.
55. Preston (2004), Luddy (1995).
56. Luddy (2004).
57. Cox (2012, p. 19).
58. Twenty-Ninth Report on the District, Criminal, and Private Lunatic Asylums in Ireland [C 2621], H.C. 1880, xxix, 459, p. 22.
59. Malcolm (1989, p. 319). The remainder in both periods were Catholic.
60. 'Census of Ireland 1901.' Accessed 6 Jan. 2012, http://www.census.nationalarchives.ie.
61. *Annual Report of the State of the Retreat, 1821*, p. 5; *Annual Report of the State of the Retreat, 1822*, p. 4; *Annual Report of the State of the Retreat, 1832*, p. 5; *Annual Report of the State of the Retreat, 1833*, p. 5.
62. Digby 1985, pp. 180–181.
63. Report into the State of Lunatic Asylums, Part II, p. 162.
64. Eighth Report on the District, Criminal, and Private Lunatic Asylums in Ireland [2253], H.C. 1857, vvii, 67, p. 24; Fortieth Report of the Inspectors of Lunatics (Ireland), H.C. 1890–1891, p. 17; Fiftieth Report of the Inspectors of Lunatics (Ireland), H.C. 1901, p. 487.
65. Twenty-First Report on the District, Criminal, and Private Lunatic Asylums in Ireland, H.C. 1872, p. 33.

66. The Forty-Fifth Report of the Inspectors of Lunatics (Ireland), H.C. 1896, p. 186.
67. O'Brien and Lunney (2002).
68. The Eighteenth Report on the District, Criminal, and Private Lunatic Asylums in Ireland, H.C. 1868–1869, p. 37.
69. Luddy (2004, p. x).
70. Preston 2004, pp. 52–55. For twentieth-century Ireland, see Earner-Byrne (2007, pp. 75–82).
71. Whelan (1995, p. 135).
72. Preston (2004, pp. 52–55).
73. Report into the State of Lunatic Asylums, Part II, p. 195.
74. Crossman (2010, pp. 138, 141).
75. Walsh (2005, pp. 108–109), Luddy (1995, p. 176).
76. Luddy (1995, p. 191).
77. 'Middle Class Lunatic Asylums,' *Irish Times*, 23 Sep. 1874.
78. Malcolm (1989, pp. 118–120, 130–131, 176–178, 187).
79. *Annual Report of the State of the Retreat* (Dublin, 1811), p. 23.
80. Report into the State of Lunatic Asylums, Part II, p. 160.
81. Digby 1985, p. 181.
82. Eighth Report on the District, Criminal, and Private Lunatic Asylums in Ireland, H.C. 1857, p. 24.
83. Tenth Report on the District, Criminal, and Private Lunatic Asylums in Ireland [2901], H.C. 1861, xxvii, 245, p. 12.
84. 'Middle Class Lunatic Asylums,' *Irish Times*, 23 Sep. 1874.
85. Report into the State of Lunatic Asylums, Part II, p. 197.
86. 5 & 6 Vic., c. 123, s. 49.
87. Forty-Sixth Report of the Inspectors of Lunatics (Ireland), H.C. 1897, p. 209.
88. Malcolm (1989, pp. 175, 200).
89. Forty-Ninth Report of the Inspectors of Lunatics (Ireland), H.C. 1900, p. 217.
90. Malcolm (1989).
91. Smith (1999b, pp. 35, 37, 43).
92. Smith (1999b).
93. The Chief Secretary of Ireland was subordinate to the Lord Lieutenant. He was responsible for the British administration of Ireland and often sat in the British Cabinet.
94. John Hitchcock to the Chief Secretary of Ireland, 1835 (NAI, CSORP, 1835/3365).
95. Cox (2003, p. 78). See also Cox (2012, p. 21).
96. Eighth Report on the District, Criminal, and Private Lunatic Asylums in Ireland, H.C. 1857, p. 12.

97. Cox (2003, p. 78).
98. Cox (2012, pp. 19–21).
99. For the English context, see Smith (1999b).
100. Report on District, Local and Private Lunatic Asylums in Ireland [820], H.C. 1847, xvii, 355, p. 12. See also Cox (2003, pp. 78–79).
101. See also Finnane (1981, p. 33), Cox (2012, pp. 18–20, 34–53).
102. Sixth General Report on the District, Criminal, and Private Lunatic Asylums in Ireland [1653], H.C. 1852–1853, xli, 353, p. 11.
103. A Bill to explain and amend the Acts relating to Lunatic Asylums in Ireland (149), H.C. 1856, v, 83, p. 3.
104. Finnane (1981, p. 38).
105. A Bill to explain and amend the Acts relating to Lunatic Asylums in Ireland, H.C. 1856, p. 3; Cox (2012, p. 22).
106. Cox (2012, p. 22), Finnane (1981, p. 38).
107. Redington was also actively involved in the Famine Relief Commission and received a knighthood for his services during the Famine.
108. Cox (2012, pp. 20–21).
109. Report into the State of Lunatic Asylums, Part II, p. 12.
110. Ibid., p. 215.
111. Ibid., p. 226.
112. Finnane (1981, p. 33). See also Cox (2012, pp. 18–20).
113. Report into the State of Lunatic Asylums, Part II, p. 346.
114. Cox (2003, p. 80).
115. See also Cox (2012, p. 23).
116. Report into the State of Lunatic Asylums, Part II, pp. 318–319.
117. Finnane (1981, p. 57).
118. Report into the State of Lunatic Asylums, Part II, p. 36.
119. Ibid., p. 226.
120. Ibid., pp. 474, 480.
121. Ibid., p. 443.
122. Ibid., p. 397.
123. Ibid., pp. 486–487.
124. Ibid., p. 244.
125. Ibid., p. 382.
126. Report into the State of Lunatic Asylums, Part I, pp. 4–5.
127. Corrigan's key concern was that asylums should have visiting physicians. See Communication of Doctor Corrigan, dissenting from portion of Report of Commissioners of Lunatic Asylums, Ireland (95), H.C. 1859, xxii, p. 203; Correspondence relating to alleged Errors in Report of Commissioners of Inquiry into State of Lunatic Asylums of Ireland regarding Belfast Asylum (178), H.C. 1859, xxii, p. 237.

128. Letter by Doctor Nugent, Inspector of Lunatic Asylums, in reply to Statements in Report of Commission on Lunatic Asylums in Ireland (147), H.C. 1859, xxii, p. 209.
129. 'Editorial Article 2,' *Irish Times*, 12 June 1860.
130. 'Lunacy and Lunatic Asylums,' *Nenagh Guardian*, 13 June 1860.
131. '"Middle-Class" Hospitals for the Insane,' *Freeman's Journal*, 20 Sept. 1864.
132. The Lord Lieutenant and the Privy Council were responsible for the formulation of asylum regulations.
133. Cox (2003, p. 81).
134. Twentieth Report on the District, Criminal, and Private Lunatic Asylums in Ireland [C 440], H.C. 1871, xxvi, 427, p. 163; Cox (2012, p. 22).
135. Cox (2003, p. 81), Cox (2012, pp. 22–23).
136. Eighteenth Report on the District, Criminal, and Private Lunatic Asylums in Ireland, H.C. 1868–1869, p. 38; Twentieth Report on the District, Criminal, and Private Lunatic Asylums in Ireland, H.C. 1871, p. 6.
137. Thirty-Second Report on the District, Criminal, and Private Lunatic Asylums in Ireland [C 3675], H.C. 1883, xxx, 433, p. 8.
138. Cox (2012, p. 23).
139. Trench Commission Report, p. 86.
140. Ibid., pp. 56, 230–231.
141. See, for example Ibid., pp. 56, 67, 87.
142. A Court of Summary Jurisdiction usually comprised two or more justices of the peace sitting in petty sessions. These assets included money, goods, possessions, rents and profits of the lands and tenements, and any other part of the patient's income.
143. 38 & 39 Vic., c. 67, s. 16.
144. Trench Commission Report, pp. 62, 67, 233.
145. Ibid.
146. Thirty-Second Report on the District, Criminal, and Private Lunatic Asylums in Ireland, H.C. 1883, pp. 8–9. Cox (2012, p. 22).
147. Fortieth Report of the Inspectors of Lunatics (Ireland), H.C. 1890–1891, p. 6.
148. For more on the impact of this rule on asylums and ratepayers see Finnane (1981, pp. 57–58). See also Melling and Forsythe (2006, p. 22).
149. Forty-Second Report of the Inspectors of Lunatics (Ireland), H.C. 1893–1894, p. 5.
150. Forty-Sixth Report of the Inspectors of Lunatics (Ireland), H.C. 1897, p. 9.
151. Cox (2003, p. 81).

152. In his study of Australian asylums, Stephen Garton has cited the stigma associated with institutional confinement as a cause of the relatively poor rates of maintenance fee recovery. Garton (1988, p. 115).
153. Trench Commission Report, pp. 86–87.
154. Ibid., p. 86.
155. Ibid., p. 231.
156. Forty-Sixth Report of the Inspectors of Lunatics (Ireland), H.C. 1897, p. 39.
157. Forty-Fifth Report of the Inspectors of Lunatics (Ireland), H.C. 1896, p. 29.

REFERENCES

Bartlett, Peter. 'The Asylum and the Poor Law: The Productive Alliance.' In *Insanity, Institutions and Society, 1800–1914*, edited by Joseph Melling and Bill Forsythe, 48–67. London and New York: Routledge, 1999.
Cox, Catherine. 'Managing Insanity in Nineteenth-Century Ireland.' PhD diss., University College Dublin, 2003.
Cox, Catherine. *Negotiating Insanity in the Southeast of Ireland 1830–1900*. Manchester: Manchester University Press, 2012.
Crossman, Virginia. 'Middle-Class Attitudes to Poverty and Welfare in Post-Famine Ireland.' In *Politics, Society and the Middle Class in Modern Ireland* edited by Fintan Lane, 130–147. Basingstoke: Palgrave Macmillan, 2010.
Duncan, James Foulis. *Popular Errors on the Subject of Insanity Examined and Exposed*. Dublin: Fannin & Co., 1853.
Earner-Byrne. Lindsey. *Mother and Child: Maternity and Child Welfare in Dublin, 1922–1960*. Manchester: Manchester University Press, 2007.
Finnane, Mark. *Insanity and the Insane in Post-Famine Ireland*. London: Croom Helm, 1981.
Garton, Stephen. *Medicine and Madness: A Social History of Insanity in New South Wales, 1880–1940*. Kensington, New South Wales, Australia: New South Wales University Press, 1988.
Kelly, Brendan D. 'Dr. William Saunders Hallaran and Psychiatric Practice in Nineteenth-Century Ireland.' *Irish Journal of Medical Science*, 117, no. 1 (2008): 79–84.
Kelly, Brendan. *Hearing Voices: The History of Psychiatry in Ireland*. Newbridge: Irish Academic Press, 2016.
Luddy, Maria. *Women and Philanthropy in Nineteenth-Century Ireland*. Cambridge: Cambridge University Press, 1995.
Luddy, Maria. Foreword to *Charitable Words: Women, Philanthropy and the Language of Charity in Nineteenth-Century Dublin*. Westport, Conn.: Praeger, 2004.

MacDonagh, Oliver. 'Ideas and Institutions, 1830–1845.' In *A New History of Ireland V: Ireland under the Union, I, 1801–1870*, edited by W. E. Vaughan, 193–217. Oxford: Oxford University Press, 1989.

Malcolm, Elizabeth. *Swift's Hospital: A History of St Patrick's Hospital, Dublin, 1746–1989*. Dublin: Gill and Macmillan, 1989.

Mauger, Alice. '"Confinement of the Higher Orders": The Social Role of Private Lunatic Asylums in Ireland, c. 1820–1860.' *Journal of the History of Medicine and Allied Sciences* 67, no. 2 (2012): 281–317.

Melling, Joseph and Bill Forsythe. *The Politics of Madness: The State, Insanity and Society in England, 1845–1814.* London and New York: Routledge, 2006.

O'Brien, Andrew and Linde Lunney. 'Henry Hutchinson Stewart.' In *Dictionary of Irish Biography*, edited by James McGuire and James Quinn. Cambridge: Cambridge University Press, 2002.

Parry-Jones, William Ll. *The Trade in Lunacy: A Study of Private Madhouses in England in the Eighteenth and Nineteenth Centuries.* London: Routledge & Kegan Paul, 1972.

Preston, Margaret H. *Charitable Words: Women, Philanthropy and the Language of Charity in Nineteenth-Century Dublin.* Westport, Conn.: Praeger, 2004.

Smith, Leonard D. 'Close Confinement in a Mighty Prison: Thomas Bakewell and his Campaign against Public Asylums, 1810–1830.' *History of Psychiatry*, 5, no. 18 (1994): 191–214.

Smith, Leonard D. *Cure, Comfort and Safe Custody: Public Lunatic Asylums in Early Nineteenth-Century England.* London and New York: Leicester University Press, 1999a.

Smith, Leonard D. 'The County Asylum in the Mixed Economy of Care, 1808–1845.' In *Insanity, Institutions and Society, 1800–1914*, edited by Joseph Melling and Bill Forsythe, 33–47. London and New York: Routledge, 1999b.

Walsh, Oonagh. *Anglican Women in Dublin: Philanthropy, Politics and Education in the Early Twentieth Century.* Dublin: University College Dublin Press, 2005.

Whelan, Irene. 'The Stigma of Souperism.' In *The Great Irish Famine*, edited by Cathal Póirtéir, 135–154. Dublin: Mercier Press, 1995.

CHAPTER 3

An Institutional Marketplace

Family members tend to be powerful lay voices in the process of institutionalisation. Historians of psychiatry have long recognised the centrality of families in dialogues with medical and legal authorities during certification and discharge.[1] In nineteenth-century Ireland, it was usually they who covered the cost of asylum care for paying patients, though less often patients with a pension, legacy or some other means paid their own fees. By the 1870s, those with means could select between public, voluntary or private care depending on how much they could—or were willing to—spend. This had implications for asylum managing bodies who were under pressure to secure fees. As we have seen, during the 1890s, the inspectors censured district asylum boards for repeatedly failing to identify patients with means. Even when they did, the inspectors complained that boards were overly lenient in the amounts requested because they tended to sympathise with ratepayers. Despite this criticism, there is evidence that boards went to great lengths to obtain fees from those they believed could afford them. Nonetheless, the revenue they collected tended to be small.[2] This chapter explores the networks through which boards gathered financial information about patients and their families, their motivations for chasing fees and the inherent difficulties surrounding their negotiation and payment. As will be seen, relatives were crucial mediators in this process.

Relatives in negotiations with voluntary and private asylums enjoyed comparatively greater influence as both asylum models depended heavily

© The Author(s) 2018
A. Mauger, *The Cost of Insanity in Nineteenth-Century Ireland*, Mental Health in Historical Perspective,
https://doi.org/10.1007/978-3-319-65244-3_3

on patient fees. While the managing committees of voluntary asylums struggled to balance providing charity for the 'respectable' against attracting a wealthier clientele, private asylum proprietors made their livelihood from profits. Although voluntary asylums were not kept for profit, this chapter contends that by the later nineteenth century, many were forced to compete with private asylums. By the 1890s, this professional competition, together with the depressed economy, had come to inform their strategies for advertising and securing fees.[3] Contrary to public criticisms of the private asylum system, examination of the outcome for patients admitted to the asylums studied reveals that private asylum patients were more likely to be discharged cured than those admitted to district asylums. Evidence of high levels of patient transfers between the three asylum sectors further underscores that the existence of a 'mixed economy of care', particularly after 1870, gave rise to an institutional marketplace for the insane.[4]

'A GROSS ABUSE ON THE TAX PAYING PUBLIC'[5]

Calculating maintenance fees was a convoluted process. Investigations into families' financial circumstances were thorough, even intrusive, and could draw on a range of sources within the local community, including the asylum board and resident medical superintendent (RMS), neighbours, friends, landlords and agents, the lunacy inspectors, solicitors, pensions offices, banks and parish priests. The intricacy of the whole process defies reasoning. In some instances, families were left with little choice but to call on their bank manager, who they insisted could attest to their inability to contribute towards asylum fees.[6] District medical officers were also known to intervene on behalf of relatives, signifying their rising position of authority within local communities.[7]

At local level, the admission of paying patients into district asylums placed new administrative burdens on asylum authorities. Although the 1870 Privy Council rules had specified rates for paying patients, they fell short of detailing how patients, families and asylum boards should agree these amounts. Since fees were based on the cost of maintaining a pauper patient (between one-quarter and the total average cost), they varied from district to district. For example, in 1890, the average cost of a pauper patient (not including casual receipts) was £20 4s 4d at Ennis, £21 12s 2d at Belfast, £24 3s 10d at Enniscorthy and £25 16s 10d at Richmond.[8] The average also changed from one year to the next. A crude estimate suggests that the average for the period 1868 to 1900 was £24 per annum, meaning that paying patients could legally be charged between £6 (one-quarter) and £24 (total) annually. This wide variation demonstrates the room for negotiation between the friends and relatives of paying patients and the asylum. It also indicates that paying patients were drawn from assorted socio-economic backgrounds.

Due to inconsistencies in the recording process, it was possible to calculate fees for just under two-thirds of paying patients in the four selected district asylums. Once agreed, fees were often cited in the minute books as per quarter or half year and even per day. The calculation of fees per annum in these cases therefore provides only a rudimentary estimate of actual spending power. Table 3.1 divides the recorded amounts contributed into three broad categories: £12 or less, £12 to £20, and over £20. Because many patients' fees altered with each readmission, likely reflecting a shift in economic circumstances, readmissions are included.

Most paying patients at Ennis were maintained at £12 or less, suggesting that relatives in this district had fewer means available. Patients in the urban asylums Belfast and Richmond were more likely to pay higher sums, while those at Enniscorthy were almost evenly represented across the three scales. At Belfast, fees were capped at £20, suggesting that managers there adhered more strictly to the Privy Council rules than the other asylums in the sample. This was characteristically cautious of Belfast, the only asylum studied that did not admit paying patients until officially authorised to do so.

Table 3.1 Breakdown of amounts contributed to maintenance of patients at Belfast, Ennis, Enniscorthy and Richmond district asylums, 1868–1900

Fees per annum	Belfast	(%)	Ennis	(%)	Enniscorthy	(%)	Richmond	(%)	Total	(%)
£12 or less	14	33.3	114	64.8	22	36.7	29	13.9	179	36.8
£12– £20	28	66.7	31	17.6	19	31.7	79	38.0	157	32.3
Over £20	N/A	N/A	31	17.6	19	31.7	100	48.1	150	30.9

Compiled from Belfast, Ennis, Enniscorthy and Richmond Minute Books and Enniscorthy and Richmond superintendent's notices

The extent to which other asylums were willing to exceed the Privy Council limit varied greatly. If the average cost per head during the period was £24, Ennis, Enniscorthy and Richmond were clearly in breach. Richmond was particularly culpable: 41% of known maintenance fees were £25 or more, while three patients contributed £40, £51 and £57. The tendency to charge over the average was less at Enniscorthy (8%) and Ennis (7%), where the maximum sums received were £25 and £30 respectively.[9] Nevertheless, except for Belfast, the fees charged in some instances were on a par with the voluntary asylums. Richmond's ability to secure higher fees is curious given its proximity to all four of the voluntary asylums, which were generally seen as preferable sites of care.

The notification process for families was equally haphazard. While some families were told they must pay fees during the committal process, others were contacted long after patients were admitted with a view to securing payment. On the contrary, those initially admitted as paying patients could become 'paupers' following a change in economic circumstances. The first point of contact, in all cases, was usually the RMS, who was responsible for outlining the procedure. For example, in 1883, the Enniscorthy asylum's RMS, Thomas Drapes, wrote to John W., a patient's husband:

> it would be well if you would come up here on Thursday next when the Board meets: as your circumstances being above those of 'pauper', the Governor will expect you to pay something for your wife's maintenance while in the asylum. The average cost is £22 per annum and if you let me know in writing that you are prepared to pay at that rate you need not come up: but if otherwise it is advisable that you should attend at the Board and state what your circumstances will admit of you paying.[10]

This letter suggests that fees at Enniscorthy were initially fixed at the highest rate. Thereafter, relatives could attempt to agree a smaller sum. Although this practice was not required by the Privy Council rules, it was probably adopted to apply pressure on families to cover costs.

At Ennis, the board took a different approach. There, relatives were subjected to a thorough investigation of their circumstances, following which an appropriate fee was agreed.[11] Surviving correspondence books for the Ennis asylum contain letters written by families, friends and acquaintances, providing first-hand accounts of the negotiation process. The sheer volume of correspondence relating to maintenance contributions in the Ennis asylum—approximately 270 letters identified for the period 1868–1900—indicates the disproportionate amount of administration generated by the reception of paying patients in district asylums.[12] It is unclear how this practice was handled at Belfast or Richmond. In all cases, it fell upon the boards of governors to assess individuals' means and arrive at a suitable maintenance fee. Acting in a secretarial capacity for the board, the RMS continued to correspond with families until matters were resolved.

Aside from payment from relatives, the boards could apply to other sources of income.[13] At Ennis, knowledge that a patient was the beneficiary of a will could spark investigations and, in some cases, the asylum's solicitor furnished the board with copies of wills and other legal documents.[14] Some patients used their pensions to pay for their maintenance, although under the 1875 Act, this was not required when patients had dependents.[15] Asylum boards apparently adhered to this law. In the case of Joseph H., a retired telegraph clerk at Richmond, the secretary to the General Post Office informed the asylum board that 'as he has no nearer relative than a brother living … the pension due to him should be paid to the asylum'.[16] However, when Anne R., wrote to Richmond, explaining that she was 'very poor' and had 'three small children', the board resolved not to claim her husband's pension.[17] Likewise, at Enniscorthy, Drapes redirected the pension of Patrick K., to his brother Thomas, 'he being in needy circumstances and having supported [the patient] for 3 years past' at home. These passing references bring home the reality for many families struggling to support a mentally ill relative. The board's compassion on this occasion was limited, however, as once Thomas died, they swiftly applied the pension to Patrick's maintenance.[18]

In some cases, asylum boards reached agreement with a patient's previous employer or pensions office to divide pensions between the asylum and the family. In 1879, the Richmond board wrote to the chief commissioner of the Dublin Metropolitan Police concerning a patient, John M., who had a 'wife and three young daughters who have no other means of living'. The board agreed to allocate £27 out of John's annual pension to his family and the remaining £13 to his maintenance.[19] The Ennis board initially demonstrated similar lenience in the case of pensioners.[20] Having learned that a patient's father was 'a very poor man' for whom the patient had been 'the chief means of … support' prior to his illness, the board resolved to reduce his maintenance to £10 and to refund £10 8s per year of the patient's excise office pension to the man's father.[21] However, in 1890, when a different patient's father requested that the Ennis board allow him to keep part of his son's pension from the Inland Revenue Board, the board refused because allowances from pensions had been 'disallowed by the Auditor in a similar case'.[22]

Families often used the workhouse as leverage when trying to evade fees, expressing fears of ending up there if forced to pay. One patient's father pleaded with the Ennis board to let him keep part of his son's pension 'to enable me to support myself, wife and family otherwise we must become inmates of the workhouse and lie a burthen on the ratepayers'.[23] Whether this fear was genuine, or merely served to remind the board that relatives too might become a burden on the ratepayer, is hard to decipher. However, as we shall see, several relatives, particularly in the Ennis district, presented themselves as being on the borderline of pauperism. Given the harsh economic conditions for many families, particularly farmers, in this district, it is likely that at least some of these claims were justified.

At their most extreme, the Ennis board threatened to discharge patients to the workhouse, a tactic that usually provoked even the most reluctant relative to contribute fees.[24] The Privy Council rules did not offer any specific protection to paying patients in this position. Moreover, while the 1875 Act empowered RMSs to acquire maintenance fees by various means, it did not sanction the discharge of patients whose fees were not paid.[25] The Act did, however, encourage the transfer of 'harmless' asylum patients to workhouses and in these cases the lunacy authorities continued to pay maintenance costs.[26] This was not a straightforward procedure. Workhouse guardians used destitution as admission criteria, posing problems for the transfer of paying patients to the workhouse.[27]

In 1892, the clerk of Tulla Union workhouse, County Clare, wrote to Richard Phillips Gelston, the RMS at Ennis, informing him that the board of guardians had heavily criticised the asylum for transferring an ex-policeman, who had been a paying patient, terming it a 'violation of the law'. Notably, this criticism was not based on the transfer of a non-pauper to the workhouse. Instead, the board of guardians was concerned that the patient, who had been committed to the asylum as a dangerous lunatic, posed a threat to the inmates of the workhouse.[28] One explanation for the Tulla guardians' lack of concern is the 1875 Act's stipulation that any expenses in respect of lunatics transferred to the workhouse must be paid by the governors out of the applicable funds.[29] In consequence, any paying patient transferred to the workhouse was supposed to be maintained out of the asylum's finance base rather than the poor rates, although Poor Law guardians encountered difficulties when they sought payments from the asylum's authorities.[30]

The frequency in transferring patients to the workhouse for non-payment should not be overestimated. In most cases when it was threatened, it was not carried out. This was because, following admission, patients in district asylums had a legal entitlement to relief, determined by their mental condition rather than their ability to contribute towards maintenance.[31] For instance, when the Ennis board threatened to transfer William M to the workhouse, his brother-in-law wrote to the asylum on behalf of the patient's father, Michael, who he claimed was 'just as much impaired in his mind as his son'. Michael had allegedly become 'very much disturbed in his mind on account of his son being [potentially] sent to the workhouse'. As a result, his son-in-law informed the Reverend McNearmond that they had 'a small sum of money ... thought he might be able to afford to contribute a little yearly towards his son's maintenance'. Having later discovered that the father was unable to contribute, the board resolved to retain William as a pauper patient in the asylum.[32]

In rural districts like Ennis, key considerations in the assessment of families' financial circumstances were land acreage, stock, number of dependents and reputation within the community. The case of Mrs. G., whose daughter was admitted to Ennis, is typical:

> Mrs G can well afford to pay at least [£]6 annually for the support of her daughter. She holds a good well stocked farm only one boy and girl at home. Some 3 or 4 years ago she paid as much as £500 for a fine farm and some stock for one of her sons at Mount Rivers. She is reputed by her neighbours to have plenty of money on deposit therefore she ought to pay the small sum named.[33]

This emphasis on the visible trappings of wealth stemmed from the nature of the board's investigations, which relied on local knowledge from members of the community. Most of the evidence gathered by boards was based on second-hand information, though relatives sometimes disputed these channels when asked to contribute. H. Skerrett, the land agent for one patient's brother, informed the RMS that he believed 'some enemies of his [the patient's brother's] have been at work trying to make you believe that he is rich'. Skerrett insisted 'this is not true. I know the position of the D[—]s well and I assure you they have nothing to spare'.[34] Ominously, the mother of another paying patient wrote to Ennis asylum warning that 'there are malicious scribes in this locality giving false names &c of whose communications you should take no notice … My opinion is those scribes are only humbugging the governors'. As evidence, she provided the following example:

> It appears that some 'Thomas K., Kilmilhil' wrote to you lately. Well there is no such householder in this parish and a little boy of that name got your letter saying he knew nothing about the matter and gave the letter to me.[35]

In most cases, however, informants were contacted directly by the RMS, possibly to guard against the danger of 'malicious' individuals providing false accounts.

Signifying their social influence in rural communities, landlords and land agents played an important role in supplying financial evidence. For example, a letter from a land agent, R.D. O'Brien, to Gelston stated that a patient's husband, Henry P., paid him an annual 'average fair rent' of £31 15s. O'Brien urged Gelston to take into consideration that:

> the loss of a wife's help is in itself a heavy blow to a dairy farmer and as Mr P has to meet his calls and rear a young family out of the small farm he holds, I do not see how he can manage to keep his wife in the asylum. He will explain his case to you himself and I hope you will consider it passionately.[36]

Several asylum board members were also landlords and their knowledge of the locality placed them in a privileged position to comment on families' financial affairs.

It is plausible that landlords and other respected members of the community disseminated advice to relatives on how best to negotiate with the asylum. Certainly, as Cox has found in her study of dangerous lunatic certifications, magistrates, clergy, and hospital and workhouse staff all advised families who wished to commit a relative to the Carlow asylum.[37] Given the small size of many rural communities, some families would have known board members personally. Henry P.R., who had both a brother and a sister in the Ennis asylum, wrote repeatedly to the board, attempting to explain his delay in contributing towards their maintenance. A solicitor and a landlord, Henry was apparently struggling financially due to the reduction in his tenants' rents following the introduction of the 1881 Land Act.[38] Five years later, the matter had not been resolved and Henry appealed to the board for sympathy:

> I think the governors and the auditors ought to know very well how hard it is to collect rents from Tenants … I am much surprised that they would take the course in the matter they are all Landlords themselves and I think they might act as landlords are acting to one another now a days and not insist on the payment of the arrears particularly when I cannot get it myself from the tenants.[39]

Henry's difficulty in paying for his relatives' maintenance fees was by no means uncommon. Asylum boards often struggled to decide who should be compelled to pay. In 1871, the Belfast board resolved to form a Committee 'to inquire into the whole subject of pay patients, including those in the House'. The committee was intended to provide counsel on how best to distinguish between those 'able to pay' and 'entirely destitute'.[40] Two months later, the matter was found to be more complicated than anticipated. The committee reported that of the eight patients identified as being able to contribute:

> five had stated their entire inability to give any assistance … the husband of Jane H was about removing her home immediately and that the mother of Ellen T hoped soon to be able to pay for her at the rate of £15 per annum and that William A's friends would pay the average … of the general cost for him in the event of his continuing here but which would not likely be the case as other arrangements were endeavouring to be made in regard to him.[41]

Following their initial enthusiasm in setting up the special committee, the Belfast board apparently lost interest and no further action was recorded.

Even when relatives agreed to contribute, payment was not always forthcoming. In these cases, the RMS assumed the role of debt collector on the board's behalf.[42] Eventually letters took the form of demand notices, threatening to discharge patients if their fees were not paid. In 1881, Enniscorthy's RMS, Joseph Edmundson, went so far as to threaten the father of patient Mary F., if he failed to pay for her maintenance: 'in case you do not agree to these terms,' he warned, 'you will have to remove her home at once.'[43] Similarly, the Richmond board threatened to discharge Eliza H., if her brother failed to continue paying for her in full.[44] This was not strictly feasible. As we have seen, once admitted, district asylum patients were legally entitled to relief until they were deemed 'recovered'.[45] Given that this practice was illegal, it is likely the asylum authorities were simply wielding discharge as a means of intimidation rather than something they intended carrying out. Due to the greater number of paying patients at Richmond, the board for that asylum often resorted to their solicitor to recover fees.[46] The Ennis board also employed their solicitor and were particularly ruthless in their pursuit of maintenance fees.[47]

The question of whether asylum boards could charge dangerous lunatics for their maintenance created yet more confusion. Several district asylums admitted non-paupers under the 1838 and 1867 dangerous lunatic acts, which did not require proof of poverty.[48] While Finnane has suggested there was little asylum boards could do to enforce payment of fees in these cases,[49] at local level they proved exceptionally vigilant when inquiring if dangerous lunatics were possessed of means. From the 1870s, numerous patients admitted to Belfast, Ennis and Enniscorthy as dangerous lunatics were quickly redesignated as paying patients.[50] Nonetheless, as late as 1891, Enniscorthy's board of governors wrote to the lunacy inspectors inquiring whether dangerous lunatics could be charged maintenance.[51] Although no reply is documented in the Enniscorthy records, in the same year, the inspectors wrote to Ennis' RMS, Gelston, about the same issue. The inspectors stated that those committed as dangerous lunatics could not be named paying patients 'until they are duly certified to be no longer dangerous … and removed from the class of dangerous lunatics in the asylum'.[52] Subsequently, there is no record of dangerous lunatics being automatically renamed as paying patients in any of the four case studies.

Despite the rigorous pursuit of maintenance fees, boards of governors were sensitive to a change in relatives' financial circumstances and renegotiated fees in line with new developments. This worked in both directions and fees were raised and lowered. In 1877, Enniscorthy's RMS, Joseph Edmundson, wrote to Miss K., with a view to raising her father's maintenance as the board 'consider it much too small'.[53] In 1890, the asylum's solicitor, John A. Sinnott was instructed to apply to the next Quarter Sessions in Gorey, County Wexford, for an increase in a patient's maintenance fee, 'there being reason to believe that the lunatic's property is able to contribute that amount'.[54] Patients at Richmond were granted a reduction in maintenance fees if their case was approved.[55] In 1878, having inquired into the financial affairs of Philip B's family, his maintenance was reduced from £16 to £12 per annum. The following year, the board found Philip's father unable to pay and at this point the patient was renamed a 'pauper' patient.[56] Likewise, in 1897, in the case of Edward C., the Enniscorthy board, 'taking into consideration [his] large family', did not request payment.[57] At Belfast, patients could also be changed from paying to pauper status when evidence was provided that the family had suffered a 'reversal in fortune'.[58] These examples illustrate that in cases where the relatives of patients were genuinely unable to contribute towards maintenance, district asylums retained their primary function as 'asylums for the lunatic poor'.

While it is conceivable that patients' relatives exaggerated their financial despair to avoid paying fees, some went to great lengths to contribute, hoping that the patient would recover before their limited means were exhausted. In 1892, the mother of Ennis paying patient Mary F., wrote to Gelston:

In the full hope and expectation that my poor daughter would recover under your skill and management, I strove by every means in my power to pay [£]20 a year and actually borrowed the money at high interest and deprived myself and family of the necessaries of life to enable me to do so. Now, however, I deeply regret to say that owing to my present embarrassments it is utterly out of my power to pay any greater sum than £10 yearly.[59]

Patients who remained in the asylum longer than expected were a considerable source of financial strain for their relatives. In 1899, James K. wrote to the Ennis board of governors concerning his sister Margaret's maintenance:

As the doctor of my district told me she would be well after a few months but as there is no improvement I cannot continue to contribute as I live on the side of a poor wet mountain and I have plenty to do to pay rent and many other calls besides this. This girl has a room in my house. And beyond this I am not bound to maintain her, so I hope gentlemen you will be considerate for a poor man. And anytime she is fit to be discharged I will receive her back.[60]

The parish priest also wrote on James' behalf:

> he tells me he only consented to pay towards the maintenance of his sister referred to on the representation of the medical attendant who said his sister's ailment was only a nervous attack from which she would be well in a few months.[61]

Margaret remained in the asylum free of charge and was discharged 'relieved' five months later.[62] Another patient's husband wrote that 'the last instalment which I paid I had to raise it in the bank where I am still paying interest for it. Besides I am greatly involved in debt. I have 10 in family and three of them in a delicate state of health'.[63] In this case, the board resolved that the payment was 'to be confirmed'.[64]

Several of the letters the Ennis asylum received from families chronicled the deterioration of their financial circumstances and the hardship and struggles endured by many in the Ennis district. In 1889, one paying patient's brother explained how their father had 'lost about £1200 by the failure of the Munster Bank, the cottages specified have fallen much below the former estimated value between reduction in rent and other losses in the line of non-payment and constant requirements for repairs &c'.[65] The following year, the father of patient Patrick McM complained of being 'destitute. I lost 9 head of cattle, a horse, 6 breeding ewes and a ram in the years 86, '7 and '8 ... I owe a lot of rent which I cannot pay'.[66] In addition to outlining their financial problems, relatives sometimes appealed to asylum boards for compassion on the grounds of their own poor health. One father described himself as 'old and feeble' and subsequently had his son's maintenance reduced, while another described his 'own direful affection on a crutch with only one leg'.[67]

Friends and relatives also invoked the boards' sympathy on patients' behalf. In 1889, D. Flannery, a parish priest, wrote of a patient:

> he is deeply in debt and has little or no stock on a wretched farm. He belongs to a class of man who are poorer than the beggars and more to be pitied – struggling farmers. Of course, now that there is no one able to look after the place properly things will become worse.[68]

Although chiefly concerned with outlining their poverty, friends frequently underscored families' 'respectability', reflecting contemporary anxieties about the undeserving poor gaining charity or state aid.[69] In 1899, parish priest, James Cahir wrote of John K's family:

> The children have behaved themselves most sensibly and through their hard work and good sense are improving their condition but they are not yet able to stock their land and they owe a years' rent. Under these circumstances if the Governors press K[...] on the maintenance of his mother the consequences will be that the family will be broken up and eventually they will have to abandon the farm and seek some other mode of livelihood.

On this occasion, the payment was 'remitted for the present'.[70] Writing of another family, seven years earlier, the same priest described a patient's father as a 'quite honest, industrious but yet struggling poor man ... general honesty of character and truthfulness give entire credit to his statement'.[71]

Notwithstanding the painstaking pursuit of fees, the proportion of money generated was negligible.[72] Table 3.2 provides a detailed breakdown of the four selected asylums and indicates that from 1875 to 1895 the proportion of revenue from admission fees was between

Table 3.2 Proportion of contributions towards patients' maintenance at Belfast, Ennis, Enniscorthy and Richmond district asylums, 1875–1895

Asylum	% District	% Treasury Grant	% Paying Patients
1875			
Belfast	71.7	27.4	0.9
Ennis	69.2	28.9	1.9
Enniscorthy	68.9	29.6	1.5
Richmond	71.4	27.3	1.3
1885			
Belfast	60.1	37.8	2.0
Ennis	51.5	43.3	5.1
Enniscorthy	51.9	46.4	1.6
Richmond	50.3	46.8	2.8
1895			
Belfast	58.4	38.8	2.7
Ennis	54.1	41.8	4.1
Enniscorthy	55.8	41.3	2.9
Richmond	65.2	32.8	2.0

Compiled from *Reports on District, Local and Private Lunatic Asylums in Ireland, 1877, 1887, 1897* approximately 1 and 5%. Ennis' figures are higher than those of the other asylums, suggesting that this board managed to extract more fees, despite the poverty in that district. Nonetheless, while these figures are slightly higher than the national average of about 1%, they clearly demonstrate that the admission of paying patients did little to alleviate the financial burden placed on the ratepayers and the treasury by the district asylum system.

Given the lack of legislative guidance, the frequent expressions of borderline poverty from relatives and the limited revenue generated, it is difficult to ascertain the boards' motivation in chasing maintenance fees. A letter from a W.S. Studdert, possibly a governor's relative,[73] to Gelston in 1888 offers one explanation:

> I consider it a gross abuse on the tax paying public to subscribe anything towards James W's daughter even though the government do contribute £10.8.3 towards her support he could afford to pay for her in Dublin – why not in Clare? Her parents are considered to be in most affluent circumstances, he could in my opinion better or as well afford to pay for her as perhaps some of this Board for this child. Yesterday he buried his son, he had the best hearse and mourning coach out from Limerick, he had a draper from Killaloe pairing out linen and crape hat bands.[74]

This excerpt illustrates contemporary concerns that those who could afford to contribute might instead become a burden on the rates. It also goes some way towards explaining the exertions of asylum boards to collect fees. Studdert concluded that 'under these circumstances I decline paying for James W's daughter … I shall not pay if I can, so will not let the matter rest here'.[75] The £10 8*s* 3*d* referred to was the annual sum received per patient in Ennis from the 'four shillings' Treasury grant, which, as Chap. 2 discussed, subsidised the maintenance of part-paying patients out of the Treasury.[76] If Studdert's sentiments were representative of the board's motivations, then they too were concerned with the protection of the ratepayer. Certainly, Cox has argued that governors were 'generally anxious to reduce the local taxation burden' created by district asylums.[77] This echoes the lunacy inspectors' criticism of asylum boards in 1895, for not putting pressure on relatives to contribute more than a certain amount in order to avail of the four shillings rule.[78]

Some relatives were aware of the Treasury grant and even appealed to the asylum board to reduce their fees to become eligible for subsidisation. In 1883, Mary C., wrote to Ennis' RMS, Daxon, asking for her son's maintenance to be reduced from £24 to £10 per annum 'at which rate I understand you will be entitled to receive a yearly contribution from the Government nearly equal to the reduction'.[79] Likewise, in 1889, James K., requested a reduction of £2 for his sister's maintenance 'to obtain the Government in aid for her maintenance as indeed I could not afford to pay more than £10 for her maintenance'.[80] The fact that boards did, on a number of occasions, reduce maintenance fees lends credence to the lunacy inspectors' criticism and suggests that boards were, in fact, 'best consulting the interests of the rate-payer'.[81]

'NOT KEPT FOR PROFIT'[82]

During the nineteenth century, the managing committees of voluntary asylums became progressively intent on promoting their establishments and attracting patient fees. This section examines how the two case studies, Bloomfield and Stewarts, ensured their survival within the institutional marketplace. As we have seen, Bloomfield's managing committee became increasingly willing to admit non-Quaker patients but charged these patients much higher rates than their Quaker counterparts. The admission of these wealthy patients not only supplied surplus funds but also made Bloomfield respectable and socially inviting. This was important to Bloomfield's ethos of providing aid for Quakers who had 'fallen on hard times'. Stewarts embodied a more complex form of voluntary care. While the government continued to cover the costs of Stewarts' dwindling 'government patient' population, an increasing number of paying patients came to occupy the lunatic branch. Excluding the government patients, these patient fees were the sole financial base for the lunatic branch, while the managing committee repeatedly identified them as the most significant source of funding for the imbecile branch.[83]

As Chap. 2 discussed, voluntary asylums charged higher rates of maintenance than district asylums. From 1858 to 1900, more than half of the documented Stewarts' patient fees were between £41 and £60. At Bloomfield, almost half of recorded fees were over £100 (see Table 3.3). While Bloomfield's fees were mostly on a par with the private asylums, some patients were kept at lower rates. Like St Patrick's, Bloomfield provided relief for the 'respectable poor' as well as the wealthy. Although by the second half of the nineteenth century St Patrick's lowered its fees, restating its original intention of providing for the poor,[84] Bloomfield

Table 3.3 Documented maintenance fees, Stewarts and Bloomfield, 1858–1900

Fees (to nearest £)	Bloomfield	(%)	Stewarts	(%)	Both	(%)
Identified as free	7	1.7	0	0.0	7	0.7
Under £20	0	0.0	2	0.4	2	0.2
£20–£25	3	0.7	8	1.5	11	1.8
£26–£40	16	3.8	30	5.7	46	4.9
£41–£60	30	7.1	278	53.3	308	32.7
£61–£100	62	14.8	33	6.3	95	10.1
£101–£150	99	23.6	2	0.4	101	10.7
£151–£200	97	23.1	1	0.2	98	10.4
£201–£240	2	0.5	0	0.0	2	0.2
Not documented	104	24.8	168	32.2	272	28.9
Total	420	100.0	522	100.0	942	100.0

Compiled from Patient Accounts (Stewarts, Stewarts Patient Records) and Bloomfield Ledgers, 1858–1900 (FHL, Bloomfield Records)

continued to charge high fees for the remainder of the century. This is because, unlike St Patrick's, Bloomfield was not founded from the bequest of an individual and its managing committee had the freedom to set terms as they saw fit. Bloomfield's only limitation was to provide for the small number of Quakers who could not afford private asylum care.

The much lower fees at Stewarts reflect its managing committee's ethos of caring for the 'middle classes', a preoccupation which was reflected in the institution's name: 'Asylum for Lunatic Patients of the Middle Classes'.[85] In addition to a strong emphasis on providing free or affordable care for the training of imbecile children, accommodating patients at low rates was considered paramount. In 1872, at the annual meeting of the committee that had established Stewarts, Stewart stated that he had been managing the asylum for twelve years 'for the maintenance of middle-class lunatics'. Stewart professed that it was the only asylum in Ireland catering for that class and that its existence was a 'great boon to the middle-classes of this country'.[86] The terms of admission included in each annual report reflected this ethos. The earliest extant annual report, published in 1871, stipulated that the asylum branch was:

> intended for patients whose means will allow of their paying for the use of all appliances necessary for restoration to health and for protection, but not for the luxurious accommodation of first class private asylums.[87]

Fees at Stewarts were on a graded scale (see Table 3.4) and in 1871 were £36 per annum. Those requiring a 'special attendant' were charged extra, while additional charges were incurred when friends or relatives did not supply clothing. 'Accommodation of a superior kind' was available for a 'few female patients' at the rate of £52 per annum.[88] Two years later, the upper limit of £52 was abolished.[89] In 1874, the minimum rate of maintenance was raised to £40 per annum and in 1878, to £50 where it stayed for the remainder of the century.[90] Yet, some patients were maintained at lower rates than those specified. In 1872, one patient was admitted at just £12 per annum and in 1900, two patients were charged just £30 each.[91] Overall, these rates were much higher than district asylum fees, revealing a gap between public and voluntary care. Nonetheless, those who could afford the highest rates at district asylums might also avail of the lowest fees in voluntary asylums such as Stewarts, suggesting that some families could select between the two forms of care.

Although voluntary asylums were not kept for profit, the managing committees for both Stewarts and Bloomfield were compelled to compete with private asylums for their clientele. In a bid to disassociate themselves from the district asylums, the managing committees stressed the enhanced privacy their asylums could provide. Privacy was an important consideration for the relatives of the mentally ill. In the English context, Charlotte MacKenzie has found that families desired confidentiality when committing patients to Ticehurst, a private asylum located in the South of England.[92] In a similar vein, Suzuki has argued that the families of the mentally ill in England were particularly troubled by the public exposure of their relatives' disruptive behaviour, which often determined decisions to commit them to an institution.[93]

Table 3.4 Maintenance fees at Stewarts

Year	Minimum fee per annum	Alternative rates
1871	£36	Superior accommodation (females) £52
1873	£36	No upper limit
1874	£40	No upper limit
1878	£50	No upper limit
1890	£50	£5 for one month, no upper limit
1897	£50	No upper limit

Compiled from *The Stewart Institution and Asylum Report* 1871, 1873, 1874, 1878, 1890, 1897

This had long been the case in Ireland. As early as 1814, Bloomfield's managing committee stated that much care has been taken to keep the patients 'in a due degree of privacy'.[94] The committee was concerned that 'fear of publicity' was deterring families from committing their relatives to Bloomfield.[95] However, by the 1860s, Bloomfield's visiting physician, Dr. Valentine Duke, reported that:

> the public seem now to look upon the affliction of lunacy, less as a disgrace to be carefully concealed from all outside the family circle, than they have been in the habit of doing heretofore and that they are more ready to avail themselves promptly of the many resources and advantages which are afforded in a well regulated Asylum.[96]

Despite this alleged shift in public attitudes, in 1884 Stewarts' managing committee was still appealing to families' desire for confidentiality. The committee was keenly aware that Stewarts offered an alternative to 'respectable families' who might otherwise be forced to commit relatives to a district asylum, a far more public procedure. This latter solution, the managing committee insisted:

> would be in many cases most disagreeable, as although the District Asylums are, as a rule, extremely well managed the greater degree of publicity, combined with the comparative inferiority of the dietary, would render such places objectionable to all who could resort to a more private establishment whose rates were not prohibitive.[97]

The managing committee routinely emphasised the shortcomings of district asylum care. In 1896, they claimed:

> no greater hardship can exist for people of respectable position, but with very small means, than to be obliged to place their insane relatives in the district asylums often by passing through a disagreeable public ordeal and by the foundation of this Asylum it was intended to mitigate this inconvenience to some extent by providing accommodation suited in degree to the ailment and the means of the patient.[98]

This 'disagreeable public ordeal' was most likely committal as a dangerous lunatic. Cox has highlighted the very 'public nature' of dangerous lunatic certifications which were heard at the petty sessions throughout Ireland.[99] Where no places existed for paying patients in district asylums, which was particularly likely at the over-crowded, neighbouring Richmond asylum, prospective patients and their families would almost certainly have faced dangerous lunatic certification. This contrasted with admissions to asylums in Britain whose examination and certification often took place in their own or their relative's home.[100] There were some exceptions, however, such as in cases of infanticide.[101] Alternatively, Stewarts' committee may have been hinting at the intrusive nature of testing paying patients' means. Either way, Stewarts' committee was appealing to the high value the wealthier classes placed on confidentiality. In 1886, the managing committee stressed that although the asylum had an 'ample extent of ground suited for exercise' and 'every reasonable liberty consistent with safety is afforded to patients ... every precaution to ensure the necessary privacy is taken'.[102]

The language used to describe Stewarts asylum branch was also that of the domestic or private sphere and the institution was characterised as 'a comfortable home for ladies and gentlemen of limited means'.[103] The managing committee proudly boasted that a number of patients preferred to remain voluntarily at Stewarts, 'regarding it as a comfortable home'.[104] In relation to the eighteenth century, Joan Busfield has also noticed a tendency for private asylum advertisements to use this language, where an underscoring of the 'residential' nature of private asylum care sought to detract from the wealthier classes' reluctance to institutionalise their relatives.[105] This was also the case in nineteenth-century Ireland. Relatives faced with selecting between public and voluntary care could draw comfort from the enhanced privacy afforded by institutions like Stewarts. Meanwhile, those able to afford private care might settle for cheaper accommodation in voluntary asylums, based on the assumption that these establishments could offer 'domestic' and private accommodation which rivalled the more expensive private ones.

While providing accommodation at lower rates than private asylums, and dissociating themselves from district asylums, both the Bloomfield and Stewarts managing committees worked hard to attract patients who could pay higher rates. In the 1840s, Bloomfield's managing committee decided to make an 'addition of several commodious apartments' to the existing building, which they expected would 'afford ample accommodation and every requisite for those who have moved in more affluent circles'.[106] Although the committee had evidently widened its target market, in 1856, they complained that large numbers of patients were paying 'but low rates'.[107] By this point, Bloomfield housed approximately twenty-five patients. A decade later, members of a general meeting of the Society of Friends encouraged the committee to lease the adjoining premises of Swanbrook in Donnybrook, which consisted of a house on about three acres of ground and was 'thoroughly remodelled and furnished and the pleasure ground of both suitably laid out'. The committee intended this house not only to allow for a 'much more perfect classification' and in turn segregation of patients by condition, but also supplied 'superior apartments' for first class patients.[108]

Stewarts' managing committee took similar steps. In the late 1880s, when Stewarts housed approximately 115 patients, the managing committee decided to extend the accommodation in the lunatic branch. By then, the committee had stopped framing this branch with its charitable contribution to the imbecile branch, instead placing more emphasis on its 'general usefulness to society' in caring for those unable to afford accommodation elsewhere. The committee now applied a portion of the profits from the lunatic branch to building work. Apparently anticipating a negative response from subscribers, they took pains to justify their departure from previous practice:

> though the intention of the late Dr. Stewart was that any profit arising from it [the asylum branch] should be applied to assist the [Imbecile] Institution, the Committee are better satisfied in seeing the Asylum fulfil its own mission usefully to the community than become a permanent source of any large income, as they are confident that any deficiency in the funds would ultimately be made good by those interested in the support of the [Imbecile] Institution.[109]

By seeking patients from the wealthier grades of society, Stewarts and Bloomfield were entering into direct competition with private asylums. This was not originally envisaged. In 1885, the Stewarts' committee stated they did not 'seek to interfere with other Private Asylums', proclaiming themselves satisfied to be 'found useful to patients of limited means'. At this point, the committee insisted, they aimed to 'studiously avoid the principle of competition with other Asylums'.[110] However, the committee was eager to point out that many patients were transferred to Stewarts 'from more expensive establishments and neither themselves nor their friends have found any occasion to regret the change'.[111]

By 1891, the number of patients in Stewarts' asylum branch had decreased. Although the committee reported that several 'very aged residents' had died, they recognised that asylum care had been 'largely extended elsewhere of late'.[112] This was presumably a reference to expanding private asylums such as St John of God's, which was providing accommodation at competitive rates, though St John of God's accommodated primarily Catholics, while Stewarts catered mostly for members of the Church of Ireland. It was at this point that the Stewarts' managing committee decided to alter the internal accommodation and provide for those of the wealthier classes.[113] By 1893, the managing committee was openly acknowledging the competitive nature of asylum provision for paying patients, noting that 'the element of competition by other establishments of a similar character tends to render the number of patients under treatment subject to variation'.[114]

The building alterations undertaken at Stewarts greatly changed its dynamic, as the asylum now offered higher standards of accommodation for those able to afford it. The apartments previously occupied by the RMS, Frederick Pim, were converted to accommodation for 'ladies and gentlemen who were desirous of greater privacy than we were enabled to give under previously existing circumstances'. Pim, meanwhile, was moved to a separate residence nearby.[115] The larger sleeping apartments were rearranged to provide several smaller private apartments for individual patients.[116] By 1897, Stewarts' terms of admission now stated that patients 'requiring separate rooms and special attendance, with extras, such as carriage drives, &c., pay extra rates according to circumstances'.[117] Once building work was completed, the number of patients in the lunatic branch rose from fifty-five in 1898 to sixty-nine in 1899— the largest rise in any one year. The managing committee characterised this growth as a 'great advance' which enabled the hospital 'to deal with a class of patients previously sent elsewhere for treatment'.[118]

Another stark indicator of mounting competition was the decision to advertise.[119] Both Bloomfield and Stewarts were advertised in the *Medical Directories for Ireland*, Bloomfield first appearing in 1889 and again in 1898, and Stewarts appearing from 1899. As we shall see, private asylums had been advertising in the *Medical Directories* from the early nineteenth century, a practice which increased swiftly in the late nineteenth century, pointing towards the economic pressures on the voluntary and private sectors. In 1901, Bloomfield's managing committee circulated copies of an 'illustrated prospectus' for Bloomfield and Swanbrook 'with the view of making Bloomfield better known'.[120]

The annual reports for voluntary asylums were also used as a means of publicity. In them, managing committees not only reassured subscribers their charity was being put to good use but also assuaged any fears concerning abuses, providing a transparency that private asylums lacked. The guarantee of a socially significant readership—the asylum's philanthropic subscribers—meant that annual reports were an excellent platform for stimulating sympathy, sensitivity and, perhaps most importantly, awareness among those who could afford to donate. Stewarts' annual reports only came to be utilised in this way from the 1890s. Previously they had contained only snippets about the workings of the asylum branch. Yet, by 1899, Stewarts' terms of admission read almost like an advertisement for the asylum: 'It is situated within a handsome demesne of nearly 100 acres in a most salubrious district and commands beautiful views.'[121] Voluntary asylums were now very much part of the institutional marketplace.

'THE TRADE IN LUNACY'?[122]

It is difficult to escape associations with the trade in lunacy when exploring the history of private asylums. This model, which traditionally emphasises proprietors' profiteering over any real concern for patient welfare, immediately distinguishes private asylums from their public or voluntary counterparts. In the English context, Parry-Jones has largely dismissed derogatory public characterisations of private asylums as sensationalist and prejudiced.[123] Yet these institutions did generate profits and were often a lucrative commercial enterprise for medical men.[124] This also held in Ireland, so long as proprietors attracted a wealthy clientele, competed well with other establishments and weathered any economic downturns that arose. However, given the development of the private sector prior to the introduction of the Poor Law, parishes did not maintain destitute lunatics or idiots in private asylums, as was the tendency in England. As a result, a 'trade in lunacy' on the scale of its English equivalent did not exist in Ireland's relatively modest network of private asylums.[125]

Like any business venture, establishing a private institution entailed personal financial risk. This was true for Drs. John Eustace and Richard Grattan, whose partnership contract for the joint ownership of Hampstead in 1826 highlights the magnitude of their investment:

we each agree to pay one half of the expenses which shall be incurred in any manner for conducting the said Establishment and we likewise agree to divide equally between us whatever profit may arise from said Establishment and in all matters relating to or connected with the management of the said Establishment we consider ourselves equally bound and responsible.[126]

If the venture proved a failure, the doctors would have been liable for any debts incurred. While Grattan left the partnership in 1830, for Eustace, Hampstead House was a success and in 1857, his sons John II and Marcus joined him.[127]

The continued success and prosperity of private asylums was dependent on the proprietor's personal reputation and the public confidence he held.[128] Eustace was a Quaker who had begun his career as a visiting physician to Bloomfield in 1815. He also had a private practice and from 1822 was a temporary physician to the Cork Street Fever Hospital in Dublin.[129] The 1842 Act favoured medical men as private asylum proprietors. If the proprietor was not a physician, surgeon or apothecary, the licensed house in question must be visited by a 'medical man' at least every fortnight who would sign a statement of health for each patient, which was entered into the asylum's books for the inspectors' perusal.[130] The position in Britain was similar, where lay proprietors were often considered 'more likely to be corrupt, negligent and avaricious than their medical colleagues'.[131] Advertisements for private asylums in England and Ireland therefore often specified the qualifications of their proprietors.[132] For example, one advertisement for Hampstead House simply listed the names of the proprietors and the consulting physician, their qualifications and the cost of maintenance, implying the doctors' reputations alone superseded any need for further embellishment (see Fig. 3.1).

Because patient fees were the sole source of funding for private institutions, they tended to be high. Between 1820 and 1860, the average private asylum fee was approximately £80 per annum.[133] Minute

---

Conducted by the Proprietors – John Eustace, Jun., M.B.T.C.D. and L.R.C.S.I.; Marcus Eustace, L.R.C.S.I., &c.
Consulting Physician – John Eustace, M.D., Fellow of the College of Physicians, 14, Montpelier Parade, Monkstown.
Terms   .   .   .   .   £20 a Quarter.

Fig. 3.1 Advertisement for Hampstead House, Glasnevin, Dublin, 1858. Source *Medical Directory for Ireland,* 1858

books for Hampstead offer the earliest indication of fees in the nine-teenth century. From its opening in 1826 until 1831, the lowest rate was fifty-two guineas (£54 12s) per annum.[134] For the first thirty-four patients admitted, the average annual fee was £61. Not unlike patients in voluntary asylums, several patients were maintained at less than the minimum rate of maintenance (almost half). Fees varied greatly from £26–£100 per annum plus an extra £40 where a servant was to accom-pany the patient. Evidence supplied by private asylum proprietors at the 1857–1858 inquiry demonstrates that this wide variation in fees con-tinued. By then, the lowest fees at Hampstead were £40 per year and the highest £150, excluding patients kept at low rates on charitable grounds. Despite the 'low rate' of maintenance offered, John Eustace II (1827–1899) informed the commissioners that he had been obliged to refuse 'patients of the middle class' who were unable to pay sufficient sums. He reasoned that these cases were probably taken into other pri-vate asylums, at low rates of maintenance, or into the district asylum.[135] Surprisingly, Eustace did not apparently consider that voluntary asylums received these patients, though he may have included these under 'pri-vate' asylums.

Several other private establishments received patients at lower rates. Maintenance fees at Eagle House in Finglas, Dublin, ranged from £25–£100. Fees at Belleview in Dublin also varied widely. While Belleview's proprietor, Richard Gregory, claimed that one patient was maintained at the staggering sum of £270 per annum, he stated that other patients were accommodated at as low as £25. Despite this disparity, Gregory maintained that the 'average' rate was £80 per annum, revealing that fees at Belleview were not dissimilar to most other Irish private asylums during the period. Nonetheless, Gregory and other proprietors claimed to have received a 'good many' applications for admissions at reduced sums, who could not be accommodated.[136] Meanwhile, fees at Hartfield in Dublin ranged from £20–£120. Hartfield's proprietor, Dr. William Lynch, remarked that only one patient paid this low rate; the lowest charge was ordinarily thirty guineas (£31 10s) and even then, very few patients were maintained at this.[137] As Chap. 2 demonstrated, the private asylums that offered lower rates were eventually criticised for their inabil-ity to provide adequate care for their patients.

At the other end of the fee scale, Farnham House in Dublin charged between 80 (£84) and 120 (£126) guineas per year. Where 'special attendance' was deemed necessary, patients were charged £50 per quarter (£200 p.a.).[138] The practice of listing maintenance fees in guineas underscored the exclusivity of institutions like Farnham House, in an era when items and services intended for the wealthier classes were often priced in this style.[139] A series of advertisements for Farnham House, published in *Medical Directories* during the 1860s, further supports this, in proclaiming 'none but patients of respectability admitted'.[140] Yet even asylums that clearly espoused an exclusive character 'very often' received applications to admit patients at lower rates. Farnham House's proprietor, Dr. James Duncan, stated that these applicants would generally go to St Patrick's Asylum or 'some other such establishment'. While Duncan claimed there existed 'at large' a considerable proportion of lunatics above the rank of pauper who could not afford to pay the lowest sum in a private asylum, he also cautioned that some who could pay would attempt to secure reduced rates, or even free accommodation, if possible.[141]

After the 1860s, there is little evidence concerning Irish private asylum fees. An account book for Hampstead and Highfield in the 1890s sheds some light on the fees charged in that decade, detailing the monthly contributions made towards patients' maintenance. Figures for individual patients differed from year to year, suggesting payments were made at irregular intervals. The presence of very small amounts, as well as large ones, implies patients were also charged for extras. The figures listed suggest that the yearly amount contributed per patient ranged from £39 to £585. However, more than 90% of fees were over £100 and the average fee during this period was £215 per annum.[142]

In 1894, the lunacy inspectors reported that the maintenance fees at Lindeville in Cork ranged from £60 to £150.[143] This isolated reference suggests that other private asylums also continued to admit patients on a graded scale of maintenance. Advertisements during this period indicate that proprietors were willing to negotiate fees with the families of potential patients, a practice which reflected the increased competition with voluntary asylums in this era. Several advertisements directed applications to be made to the proprietor or resident superintendent, who would furnish the relatives and friends of potential clients with a prospectus, terms of pay and admission forms.[144] Those wishing to apply for admission to Hampstead and Highfield could simply call into the offices of the Drs. Eustace, located conveniently on Grafton Street in Dublin's city centre.[145]

Irish private asylum fees were high compared with England. This is striking, given that the cost of living, as well as wages, in Ireland was lower than in England. Parry-Jones has estimated that, in 1850, fees at a typical middle-class establishment ranged from 15 shillings to two guineas per week (approx. £39–£109 p.a.).[146] England also possessed private asylums that charged high rates. At Ticehurst, patients were charged between £50 and £500 per annum, or an average of £150 in 1845, a figure that tripled to between £400 and £500 by 1875. MacKenzie attributes this rise to the 'general increase in retail prices associated with the growth of consumerism generated by the expansion of the middle classes in the 1850s–1870s'. After 1875, fees in the middle range plateaued, while those on the higher scale continued to rise.[147] It is unclear whether private asylum fees in Ireland underwent a comparable increase during the mid-Victorian period. However, many proprietors may have been forced to reduce fees in the latter part of the century due to the economic depression that began in Ireland in 1879 and lasted until the middle of the 1890s. Indeed, MacKenzie suggests that a combination of economic downturn and therapeutic pessimism impacted negatively on business at Ticehurst. Although fees at that asylum remained at a similar level, during the last decades of the nineteenth century patients obtained larger lodgings, suggesting better value for money.[148] As with voluntary asylums, increased advertising for Irish private asylums in the *Medical Directories* indicates a mounting need to generate more business. While in the 1860s only one or two proprietors advertised there, by the turn of the century, the majority were doing so.

By the 1880s, several private asylums were in financial difficulty. The lunacy inspectors frequently referred to 'the depressed state of the country', noting an increase in applications for private patients to be transferred to public institutions.[149] The inspectors also referred to 'an irregular system of payment, even of small stipends'.[150] Difficulties in obtaining maintenance fees were not confined to the late nineteenth century. During the 1857–1858 inquiry, private asylum proprietors expressed frustration at being unable to recover payment from patients' relatives. Duncan informed the commissioners that in one or two cases he had received neither clothing nor maintenance fees and was obliged to maintain some patients at his own personal cost. These cases cost him from 20 to 30 guineas per quarter (£84–£126 p.a. each).[151]

During the 1857–1858 commission, Hartfield's proprietor, Dr. William Lynch, outlined his difficulties in obtaining Chancery patients' maintenance fees. The committees established by Chancery to manage patients' affairs allegedly made a 'hard bargain with the asylum proprietor and at times would not pay regularly', even when patients had been awarded a maintenance of about £150 per annum. In these cases, Lynch claimed he sustained heavy losses. Fees were not paid regularly during the patient's residence in the asylum and, following the patient's death, were generally not paid at all.[152] In another instance, Lynch complained, a female patient with 'upwards of £2000 in the bank and a nice property besides' was neglected by her Chancery committee. She was reportedly 'in a most disgraceful state' and the cloak eventually supplied for her would have 'scarcely fit a child'. Although Lynch stated he had written frequently to the Committee, arrears of maintenance were still due to him for this patient.[153]

The fact that these proprietors kept patients at their own expense might be attributed to motives of philanthropy. In England, certain private asylum proprietors were 'remarkably charitable', keeping some patients at especially low rates or allowing them to remain free of charge.[154] It is equally possible, however, that proprietors were anxious to safeguard their asylums' reputation of care. The 1842 Act offered no protection for proprietors who were unable to recover maintenance fees. While suing for fees was an option, the legal costs probably deterred proprietors from entering a conflict which might impact negatively on their own and the institution's reputation. In 1855, when Lynch attempted to sue for outstanding fees, the expense of the application and legal proceedings equalled the balance due to him.[155] While these legal proceedings do not appear to have attracted any media attention, the matter was listed under 'insolvent debtors' in the *Nation* newspaper and both Lynch and his asylum were explicitly named.[156]

Given the futility of attempts to recover arrears legally, it is notable that proprietors did not simply expel patients whose fees were not paid. When the governors at St Patrick's Hospital confronted comparable difficulties in the 1870s, they resolved to remove any patient who was more than six months in arrears. However, Malcolm argues that the board seemed hesitant to carry out this threat, presenting multiple reasons for their reluctance:

Expulsion was not a pleasant procedure and usually meant the end of hope of recovery of arrears. Also frequently patients had been in the hospital for decades and the relatives or guarantors who had originally signed the bond for the fees were dead or untraceable ... In these circumstances the governors did not have any very strong legal grounds for demanding payment. If families flatly refused to accept elderly relatives, whom they may never have even seen, the hospital authorities could hardly leave the patients on their doorstep.[157]

Malcolm also suggests the transfer of patients to either the Richmond asylum or the workhouse would reflect poorly on the reputation of a supposedly charitably institution,[158] although this may have been less concerning for those conducting private enterprises. Nonetheless, whether for motives of altruism or for fear of attracting hostility from patients' relatives and potentially putting off new clients, both Duncan and Lynch demonstrated a similar hesitance in discharging patients who were in arrears. Given the nature of record keeping for the private asylums studied, it is impossible to ascertain either how many patients were not supported financially or for how long.

The boundaries between who could afford voluntary and private asylum care and who could not became further blurred after the establishment of Belmont Park in Waterford in 1884 and the St John of God's in Dublin in 1885. The 1884 prospectus for the St John of God's specified fees of one guinea, £1 10s and £2 per week (£54 12s, £78 and £104 p.a.) for permanent boarders in good health and between £2 and £3 per week (£104 and £156 p.a.) for the sick. These rates included the 'ordinary requirements' of a separate furnished bedroom, general sitting room, billiard and smoking room, board but no stimulants, ordinary medical attendance, ordinary nursing and attendance by Brothers. Further private arrangements could be made to have special attendance. Extras included additional consultations, medicines, stimulants and the washing of boarders' linen.[159] These rates correspond to the lunacy inspectors' statement that the hospital offered low rates for middle-class patients. Although the inspectors referred to St John of God's as a private asylum, it is probable, given the religious ethos of the hospital's founders, that it was not kept for profit. In fact, the hospital's only distinguishing feature from the voluntary asylums was that it did not provide for charity patients. The religious and philanthropic elements of St John of God's was clearly popular with prospective clients, shown by the asylum's dramatic expansion in the twentieth century. As Chap. 2 argued, this meant that asylums like St John of God's created a bridge between the cost of accommodation in a voluntary asylum and a more expensive private establishment.

LENGTH AND OUTCOME OF STAY

As we have seen, there was some debate over whether private asylums offered a greater likelihood of curing insanity than the district sector. Those attempting to appease contemporary public alarm over wrongful or prolonged confinement in private asylums maintained that it was in the financial interest of proprietors to cure as many patients as possible in as short a time as possible. The strategy of treating insanity both promptly and successfully was also aspired to in English contexts, where, as Parry-Jones has found, it could serve as an 'effective advertisement' for a private asylum.[160] Critics' claims that private asylums provided little more than custodial care, rather than cure, were therefore often misleading.[161] In reality, those investing high sums in the care of their relatives would have anticipated fast, effective results. When such an outcome was not forthcoming, patients were frequently removed to alternative places of care.

Evidence abounds that private asylums tended to achieve high rates of discharge and even cure for private patients. Between 1826 and 1867, most patients whose length of stay at Bloomfield (63.5%) and Hampstead (69.9%) is known stayed for less than one year. These figures are almost identical to those for the two Oxfordshire private asylums at Hook Norton and Witney (62% and 66% respectively) and higher than the York Retreat (approx. 40–50%) in this period.[162] Digby has interpreted such high patient turnover as evidence against contemporary anxieties about the silting up of asylums with chronic, long-stay cases, while Parry-Jones contends that it goes some way towards refuting accusations of the prolonged confinement of private patients for corrupt motives including financial gain.[163] These arguments also apply in the Irish context. As shown in Table 3.5, from 1868 to 1900, the majority of patients admitted to the asylums studied spent short periods there. Not unlike patients admitted to the York Retreat,[164] Irish private asylum patients, in particular, tended to stay for less than one year (67.1%), as did two-thirds of male and over one-half of female paying patients admitted to the district asylums. This compares favourably with district asylums in this period. For example, in her study of the Armagh, Belfast, Omagh and Sligo asylums, Malcolm has found that at most, half of the patients admitted stayed for twelve months or less.[165] Meanwhile, longer stays of five years or more were slightly less common among paying patients than total district asylum populations.[166]

Table 3.5   Known length of stay for patients admitted to the district, voluntary and private asylums studied, 1868–1900[a]

	District			Voluntary			Private		
	F (%)	M (%)	T (%)	F (%)	M (%)	T (%)	F (%)	M (%)	T (%)
Less than 1 year	52.9	66.3	60.9	59.4	56.3	58.3	62.2	67.6	67.1
1–5 years	22.8	17.0	19.3	22.3	22.0	22.2	20.3	20.0	20.0
5–10 years	9.1	4.9	6.6	7.0	10.8	8.4	6.8	3.0	3.4
10 + years	15.2	11.8	13.2	11.3	10.8	11.1	10.8	9.4	9.6
Total	100.0	100.0	100.0	100.0	100.0	100.0	100.0	100.0	100.0
N =	276	407	683	471	277	748	74	700	774

Compiled from Belfast, Ennis, Enniscorthy, Richmond, Stewarts, Bloomfield, St John of God's, Hampstead and Highfield admissions registers
[a]The first admission to St John of God's was in 1885

The likelihood of dying in the asylum was less for private and voluntary asylum patients than for paying patients sent to district asylums. Like patients at the Witney asylum, in the earlier period, one-tenth of patients admitted to Hampstead and Bloomfield died in the asylum.[167] While a larger proportion of Hook Norton patients (21.9%) died there, Parry-Jones has related this disparity to the reception of paupers to this institution, among whom a number were admitted suffering with chronic or intractable physical and mental conditions.[168] This reasoning also explains the differences in mortality rates in Irish asylums. While between 1868 and 1900, 20.1% of patients admitted to the private asylums and 30% of those admitted to voluntary asylums died there, 40.9% of paying patients admitted to the district asylums suffered a similar fate (see Table 3.6). References to poor bodily health were far more frequent in the case notes for paying patients admitted to Enniscorthy and Richmond than to the voluntary and private asylums studied. In fact, district asylum paying patients seemed especially vulnerable, even compared with some 'pauper' populations, such as the Sligo asylum, where one-third of admissions between 1855 and 1893 died.[169] Yet, while death rates among the district asylum paying patients decreased slightly over the period examined, Finnane has found that, by 1901, nearly half of district asylum patients were dying.[170]

The most notable difference in outcome in the Irish context was the proportion of cures, which was reportedly significantly higher in Irish private asylums than in English ones. Between 1826 and 1867, half of patients admitted to Bloomfield and Hampstead were discharged cured and a further fifth improved or relieved. By comparison, 27% of private patients admitted to Hook Norton, 35% to Witney and between 35 and 44% to the York Retreat were 'cured' during the same period.[171] As was the trend in other asylums, most of those recorded as cured were released within one year of admission (78.7% at Bloomfield and 82.1% at Hampstead). In the later period, almost half of the private asylum patients were discharged cured, while one in three were discharged from the voluntary and district asylums under this description (see Table 3.6). In her discussion of patient outcomes at Ticehurst, MacKenzie has challenged Scull's contention that private asylum cure rates were 'abysmally low', showing that some 60–80% of admissions were discharged, while 16–39% were discharged recovered. However, as MacKenzie concedes, this was low compared with recovery rates at less expensive asylums including the Retreat, lending some credence to Scull's argument that 'money could not buy health'.[172] At the Retreat during the same era, recovery rates were roughly one-third of admissions.[173] This reveals that

Table 3.6 Known outcome of stay for patients admitted to the district, voluntary and private asylums studied, 1868–1900[a]

	District Asylums			Voluntary Asylums			Private Asylums		
	F (%)	M (%)	T (%)	F (%)	M (%)	T (%)	F (%)	M (%)	T (%)
Cured/ Recovered	31.6	33.4	32.7	33.1	31.2	32.4	46.1	48.6	48.3
Improved/ Relieved	17.4	20.0	18.9	26.9	20.8	24.7	19.7	13.4	14.1
Not Improved/ Not Relieved	6.7	7.9	7.4	13.3	12.3	12.9	0.0	3.8	3.4
Not Cured/Not Recovered	0.0	0.0	0.0	0.0	0.0	0.0	10.5	5.6	6.1
Died	44.3	38.6	40.9	26.7	35.7	30.0	23.7	28.6	28.1
Total	100.0	100.0	100.0	100.0	100.0	100.0	100.0	100.0	100.0
N =	253	365	618	465	269	734	76	640	716

Compiled from Belfast, Ennis, Enniscorthy, Richmond, Stewart's, Bloomfield, St John of God's, Hampstead and Highfield admissions registers
[a]The first admission to St John of God's was in 1885

Irish private asylum patients had better chances of being cured, or at least of being described as cured, than their English counterparts. Irish voluntary and district asylums, meanwhile, were keeping pace with, if not outperforming, the renowned York Retreat when it came to cure rates for paying patients.

Of course, discharge did not always signal the end of institutionalisation for patients. Of the 2368 patients admitted to the asylums studied between 1868 and 1900, 284 (12.0%) were identified as readmissions. In contrast to Malcolm's finding that patients readmitted to district asylums were commonly committed several times before being committed permanently to die in the institution, the outcome for readmissions in this study tended to be more positive than that for first admissions.[174] Overall, half (50.8%) were cured compared with 36.3% of first admissions, while fewer died (22.7% of readmissions; 33.9% of first admissions).

As Cox has pointed out, discharge rates have been largely neglected in the Irish context.[175] Her finding that 42.8% of admissions to the Carlow asylum between 1832 and 1922 were discharged 'recovered' thus provides the only point of reference.[176] While recovery rates for paying patients admitted to the district and voluntary asylums are comparably low, the proportion of patients discharged as 'relieved' is much higher (18.9 and 24.7% respectively) than the 6.9% at Carlow.[177] Moreover, given the higher death rates in district asylums, it is plausible that the private and voluntary asylums tended to produce more cures or partial improvement than the district ones.

The large proportion of those discharged 'relieved', 'not relieved' or 'not recovered' in this study suggests that the families of fee-paying patients tended to withdraw them prematurely, probably to lessen the financial burden of asylum care.[178] As we have seen, families often went to great lengths to pay for relatives' care in these institutions, while for many a fast recovery was all their limited means could afford. This echoes Walsh's suggestion that relatives viewed asylums as a resource to be used when needed.[179] For families with greater disposable funds who were displeased with the outcome of care in one asylum, the institutional marketplace offered many alternatives.

The transfer of patients to other institutions was not uncommon. Despite wide disparities in maintenance fees and standard of accommodation, the boundaries between district, voluntary and private asylums were extremely permeable and patients were transferred between the three sectors. Reasons for transfer varied. Understandably a change in economic circumstances could prevent continued accommodation at a private or voluntary asylum and result in a patient being moved to an institution charging lower rates. Although data on transfers in the asylum records is patchy, case notes for both Stewarts and Bloomfield patients, resident during the 1890s, contain a field marked 'where and when previously under care', allowing for some analysis. The information provided also takes into account patients who had been discharged from one institution and then later admitted to another.

The Stewarts case notes reveal that a number of patients admitted there had previously spent time in district asylums. This cohort tended to pay lower sums (£30–£60 p.a.) in the voluntary asylums, although not exclusively. For example, three women were transferred from Richmond, where they had been contributing £14, £15 and £24 17s. 8d. per annum respectively, to Stewarts, where they were charged between £50 and £52 per annum each. However, patients admitted to Bloomfield and Stewarts were most likely to be transferred from a private asylum, suggesting reduced circumstances or simply decreased confidence in the efficacy of private asylum care were reasons for the move. Patients transferred from private asylums usually paid between £50 and £100 at the voluntary asylums, although some were maintained at higher rates on a par with private asylum fees. For example, four years after his discharge from Hampstead House, Cecil W.W., a twenty-two year-old, single, ship-builder's apprentice was admitted to Bloomfield in September 1896. There he was charged £160 per annum but after one year it was recorded that Cecil had 'been visited lately a good deal by his sisters and uncle, and yesterday was removed to Dr. Eustace's'.[180] Similarly, Henrietta Sophia M., a forty year-old single woman was sent by her brother to Bloomfield in April 1893 at £100 per annum. She had previously been a patient in the Crichton Royal Institution in Dumfries from September 1891 to 1892. This case was not unusual. Several voluntary asylum patients had previously been accommodated in asylums in Britain, including Morningside, West Riding and Crichton. These patients tended to pay average rates in the voluntary asylums, lending weight to the lunacy inspectors' claims that wealthier families often chose to send relatives to Britain where private asylums charged more competitive rates.[181] After she was discharged from Crichton, Henrietta had stayed 'in various places' where she was reportedly 'excited, crying much and talking incessantly of herself and her misfortunes'. Henrietta gave an account of her experience at Crichton:

> Whenever I see her she talks about herself constantly, saying she is quite sane and that her troubles and the bad treatment she says she got at Dumfries have made her nervous and excited ... Is very unhappy. Says she was ruined by the cruelty she received in Dumfries and that she needed lively and happy society and was just improving when sent here.

While in Bloomfield, the physician reported that:

> Some days she stays in bed. Others gets up, but would not go out except once for a few minutes. She says she cannot work, read, or do anything as long as she is here, and that the sight of a lunatic would make her die... She cries loudly. She tears her fingers till they bleed and is dirty in habits, wetting her things frequently. She wants to leave, but when at liberty before coming here she says she was in much the same state as now.

By November, it was reported that Henrietta was to be moved to a private asylum in Finglas.[182] In these instances, the high fees paid for Cecil and Henrietta confirm that families with considerable disposable income had the luxury of selecting between institutions.

CONCLUSIONS

This chapter has shown that district, voluntary and private asylums operated in an institutional marketplace. Within this marketplace, families held the purse strings. Of the three groups, relatives negotiating with district asylums exerted the least influence and were subject to thorough and sometimes intrusive investigations into their financial circumstances. Although the lunacy inspectors criticised asylum boards for failing to identify patients with means, this chapter has revealed that the boards went to great lengths to identify those who could afford to contribute. The boards did, however, demonstrate compassion for those genuinely in need of relief, as these patients were legally entitled to accommodation based on their mental condition rather than their ability to pay fees. This conforms to Cox's findings in the context of the Carlow and Enniscorthy districts.[183] Ultimately, however, and as Cox has found for Carlow and Enniscorthy, the proportion of revenue generated from patient contributions was small.[184]

Families possessed of greater means had more influence in the marketplace and the managing bodies of voluntary and private asylums were compelled to tailor accommodation and maintenance fees to the needs of their clientele. This eventually resulted in competition between the voluntary and private sector in the 1890s, as evidenced by the decision of Stewarts' and Bloomfield's managing committees to provide more expensive and luxurious accommodation and to advertise. This resulted in part from the establishment of less expensive private asylums including St John of God's. It was also a consequence of the economic downturn of the 1880s and 1890s: families who might once have availed of private care were now forced to consider less expensive options. These developments in turn affected private asylums. Although the lunacy inspectors frequently criticised private asylum proprietors who charged lower fees, the combined effects of the economy and competition from voluntary asylums meant that they were increasingly under threat of closure. This is in spite of the higher proportion of patients cured at the private asylums studied, which would have sat well with contemporary private asylum proprietors anxious to guard against accusations of wrongful or over-lengthy confinement. While in the English context Parry-Jones has characterised private asylum proprietors as 'remarkably charitable' for charging some patients low rates, this chapter has highlighted that, at least in Ireland, proprietors were anxious to safeguard their asylums' reputation of care.[185] Thus, by 1900, many of the more prestigious asylums had shifted their target market to encompass less affluent socio-economic groups.

NOTES

1. Cox (2012), pp. 97–132, 148, 154–159, Wright (1998), Finnane (1981), pp. 175–220; Walton (1979–1980), pp. 1–22.
2. Cox (2012), p. 23.
3. Malcolm has traced similar developments in the history of St Patrick's: Malcolm (1989), pp. 118–120.
4. Smith (1999a), (1999b). See also Melling and Forsythe (2006).
5. W.S. Studdert to R.P. Gelston, 26 Jul. 1888 (CCA, Our Lady's Hospital, OL1/7 Letter 1489).
6. For example, James K. to R.P. Gelston, 10 Jan. 1893 (CCA, Our Lady's Hospital, OL1/7 Letter 1883).
7. For example, J. Coffey Ryan to R.P. Gelston, 18 Jun. 1894 (CCA, Our Lady's Hospital, OL1/7 Letter 2025b). For more on the role of medical officers in the Irish medical dispensary system see Cox (2010), pp. 57–78.

8. Fortieth Report of the Inspectors of Lunatics (Ireland), H.C. 1890–1891, p. 521.

9. Minute Books (CCA, Our Lady's Hospital, OL1/1); Medical Superintendent Memorandum Books (WCC, St Senan's Hospital, Enniscorthy); Minutes of the Governors of Enniscorthy District Lunatic Asylum (WCC, St Senan's Hospital, Enniscorthy).

10. Medical Superintendent Memorandum Books, 1868–1889 (WCC, St Senan's Hospital, Enniscorthy, p. 239).

11. For example, Rough Minute Book, 1867–1871 (CCA, Our Lady's Hospital, OL1/24/4, 14 Sep. 1871); Minute Book, 1878–1881 (CCA, Our Lady's Hospital, OL1/1/2, pp. 246, 378); Minute Book, 1888–1891 (CCA, Our Lady's Hospital, OL1/1/5, p. 216).

12. Some correspondence books for this period are not extant.

13. 38 & 39 Vic., c. 67, s. 16.

14. For example, Fred G. Kerin, Solicitor to RMS, Ennis, 26 Aug. 1898 (CCA, Our Lady's Hospital, OL1/7 Letters 2504a and 2504b).

15. For example, Medical Superintendent Memorandum Book, 1868–1889 (WCC, St Senan's Hospital, Enniscorthy, pp. 48, 389, 436), 38 & 39 Vic., c. 67, s. 16.

16. Minute Book No. 13, 1872–1877 (NAI, Richmond District Lunatic Asylum, p. 80).

17. Ibid., p. 343.

18. Minutes of the Governors of Enniscorthy District Lunatic Asylum, 1883–1898 (WCC, St Senan's Hospital, Enniscorthy, pp. 16, 50).

19. Minute Book No. 14, 1877–1881 (NAI, Richmond District Lunatic Asylum, pp. 185–186).

20. For example, Minute Book, 1874–1880 (CCA, Our Lady's Hospital, OL1/1/1, p. 218).

21. Minute Book, 1880–1885 (CCA, Our Lady's Hospital, OL1/1/3, p. 331).

22. Michael B. to Governors of the Lunatic Asylum, Ennis (CCA, Our Lady's Hospital, OL1/7 Letter 1657); Minute Book, 1888–1891 (CCA, Our Lady's Hospital, OL1/5, p. 286).

23. Michael B. to the Governors of the Lunatic Asylum Ennis, 13 Jun. 1890 (CCA, Our Lady's Hospital, OL1/7 Letter 1657).

24. See Minute Book, 1898–1902 (CCA, Our Lady's Hospital, OL1/1/8, pp. 17, 27, 216); Letter from J. Garry to Dr. O'Mara, 21 Dec. 1899 (CCA, Our Lady's Hospital, OL1/7 Letter 2706).

25. 38 & 39 Vic., c. 67, s. 16.

26. Cox (2012), p. 181.

27. Ibid., p. 182.

28. Clerk of Union, Workhouse, Tulla to R.P. Gelston, 14 Sep. 1892 (CCA, Our Lady's Hospital, OL1/7 Letter 1857).
29. 38 & 39 Vic., c. 67, s. 9.
30. See Cox (2012), pp. 181–183.
31. Ibid., p. 22.
32. Pat F. to R.P. Gelston, 3 Nov. 1892 (CCA, Our Lady's Hospital, OL1/7 Letter 1866).
33. J. Culligan JP to Ennis District Asylum, 29 Nov. 1894 (CCA, Our Lady's Hospital, OL1/7 Letter 2054).
34. H.S. Land Agency Office, Galway to R.P. Gelston (CCA, Our Lady's Hospital, OL1/7 Letter 2469).
35. Ellen D. to The Secretary, Asylum, Ennis, 3 Dec. 1883 (CCA, Our Lady's Hospital, OL1/7 Letter 984).
36. R.D. O'Brien to R.P. Gelston, 17 Nov. 1888 (CCA, Our Lady's Hospital, OL1/7 Letter 1519).
37. Cox (2012), pp. 99, 102.
38. Henry P.R to Governors of Ennis Asylum, 3 Jun. 1884 (CCA, Our Lady's Hospital, OL1/7 Letter 1045).
39. Henry P.R to R.P. Gelston, 28 May 1888 (CCA, Our Lady's Hospital, OL1/7 Letter 1471); Henry P.R., to R.P. Gelston, 27 Apr. 1889 (CCA, Our Lady's Hospital, OL1/7 Letter 1560).
40. Minute Book, 1870–1882 (PRONI, Purdysburn Hospital, HOS/28/1/1/4, p. 101).
41. Ibid., p. 111.
42. For example, Medical Superintendent Memorandum Book, 1868–1889 (WCC, St Senan's Hospital, Enniscorthy, p. 198).
43. Medical Superintendent Memorandum Book, 1868–1889 (WCC, St Senan's Hospital, Enniscorthy, p. 176).
44. Minute Book No. 14, 1877–1881 (NAI, Richmond District Lunatic Asylum, p. 206).
45. Cox (2012), p. 22.
46. For example, Ibid., pp. 37–38, 43.
47. For example, Minute Book, 1880–1885 (CCA, Our Lady's Hospital, OL1/1/3, p.158); Minute Book, 1891–1894 (CCA, Our Lady's Hospital, OL1/1/6, p. 213); Minute Book, 1894–1898 (CCA, Our Lady's Hospital, OL1/1/7, pp. 333, 393); Rough Minute Book, 1867–1871 (CCA, Our Lady's Hospital, OL1/2/4, 14 Nov. 1868, 12 Dec. 1868); Minute Book, 1874–1880 (CCA, Our Lady's Hospital, OL1/1/1, pp. 2, 17).
48. Cox (2012), p. 20.
49. Finnane (1996), p. 97.

50. For example, Minute Book, 1870–1882 (PRONI, Purdysburn Hospital, HOS/28/1/1/4, p. 120); Minute Book, 1874–1880 (CCA, Our Lady's Hospital, OL1/1/1, p. 176); Medical Superintendent Memorandum Book, 1868–1889 (WCC, St Senan's Hospital, Enniscorthy, pp. 137, 404, 487, 496).

51. Medical Superintendent Memorandum Book, 1868–1889 (WCC, St Senan's Hospital, Enniscorthy, p. 109).

52. Office of Lunatic Asylums to R.P. Gelston (CCA, Our Lady's Hospital, OL1/7 Letter 1707).

53. Medical Superintendent Memorandum Book, 1868–1889 (WCC, St Senan's Hospital, Enniscorthy, p. 138).

54. Minutes of the Governors of Enniscorthy District Lunatic Asylum, 1883–1898 (WCC, St Senan's Hospital, Enniscorthy, p. 99).

55. For example, Minute Book No. 13, 1872–1877 (NAI, Richmond District Lunatic Asylum, pp. 134–135).

56. Minutes of the Governors of Enniscorthy District Lunatic Asylum, 1883–1898 (WCC, St Senan's Hospital, Enniscorthy, pp. 138, 145).

57. Ibid., p. 183.

58. For example, Minute Book, 1882–1893 (PRONI, Purdysburn Hospital, HOS/28/1/1/5, p. 130).

59. Thelma F. to R.P. Gelston, 5 Aug. 1892 (CCA, Our Lady's Hospital, OL1/7 Letter 1845).

60. James K. to Board of Governors, Ennis District Asylum, 13 Jan. 1899 (CCA, Our Lady' Hospital, OL1/7 Letter 2569).

61. R.H. Little, Parish Priest to the Chairman, Board of Governors, District Asylum Ennis, 13 Jan. 1899 (CCA, Our Lady's Hospital, OL1/7 Letter 2569a).

62. Admissions Register (CCA, Our Lady's Hospital, OL3/1.3).

63. John C. to the Chairman and Board of Governors, Ennis Lunatic Asylum, 9 Feb 1894 (CCA, Our Lady's Hospital, OL1/7 Letter 1987).

64. Minute Book, 1891–1894 (CCA, Our Lady's Hospital, OL1/1/6, p. 336).

65. Denis O'F to the Governors of Ennis District Lunatic Asylum, 1889 (CCA, Our Lady's Hospital, OL1/7 Letter 1536a).

66. Patrick McM to R.P. Gelston, Jan. 1890 (CCA, Our Lady's Hospital, OL1/7 Letter 1624).

67. James W. to R.P. Gelston, Nov. 1889 (CCA, Our Lady's Hospital, OL1/7 Letter 1600); James K. to Board of Governors, Ennis Asylum, May 1892 (CCA, Our Lady's Hospital, OL1/7 Letter 1820).

68. D. Flannery, Parish Priest to R.P. Gelston, 6 Dec. 1889 (CCA, Our Lady's Hospital, OL1/7 Letter 1613).

69. For more on charity in nineteenth–century Ireland, see Walsh (2005), Luddy (1995); Preston (2004).
70. James Cahir, Parish Priest to RMS Ennis, 7 Apr. 1899 (CCA, Our Lady's Hospital, OL1/7 Letter 2606).
71. James Cahir, Parish Priest to Ennis Asylum, 13 May 1892 (CCA, Our Lady's Hospital, OL1/7 Letter 1815a).
72. Cox (2012), p. 23.
73. In 1888, there were a G.S. Studdert and R.M. Studdert on the Ennis board of governors.
74. W.S. Studdert to R.P. Gelston, 26 Jul. 1888 (CCA, Our Lady's Hospital, OL1/7 Letter 1489).
75. Ibid.
76. See Chap. 1.
77. Cox (2012), p. 19.
78. See Chap. 1.
79. Mary C. to William Daxon, 11 May 1883 (CCA, Our Lady's Hospital, OL1/7 Letter 922).
80. James K. to Asylum, Ennis, 7 Nov. 1889 (CCA, Our Lady's Hospital, Ol1/7 Letter 1603).
81. Forty-Second Report of the Inspectors of Lunatics (Ireland), H.C. 1893–1894, p. 369.
82. Forty-Third Report of the Inspectors of Lunatics (Ireland), H.C. 1894, p. 401.
83. *Stewart Institution and Asylum Report* (Dublin 1871), p. 8; For example, *Stewart Institution and Asylum Report* (Dublin 1879), p. 19; *Stewart Institution and Asylum Report* (Dublin 1884), p. 16.
84. Malcolm (1989), pp. 118–120.
85. Stewarts was described as an 'Asylum for Lunatic Patients of the Middle Classes' from at least 1871, in the first extant Annual Report until 1881, when it was changed to 'Asylum for Lunatic Patients'. *Stewart Institution and Asylum Report* (Dublin 1871), (Dublin 1881).
86. *Stewart Institution and Asylum Report* (Dublin 1872), p. 17.
87. *Stewart Institution and Asylum Report* (Dublin 1871).
88. *Stewart Institution and Asylum Report* (Dublin 1871).
89. *Stewart Institution and Asylum Report* (Dublin 1873), p. 5.
90. *Stewart Institution and Asylum Report* (Dublin 1874), p. 5; *Stewart Institution and Asylum Report* (Dublin 1878), p. 5.
91. Patient Accounts Book (Stewarts, Stewarts Patients' Records).
92. MacKenzie (1992), p. 130.
93. Suzuki (2006), p. 121.
94. *Annual Report of the State of the Retreat* (Dublin 1814), p. 6.
95. *Annual Report of the State of the Retreat* (Dublin 1852), p. 7.

96. *Annual Report of the State of the Retreat* (Dublin 1863), pp. 8–9.

97. *The Stewart Institution and Asylum Report* (Dublin 1884), p. 16.

98. *The Stewart Institution and Asylum Report* (Dublin 1896), p. 19.

99. Cox (2012), pp. 97–132.

100. Melling and Forsythe (2006), p. 146.

101. See Marland (2004).

102. *Stewart Institution and Asylum Report* (Dublin 1886), p. 17.

103. *Stewart Institution and Asylum Report* (Dublin 1887), p. 16.

104. *Stewart Institution and Asylum Report* (Dublin 1885), p. 16.

105. Busfield (1986), p. 176.

106. *Annual Report of the State of the Retreat* (Dublin 1849), p. 6.

107. *Annual Report of the State of the Retreat* (Dublin 1856), p. 9.

108. *Annual Report of the State of the Retreat* (Dublin 1864), p. 5; *Annual Report of the State of the Retreat* (Dublin 1865), p. 13.

109. *Stewart Institution and Asylum Report* (Dublin 1888), p. 17.

110. *Stewart Institution and Asylum Report* (Dublin 1885), p. 16; *Stewart Institution and Asylum Report* (Dublin 1886), p. 17.

111. *Stewart Institution and Asylum Report* (Dublin 1886), p. 17.

112. *Stewart Institution and Asylum Report* (Dublin 1891), p. 18.

113. Ibid., p. 18.

114. *Stewart Institution and Asylum Report* (Dublin 1893), p. 20.

115. *Stewart Institution and Asylum Report* (Dublin 1896), p. 23.

116. *Stewart Institution and Asylum Report* (Dublin 1895), p. 25.

117. *Stewart Institution and Asylum Report* (Dublin 1897), pp. 1, 9.

118. *Stewart Institution and Asylum Report* (Dublin 1899), pp. 21–22.

119. Parry-Jones has surveyed printed advertisements for private asylums in England see Parry-Jones, 1972, pp. 102–111.

120. *Annual Report of the State of the Retreat* (Dublin 1901), pp. 5–6.

121. *Stewart Institution and Asylum Report* (Dublin 1899), p. 9.

122. Parry-Jones (1972).

123. For a full discussion of the 'trade in lunacy' in eighteenth- and nineteenth-century England and Wales, see Parry-Jones (1972).

124. MacKenzie (1992), Parry-Jones (1972), p. 84.

125. Finnane (1981), p. 21; Cox (2012), p. 2.

126. Hampstead Proceedings, 1825–1831 (Highfield Hospital Group, Records, 21 Aug. 1826).

127. Ibid., O'Hare (1998), p. 5. In 2014, under the name of Highfield Hospital Group, the establishment continued to be overseen by a sixth generation of the Eustace family. See Eustace Family Tree (Highfield Hospital Group, Records).

128. Parry-Jones (1972), p. 85.

129. O'Hare (1998), p. 1.

130. 5 & 6 Vic., c. 123, s. 18.
131. Parry-Jones (1972), p. 284.
132. Ibid., pp. 106–107.
133. See Mauger (2012).
134. Hampstead Proceedings, 1825–1831 (Highfield Hospital Group, Records, 1 Nov. 1825).
135. *Report into the State of Lunatic Asylums, Part II*, p. 159.
136. Ibid., pp. 155, 159.
137. Ibid., p. 159.
138. Ibid., p. 154.
139. See Burnett (1969).
140. For example, *Medical Directories, London and Provincial, Scotland, Ireland* (London, 1862), p. 1075.
141. *Report into the State of Lunatic Asylums, Part II*, p. 154.
142. Patient Accounts (Highfield Hospital Group, Records).
143. Forty-Third Report of the Inspectors of Lunatics (Ireland), H.C. 1894, p. 168.
144. *Medical Directories, London and Provincial, Scotland, Ireland* (London, 1877), p. 1616; (London, 1887), p. 1616; (London, 1889), p. 1718.
145. *Medical Directories, London and Provincial, Scotland, Ireland* (1876), p. 1290.
146. Parry-Jones (1972), p. 125.
147. MacKenzie (1992), pp. 128, 135.
148. Ibid., pp. 167, 172.
149. Thirty-Fourth Report on the District, Criminal, and Private Lunatic Asylums in Ireland [C 4539], H.C. 1884–1885, xxxvi, 635, p. 15.
150. Thirty-Sixth Report on the District, Criminal, and Private Lunatic Asylums in Ireland [5121], H.C. 1887, xxxix, 591, p. 20.
151. *Report into the State of Lunatic Asylums, Part II*, p. 154.
152. Ibid., p. 159.
153. Ibid.
154. Parry-Jones (1972), p. 86.
155. *Report into the State of Lunatic Asylums, Part II*, p. 159.
156. 'Insolvent Debtors,' *The Nation*, June 2, 1855.
157. Malcolm (1989), p. 179.
158. Ibid.
159. Prospectus of St John of God Hospital, 1884 (SJOGH, Records).
160. Parry-Jones (1972), pp. 168, 201–202.
161. Ibid.
162. Ibid., p. 207, Digby (1985), p. 218.
163. Digby (1985), p. 219; Parry-Jones (1972), p. 208.

164. Digby (1985), p. 218.
165. Malcolm (1999), p. 180.
166. In Malcolm's study, over one-quarter stayed for five years or more, although Cox has found a smaller number of long-stay patients at the Carlow asylum in this period. Malcolm (1999, p. 180), Cox (2012), p. 141.
167. Parry-Jones (1972), p. 212.
168. Ibid. Digby has found similar in her comparison of death rates at the York Retreat and neighbouring York asylum. Digby (1985), p. 225.
169. Malcolm (1999), p. 181.
170. Finnane (1981), p. 188.
171. Parry-Jones (1972, pp. 211–212), Digby (1985), p. 231.
172. MacKenzie (1992), p. 121.
173. Digby (1985), p. 231.
174. Malcolm (1999), pp. 180–181.
175. Cox (2012), p. 153.
176. Ibid.
177. Ibid.
178. Parry-Jones (1972), p. 208.
179. Walsh (2001), p. 145.
180. Case Book (FHL, Bloomfield Records, pp. 73, 75).
181. Catherine Cox and Hilary Marland have identified a significant preponderance of Irish-born patients in a number of pauper asylums in the north-west of England. See Cox and Marland (2015), pp. 263–287.
182. Case Book (FHL, Bloomfield Records, pp. 40, 47).
183. Cox (2012), p. 23.
184. Ibid.
185. Parry-Jones (1972), p. 86.

REFERENCES

Burnett, John. *A History of the Cost of Living*. Harmondsworth, 1969.
Busfield, Joan. *Managing Madness: Changing Ideas and Practices*. London, 1986.
Cox, Catherine. 'Access and Engagement: The Medical Dispensary System in Post-Famine Ireland.' In *Cultures of Care in Irish Medical History, 1750–1970*, edited by Catherine Cox and Maria Luddy, 57–78. Basingstoke, 2010.
Cox, Catherine. *Negotiating Insanity in the Southeast of Ireland 1830–1900*. Manchester: Manchester University Press, 2012.
Cox, Catherine and Hilary Marland. '"A Burden on the County": Madness, Institutions of Confinement and the Irish Patient in Victorian Lancashire'. *Social History of Medicine* 28, no. 2 (2015): 263–287.

Digby, Anne. *Madness, Morality and Medicine: A Study of the York Retreat, 1796–1914*. Cambridge: Cambridge University Press, 1985.

Finnane, Mark. *Insanity and the Insane in Post-Famine Ireland*. London: Croom Helm, 1981.

Finnane, Mark. 'Law and the Social Uses of the Asylum in Nineteenth-Century Ireland.' In *Asylum in the Community*, edited by John Carrier and Dylan Tomlinson, 88–107. London, 1996.

Luddy, Maria. *Women and Philanthropy in Nineteenth-Century Ireland*. Cambridge: Cambridge University Press, 1995.

MacKenzie, Charlotte. *Psychiatry for the Rich: A History of the Private Madhouse at Ticehurst in Sussex, 1792–1917*. London, Routledge 1992.

Malcolm, Elizabeth. *Swift's Hospital: A History of St Patrick's Hospital, Dublin, 1746–1989*. Dublin: Gill and Macmillan, 1989.

Malcolm, Elizabeth. 'The House of Strident Shadows: The Asylum, the Family and Emigration in Post-Famine Rural Ireland.' In *Medicine, Disease and the State in Ireland 1650–1940*, edited by Elizabeth Malcolm and Greta Jones, 177–195, Cork: Cork University Press, 1999.

Marland, Hilary. *Dangerous Motherhood: Insanity and Childbirth in Victorian Britain*. Basingstoke: Palgrave Macmillan, 2004.

Mauger, Alice. '"Confinement of the Higher Orders": The Social Role of Private Lunatic Asylums in Ireland, c. 1820–1860.' *Journal of the History of Medicine and Allied Sciences* 67, no. 2 (2012): 281–317.

Melling, Joseph and Bill Forsythe. *The Politics of Madness: The State, Insanity and Society in England, 1845–14*. London and New York: Routledge, 2006.

O'Hare, Pauline. *In the Care of Friends*. Dublin: Highfield Healthcare, 1998.

Parry-Jones, William Ll. *The Trade in Lunacy: A Study of Private Madhouses in England in the Eighteenth and Nineteenth Centuries*. London: Routledge & Kegan Paul, 1972.

Preston, Margaret H. *Charitable Words: Women, Philanthropy and the Language of Charity in Nineteenth-Century Dublin*. Westport, Conn.: Praeger, 2004.

Smith, Leonard D. *Cure, Comfort and Safe Custody: Public Lunatic Asylums in Early Nineteenth-Century England*. London and New York, 1999a.

Smith, Leonard D. 'The County Asylum in the Mixed Economy of Care, 1808–1845.' In *Insanity, Institutions and Society, 1800–1914*, edited by Joseph Melling and Bill Forsythe, 33–47. London and New York: Routledge, 1999b.

Suzuki, Akihito. *Madness at Home: The Psychiatrist, the Patient and the Family in England, 1820–1860*. Berkeley and Los Angeles, 2006.

Walsh, Oonagh. 'Lunatic and Criminal Alliances in Nineteenth-Century Ireland.' In *Outside the Walls of the Asylum: The History of Care in the Community 1750–2000*, edited by Peter Bartlett and David Wright, 132–152. London: Athlone Press, 2001.

Walsh, Oonagh. *Anglican Women in Dublin: Philanthropy, Politics and Education in the Early Twentieth Century*. Dublin, 2005.

Walton, John. 'Lunacy in the Industrial Revolution: A Study of Asylum Admission in Lancashire, 1848–50.' In *Journal of Social History* 13, no. 1 (1979–1980): 1–22.

Wright, David. 'Family Strategies and the Institutional Confinement of 'Idiot' Children in Victorian England.' *Journal of Family History*, 23, no. 2 (April, 1998): 190–208.

PART II

Understanding Insanity

'A Considerable Degree Removed from Pauperism'?: The Social Profile of Fee-Paying Patients

During the 1857–1858 commission, Nugent emphasised the permeability of class boundaries among asylum patients. When asked if he considered paying patients in district asylums to be 'generally of a class little above paupers', Nugent replied:

> Very little above paupers. A man has sixty or eighty acres of ground; his beneficial interest in that will probably be £120 or £130 a-year, out of which he has to maintain himself, his wife and probably four or five children. That man cannot swear that he is a pauper and if he has a lunatic child, he offers at an asylum as much as he would expend on that child in his own house.

The commissioners pressed this point, querying whether this man would not be 'a considerable degree removed from pauperism' but Nugent clarified his statement, stressing that 'if he is obliged to pay £40 or £50 a-year for one lunatic child, he will be doing a gross injustice to his wife and other children and he will be pauperising himself and family'.[1] Nugent was suggesting that patients' financial circumstances should not be measured in isolation, but rather in terms of their family unit and the number of dependents outside, as well as inside, the asylum.[2]

Social categories such as 'higher orders', 'lunatic poor' and 'the great class which lies between' are often misleading and should not be misread as signposts of social class.[3] As Melling and Forsythe have found in their analysis of four Devon asylums, asylum populations should also be understood in relation to their occupational status, economic resources,

© The Author(s) 2018
A. Mauger, *The Cost of Insanity in Nineteenth-Century Ireland*, Mental Health in Historical Perspective,
https://doi.org/10.1007/978-3-319-65244-3_4

the social and collective resources available, their market power and employment status.[4] While examination of patients' former occupations therefore offers some indication of their socio-economic background, these data must be interpreted sensitively. This chapter's primary concern is to identify the various social groups committed to district, voluntary and private asylums. For these purposes, analysis of the socio-economic profile of paying patients, their land and business interests and their maintenance fees serves to highlight, rather than define, social diversity within asylum populations.

Based on her survey of the lunacy inspectors' reports, Walsh has argued that private asylum patients in Ireland were predominantly male and single.[5] Malcolm has found that patients admitted to St Patrick's (voluntary asylum) during the 1870s and 1880s were typically members of the Church of Ireland, female and single.[6] Building on these analyses, this chapter provides the first comparative study of paying patients admitted to nine Irish asylums: Belfast, Ennis, Enniscorthy and Richmond district asylums, Stewarts and Bloomfield voluntary asylums and St John of God's, Hampstead and Highfield private asylums. Drawing heavily on statistics gleaned from asylum records (for methodology, see Appendix A), it charts admissions in two phases: the first to Bloomfield and Hampstead between 1826 and 1867, and the second to the nine asylums studied between 1868 and 1900. In doing so, it explores patients' gender, marital status, religious denomination and former occupation.

GENDER AND FAMILY TIES

Historians of psychiatry have long placed value on surveys of asylum patients' gender. In her study of residence rates, medical texts and literature, Elaine Showalter has suggested that doctors in Victorian England considered women to be particularly prone to insanity, giving rise to its depiction as a 'female malady'.[7] Busfield has disputed this finding, attributing women's numerical predominance in English asylums to mounting numbers of female patients who tended to stay longer.[8] These findings also apply to private asylums.[9] Commenting on Ticehurst patients, MacKenzie has suggested that 'families who were dependent on a male breadwinner for a high income may have felt it worth staking a considerable proportion of their financial resources on the chance of a cure'.[10] Similarly, Walsh has posited that the higher proportion of men in Irish private asylums might reflect families' greater willingness to pay for male relatives' treatment due to their 'greater economic importance'.[11]

From 1826 to 1867, the Hampstead private asylum admitted more men (65%) than women, while the Bloomfield voluntary asylum received more women (61.1%) than men. These trends changed little over the century, despite the continued expansion of asylum care and sanctioning of paying patients in district asylums. Between 1868 and 1900, approximately 60% of paying patients admitted to the district asylums studied were male (see Table 4.1) with little regional variation. This is especially striking given that there were more women in Ireland in this period.[12] It conforms broadly to surveys of total district asylum populations (pauper and paying patients), which have identified a predominance of male admissions.[13] St John of God's asylum limited admissions to men only and, taken together, sister asylums Highfield, which admitted women only, and Hampstead, which admitted men only after Highfield was established, had a wide disparity between the sexes: 66.8% of first admissions were men. These findings support those of MacKenzie and Walsh in suggesting that families were more willing to procure expensive private asylum care for their male relatives.[14]

Although Walsh has suggested that there were fewer women in private asylums because they were easier to care for at home,[15] there is scant evidence to support this contention. The two voluntary asylums, Stewarts and Bloomfield, admitted more women than men. Moreover, the very existence of St Vincent's voluntary asylum, which catered exclusively for women, signifies the willingness of families to purchase asylum care for women. In her study of the York Retreat, Anne Digby contends that while families considered expensive medical treatment as a 'form of investment particularly suited for the male bread-winner, the subsidised treatment available at the Retreat was an inducement for women to be

Table 4.1 Gender of first admissions to the case studies, 1868–1900

Asylum	Male	(%)	Female	(%)
Paying patients in district asylums	418	60.1	278	39.9
Stewarts	177	40.1	264	59.9
Bloomfield	90	35.6	163	64.4
St John of God's[a]	405	100.0	0	0.0
Hampstead and Highfield	219	66.8	109	33.2
Total	1309	100.0	814	100.0

Compiled from Belfast, Ennis, Enniscorthy, Richmond, Stewarts, Bloomfield, St John of God's and Hampstead admissions registers, 1868–1900
[a] The first admission to St John of God's was in 1885

sent there'.[16] Digby's argument goes some way towards accounting for the larger number of women admitted to Bloomfield and Stewarts. Yet it would be mistaken to argue that families were simply unwilling to invest larger amounts in the care of their female relatives. As Table 4.2 indicates, male district asylum patients were only marginally more likely to be maintained at high rates (over £20). Stewarts and Bloomfield tended to charge comparable rates for women and men, while women were among those maintained at the highest fees in both asylums (see Table 4.3). Women and men at Highfield and Hampstead, meanwhile, had almost equal chances of being maintained at over £100 per annum

Table 4.2 Known maintenance fees by gender of paying patients admitted to Belfast, Ennis, Enniscorthy and Richmond district asylums, 1868–1900[a]

Fees per annum	Male	(%)	Female	(%)	Total	(%)
£12 or less	93	36.8	70	35.0	163	36.0
£12–£20	68	26.9	77	38.5	145	32.0
Over £20	92	36.4	53	26.5	145	32.0
Total	253	100.0	200	100.0	453	100.0

Compiled from Belfast, Enniscorthy and Richmond Minute Books, Enniscorthy and Richmond superintendent's notices and Belfast, Ennis, Enniscorthy and Richmond admissions registers
[a]Maintenance fees are recorded for 65.1% of the sample

Table 4.3 Known maintenance fees by gender of first admissions to Bloomfield and Stewart's, 1868–1900[a]

Fees per annum	Bloomfield				Stewarts			
	Male	(%)	Female	(%)	Male	(%)	Female	(%)
Free	4	4.9	2	1.4	0	0.0	0	0.0
Under 20	0	0.0	0	0.0	0	0.0	2	1.0
20–25	1	1.2	0	0.0	0	0.0	6	2.9
26–40	5	6.2	6	4.1	8	6.4	17	8.1
41–60	8	9.9	8	5.4	98	78.4	168	80.0
61–100	9	11.1	28	18.9	17	13.6	16	7.6
101–150	19	23.5	52	35.1	2	1.6	0	0.0
151–200	35	43.2	51	34.5	0	0.0	1	0.5
201–240	0	0.0	1	0.7	0	0.0	0	0.0
Total	81	100.0	148	100.0	125	100.0	210	100.0

Compiled from Bloomfield and Stewarts admissions registers and financial accounts
[a]Maintenance fees are recorded for 89.4% of first admissions to Bloomfield and 74.2% of first admissions to Stewarts

in these asylums (see Table 4.4). Maintenance fees for those admitted to St John of God's are not recorded, though as seen in Chap. 3, this asylum reportedly charged its all-male patient population between approximately £50 and £150 per annum, underscoring a market for less expensive asylum care for men. These findings highlight wealthier Irish families' readiness to pay significant sums towards the care of their female—as well as male—relatives.

Table 4.4 Known maintenance fees by gender of first admissions to Hampstead and Highfield, 1868–1900[a]

Fees per annum	Male	(%)	Female	(%)	Total	(%)
£26–£50	0	0.0	1	4.8	1	2.6
£50–£100	2	11.1	2	9.5	4	10.3
£100–£200	9	50.0	7	33.3	16	41.0
£200–£300	4	22.2	8	38.1	12	30.8
Over £300	3	16.7	3	14.3	6	15.4
Total	18	100.0	21	100.0	39	100.0

Compiled from Hampstead and Highfield admissions registers and financial accounts
[a]Maintenance fees are recorded for 11.9% of first admissions to Hampstead and Highfield

Table 4.5 Known marital status by gender of first admissions to the case studies, 1868–1900 and in the Irish census, 1871–1901

Asylum	Married (%)			Single (%)			Widowed (%)		
	Male	Female	Total	Male	Female	Total	Male	Female	Total
Paying patients in district asylums	26.0	30.9	28.0	70.0	55.6	64.2	4.0	13.5	7.8
Stewarts	22.4	25.8	24.5	73.3	57.8	63.9	4.2	16.4	11.6
Bloomfield	28.9	36.3	33.6	62.2	52.8	56.1	8.9	11.0	10.3
St John of God's[a]	27.1	0.0	27.1	67.6	0.0	67.6	5.3	0.0	5.3
Hampstead and Highfield	42.1	42.6	42.3	52.8	49.1	51.5	5.1	8.3	6.2
Irish census	27.4	27.0	27.2	68.8	63.5	66.1	3.9	9.5	6.7

Compiled from Belfast, Ennis, Enniscorthy, Richmond, Stewarts, Bloomfield, St John of God's and Hampstead admissions registers 1868–1900; *Irish Historical Statistics: Population, 1821–1971*, W.E. Vaughan and A.J. Fitzpatrick (eds.) (Dublin, 1978), pp. 88–89
[a]The first admission to St John of God's was in 1885

Table 4.6   Maintenance fees by gender by marital status of first admissions to the case studies, 1868–1900

Fees	Female (%)				Male (%)			
	Married	Single	Widowed	Total	Married	Single	Widowed	Total
Less than £50	64.0	71.1	66.2	68.3	72.4	77.4	63.6	75.5
£51–£100	9.3	10.1	14.3	10.4	11.2	7.8	9.1	8.8
£100–£200	23.8	17.6	18.2	19.6	14.7	13.2	27.3	14.2
More than £200	2.9	1.3	1.3	1.8	1.7	1.6	0.0	1.5
Grand total	100.0	100.0	100.0	100.0	100.0	100.0	100.0	100.0

Compiled from Belfast, Ennis, Enniscorthy and Richmond admissions registers, minute books and superintendent's notices

Being married or single had further implications for the amounts contributed towards maintenance. While Malcolm has found that district asylum patients of both sexes were more likely to be single, reflecting 'the trend towards celibacy strongly evident in the general Irish population after the Famine', Cox has shown that single men during this period were 'particularly vulnerable to institutionalisation' in district asylums, a trend which she identifies as pre-dating declining marriage rates in Irish society and being linked to the use of dangerous lunatic certification.[17] Between 1826 and 1867, patients committed to Bloomfield (62%) and Hampstead (62.2%) were more often single. Single men were more likely to be committed to Hampstead and single women to Bloomfield. The marital status of first admissions changed little in the second period. Table 4.5 indicates that from 1868 to 1900 there was a predominance of single first admissions to all the asylums studied. However, except for Hampstead House, these figures were close to average for the population of Ireland. In fact, bachelors were underrepresented among first admissions to Bloomfield, Hampstead and St John of God's, deviating from the profile of district asylum populations in Ireland.

The story is similar for women admitted to the asylums. Apart from Stewarts, married women were over-represented, implying wives were more vulnerable to committal, especially to expensive asylums. This predominance of husbands and wives deviates from English contexts, where there was a preponderance of single women admitted to Ticehurst and over two-thirds of woman admitted to Wonford House private asylum near Exeter were single.[18] Digby has found that wives were also less

Table 4.7 Known religious persuasion of first admissions to the case studies, 1868–1900

Asylum	Catholic	(%)	Church of Ireland	(%)	Presbyterian	(%)	Methodist	(%)	Quaker	(%)	Other^b	(%)
Belfast	8	9.4	24	28.2	42	49.4	6	7.1	1	1.2	4	4.7
Antrim (1901 census)		20.59		20.90		50.77		1.91			5.83	
Ennis	130	92.2	11	7.8	0	0.0	0	0.0	0	0.0	0	0.0
Clare (1901 census)		97.98		1.81		0.14		0.04			0.03	
Enniscorthy	81	73.6	29	26.4			0	0.0	0	0.0	0	0.0
Wexford (1901 census)		91.67		7.55		0.26		0.33			0.19	
Richmond	193	58.1	121	36.4	7	2.1	4	1.2	1	0.3	6	1.8
Dublin (1901 census)		70.37		23.91		2.27		1.47			1.98	
Ireland (1901 census)		74.21		13.03		9.94		1.39			1.43	
Stewarts	30	17.5	126	73.7	8	4.7	3	1.8	1	0.6	3	1.8
Bloomfield	1	3.6	8	28.6	2	7.1	1	3.6	15	53.6	1	3.6
St John of God's^a	65	97.0	2	3.0	0	0.0	0	0.0	0	0.0	0	0.0
Hampstead/Highfield	81	20.5	63	71.6	1	1.1	0	0.0	2	2.3	4	4.5

Compiled from Belfast, Ennis, Enniscorthy, Richmond, Stewarts, Bloomfield, St John of God's, Hampstead and Highfield admissions registers

a The first admission to St John of God's was in 1885

b Includes Baptist, Dissenter, Jesuit, Jewish, Unitarian, Exclusive Brethren, Episcopalian

Table 4.8 Former occupation of male first admissions to the case studies, 1868–1900

Occupation	District Asylums	(%)	Stewarts	(%)	Bloomfield	(%)	St John of God's	(%)	Hampstead	(%)	Total	(%)
Army	64	15.3	3	1.7	5	5.6	1	0.2	17	7.8	90	6.9
Church	4	1.0	1	0.6	3	3.3	63	15.6	12	5.5	83	6.3
Class specified	2	0.5	46	26.0	3	3.3	20	4.9	21	9.6	92	7.0
Clerk	20	4.8	20	11.3	8	8.9	33	8.1	14	6.4	95	7.3
Farmer	77	18.4	28	15.8	2	2.2	51	12.6	14	6.4	172	13.1
In trade	55	13.2	28	15.8	28	31.1	112	27.7	30	13.7	253	19.3
Labourer	12	2.9	1	0.6	0	0.0	0	0.0	0	0.0	13	1.0
Law	3	0.7	3	1.7	8	8.9	6	1.5	18	8.2	38	2.9
Medicine	1	0.2	7	4.0	4	4.4	14	3.5	12	5.5	38	2.9
Navy	3	0.7	2	1.1	0	0.0	0	0.0	3	1.4	8	0.6
No occupation	46	11.0	4	2.3	15	16.7	26	6.4	27	12.3	118	9.0
Not recorded	11	2.6	0	0.0	1	1.1	6	1.5	0	0.0	18	1.4
Other occupation	20	4.8	23	13.0	12	13.3	49	12.0	38	17.4	142	10.8
Pensioner	30	7.2	0	0.0	0	0.0	3	0.7	0	0.0	33	2.5
Police	31	7.4	1	0.6	0	0.0	3	0.7	1	0.5	36	2.8
Son of	26	6.2	5	2.8	0	0.0	0	0.0	1	0.5	32	2.4
Student	13	3.1	5	2.8	1	1.1	15	3.7	9	4.1	43	3.3
Unclear	0	0.0	0	0.0	0	0.0	3	0.7	2	0.9	5	0.4
Total	418	100.0	177	100.0	90	100.0	405	100.0	219	100.0	1309	100.0

Compiled from Belfast, Ennis, Enniscorthy, Richmond, Stewarts, Bloomfield, St John of God's and Hampstead admissions registers

Table 4.9 Known maintenance fees for male farmer first admissions to Belfast, Ennis, Enniscorthy and Richmond district asylums, 1868–1900

Fees per annum	Belfast	(%)	Ennis	(%)	Enniscorthy	(%)	Richmond	(%)	All	(%)
Less than £12	1	50.0	19	76.0	3	17.6	3	37.5	26	50.0
£12–£20	1	50.0	4	16.0	7	41.2	0	0.0	12	23.1
Over £20	0	0.0	2	8.0	4	41.2	5	62.5	14	26.9

Compiled from Belfast, Ennis, Enniscorthy and Richmond admissions registers, minute books and superintendent's notices

prone to committal to the York Retreat, possibly reflecting their responsibility for children and the household. Interestingly, Digby characterises this finding as 'a thought-provoking corrective to contemporary alarmist literature on asylums, which often emphasised the abuses of vengeful husbands wrongfully confining sane wives'.[19] By extension, it could be held that the over-representation of married women in some of Ireland's more expensive asylums reveals a tendency towards the 'wrongful confinement' of wealthy Irishmen's wives. Certainly, husbands paid the fees for 67.9% of wives committed to Stewarts.[20] However, there is no qualitative evidence to support this. Moreover, as Chap. 5 contends, spouses and other family members often demonstrated affection and care for their mentally ill relatives, casting some doubt on the extent to which wrongful confinement occurred.[21]

Male heads of families and adult relatives tended to be maintained at lower fees than female ones, reflecting men's greater economic significance in their households. With the loss of their incomes, it is plausible that remaining members of the family struggled to pay high fees. This contrasts with the arguments put forward by Walsh and MacKenzie that families were more willing to invest in the care of male breadwinners[22] and suggests that the relatives of married male patients had less disposable income to contribute towards asylum care (Table 4.6).

As we have seen, the relatives of district asylum patients sometimes went to great lengths to contribute maintenance fees, even borrowing money and falling into debt. The wealthier families of voluntary and private asylum patients also paid directly for relatives' care.[23] The financial accounts for Stewarts indicate the relationship between patients and those who paid their fees. Relatives were by far the most common creditors: a single relative contributed fees for 68.7% of first admissions, two relatives for a further 6.8%, a relative and friend for 3.7% and a relative in conjunction with a Chancery fund for 0.9%. 'Friends' accounted for another 6.8%, although this figure may be higher as a handful of the names recorded in the financial accounts did not include their relation to the patient (4.3%). In contrast, very few Stewarts patients paid their own fees out of an income. A Chancery fund alone accounted for 6.8%, one patient paid her fees from the Dublin Widow's Fund, one from the War Office and two from dividends on stock they possessed.

The predominance of relatives covering fees at Stewarts (80.2%) and the large number paying for patients at Bloomfield, Hampstead and Highfield who shared their surname, demonstrates that families in Ireland were willing to pay for their relatives' care.[24] Whether this was simply to get rid of a difficult household member or a genuine attempt to seek treatment in the hope of a cure is unclear. What can be inferred is that a large proportion of paying patients—even those who were unmarried—were part of an often large, family network. Cox has highlighted the presence of mentally ill adult offspring in family households, which, she suggests indicates that 'relatives with some legal obligation undertook a caring role'.[25] In this study, the very fact that families paid for the care of their relatives corroborates these findings.

Record linkage with the census records casts further light on the familial contexts of paying patients. Out of twenty-nine patients discharged from the asylums studied between 1898 and 1900 who could be identified in the 1901 census, none returned to an empty home.[26] Johanna R., previously a paying patient at Enniscorthy, lived with her widowed sister-in-law and this woman's eight children. More typically, when Hannah B., an unemployed schoolteacher, was discharged from Highfield, she returned to live with her father (a railway clerk), her mother, two brothers (a railway clerk and hardware merchant's clerk) and one sister. However, a minority had apparently broken ties with their previous households. Six discharged patients were no longer at their previous address in 1901 and one was in a boarding house. Margaret D., a fifty-nine-year-old retired schoolteacher, was admitted to and discharged from Richmond in 1898 from an address in Dublin. By 1901, Margaret no longer lived at the address, which housed a married couple in their fifties (sharing Margaret's surname) and their teenage niece. This implies that prior to committal, Margaret had been living with her younger brother (who is mentioned in the case notes) and his wife, who had or soon would take custody of the niece. It is plausible that this household unit found itself incapable of caring for more than one dependent, which would account for Margaret's move following discharge. A property Margaret owned had become a source of tension between herself and her brother and sister-in-law, suggesting that this may also have played a role in her change of address following discharge.[27]

This section has demonstrated that where gender and marital status were concerned, fee-paying patients were similar to total district asylum populations. There is danger, however, in discussing such diverse patient populations simply in terms of demographic trends. Rather than forming a single cohesive group, each patient emerged from a distinctive family unit—some were breadwinners, some adult dependents. That many of these families struggled to cope without their breadwinner's income or to drum up enough financial support to provide 'class-appropriate' care for a dependent is probable. In fact, evidence of the financial sacrifices families made to pay for asylum care casts doubt on the extent to which relatives tended to 'dump' their female, their single or their 'unwanted'.[28]

RELIGION, OCCUPATION AND WEALTH

Lorraine Walsh has cautioned against directly associating patients' former occupation with social status, arguing that on admission, patients were labelled and classified based purely on their own or their relatives' and friends' spending power, while their class or social status meant little.[29] In her analysis of private patients at the Dundee Royal Asylum in Scotland, Walsh highlights the difficulties in accurately constructing 'a system of commensurability' between occupation and status.[30] Analysis of patients' occupations alongside maintenance fees, however, facilitates direct correlation between particular professional groups and their families' spending power. In the Irish context, patients' religious affiliation is also of interest as it formed an integral part of social identity in this era. Patients' religious denomination therefore reveals much about the sectors of society admitted to the asylums studied. It is useful, too, to consider what parts of Ireland (or abroad) patients in the study were drawn from.

District asylums were intended to provide care for people of the same district. Paying patients were therefore usually committed to the asylum in the county in which they had lived. Thus, Belfast patients came from

Antrim, Ennis patients from Clare or less often neighbouring Limerick (9.4%) and Enniscorthy patients from Wexford. The Richmond district was larger and admitted paying patients from Dublin (85.3%) and neighbouring counties Louth (7.6%) and Wicklow (6.7%). Roughly, half of those admitted to the voluntary and private asylums studied had a previous residence in Dublin, while the other half were from various other Irish counties.[31] This indicates that these Dublin-based voluntary and private asylums served the whole of Ireland and many patients would have travelled large distances to receive care. In her study of Ticehurst, MacKenzie attributes families' willingness to send patients long distances for care to a 'desire for confidentiality'.[32] While this might be the case for Ireland, it is important to remember that there were few private asylums outside Dublin, meaning that wealthier families had little option but to send their relatives to the capital.

The religious profile of paying patients speaks volumes about the impact the religious character of institutions had on committal patterns. Apart from Belfast, paying patients committed to the district asylums studied were far more likely to be Catholic than those sent to the voluntary or private asylums (see Table 4.7).[33] This excludes St John of God's which, as we have seen, was managed by a Catholic order of brothers and therefore admitted mainly Catholics (97%). Compared with the general population of Ireland, patients in this study, except for those at St John of God's, were disproportionally members of the Church of Ireland, while Catholics were underrepresented. The reasons for this could vary. The over-representation of Church of Ireland patients admitted to most asylums in this study suggests that Protestant communities in nineteenth-century Ireland could better afford to purchase asylum care. Predictably, there was a preponderance of Quakers admitted to Bloomfield (53.6%), at odds with the number outside. Catholic admissions were in a minority at Bloomfield, equalling Methodists and Brethren and outstripped by Presbyterians. In keeping with its Protestant ethos, almost three-quarters of the patients admitted to Stewarts were members of the Church of Ireland, compared with less than one-quarter being Catholic.

As Chap. 3 outlined, varying rates of maintenance signified social diversity within and between asylum populations. Examining patients' former occupations alongside their maintenance fees further supports this position. Beginning with male first admissions to the asylums studied, Table 4.8 provides a crude breakdown of their former occupations.[34]

The most prominent category was 'in trade', which is unsurprising, given that many industries and crafts were on the rise in late nineteenth-century Ireland.[35] Among paying patients admitted to the district asylums, the highest proportion of trades-craftsmen was in Belfast (24.4%), which included dealers in unspecified goods, printers, drapers, boot and shoe-makers, businessmen, merchant tailors and linen merchants. This sits well with industrial Belfast's expanding linen and shirt-making industries in the later nineteenth century.[36] In contrast, the proportion of tradesmen in Ennis was far lower (3.4%) and comprised only one car man, three shopkeeper's sons and two of the 'trading class'. With the exception of one man whose maintenance was £20 per annum, the remainder of this cohort were charged modest sums (£6–£12).

In keeping with Wexford's stronger trade element, trade was the second most common occupation (21.3%) after farming for male paying patients in Enniscorthy. This group comprises an equally wide range of occupations including bakers, builders, carpenters, coopers, drapers, painters, printers, saddlers, shoemakers, shopkeepers and tailors. The Enniscorthy case notes often indicated that these patients were business owners. For example, one patient owned a draper's shop on Wexford town's Main Street. On other occasions, patients simply worked in a shop, as was the case with Thomas G., a baker.

For the period 1868–1900, Richmond admitted a relatively small proportion of trades-craftsmen as paying patients (12.6%). These patients represented a disparate range of trades and crafts including bakers, carpenters, cashiers, chefs, draper's assistants, grocers or shopkeepers, linen coopers, merchants and victuallers. Shopkeepers and grocers were the most prominent in this category, although even they comprised only about 2%. Similarly, only about 5% of those admitted to the private and voluntary asylums fell into this category. The absence of patients from Dublin's brewing and distilling industries is particularly noteworthy, given the rising importance of the Guinness Brewery and Powers Distillery during the period.[37] Despite the prominence of baking, textiles and, to a lesser extent, dressmaking in late nineteenth-century Dublin,[38] very few of Richmond's paying patients, or those sent to the voluntary or private asylums, had engaged with these industries, implying that the relatives of a number of Dublin's most common tradesmen could not afford asylum care.

Patients described as travellers, merchants or dealers were charged between £24 and £27 per annum at Richmond and were most commonly found in voluntary or private asylums. Out of male admissions to Bloomfield and Hampstead, 7.9% and 6.4% respectively were merchants. That a large proportion of Bloomfield's admissions were in trade may be attributable to traditional links between Quakerism and the merchant trade, although the religion of merchants in Bloomfield was not recorded in most cases. Shopkeepers and grocers also featured more prominently among patients in voluntary and private asylums, suggesting that the families of these men, together with merchants, had greater disposable income to spend on asylum care.

Farmers in this study are relatively well represented across the board. The predominance of farmers (13.1%) in the asylums studied is unsurprising, given their growing importance during the second half of the nineteenth century. After the Famine (c. 1845–1850), many Irish farmers prospered and on the whole rural incomes increased.[39] In the later nineteenth century, the number of landless labourers declined and larger farms became more common.[40] Above the grade of small farmers, who can be broadly characterised as those holding at least five acres of land, David Seth Jones has identified another group, which he terms graziers: those who occupied at least one holding of 150–200 acres.[41] Between small farmers and graziers, the smaller tenants and cottiers who decreased in number during the Famine (c. 1850) were replaced by the more successful, middle-class farmer.[42]

While the asylum records do not facilitate a full statistical breakdown of the varying grades of farmers catered for, they do allow some glimpses. Of the 172 farmers sent to the nine selected asylums, 155 were recorded simply as 'farmer'. Others under this heading included a farmer and miller, a farmer who owned a shop, seven 'gentlemen' farmers, three graziers and one small farmer. The small number of graziers probably stems from inconsistencies in the asylums' recording processes, though it is significant that they appear only in the private asylums, St John of God's and Hampstead, signalling the higher spending power of this group and their families. The only 'small farmer' in this study was admitted to Richmond, while all but one of the gentlemen farmers were admitted to private asylums, with the other admitted to Enniscorthy.

An analysis of farmers' maintenance fees further underscores the wide socio-economic variation within this group. The majority of known fees for farmers are for those admitted to the district asylums. Table 4.9 reveals that there were significant differences between each district. County Wexford was traditionally one of the wealthier farming areas in

Ireland and boasted many large estates as well as smaller holdings.[43] This is reflected in the fees paid for farmers at Enniscorthy, which are distributed quite evenly between the three categories. Enniscorthy also had the smallest proportion of farmers paying less than £12. At Ennis, more than three-quarters of farmers were maintained at less than £12, reflecting the difficult economic circumstances experienced by many in the west of Ireland.[44] While in earlier periods the landlord class was the smallest, but economically most significant, group in rural Irish society, the Land Wars of the 1880s diminished the significance of this social group, resulting in the rising importance of Catholic landowners.[45] Farmers maintained at over £20 per annum in Ennis were exclusively Catholic, suggesting that this group preferred to commit relatives to the local district asylum rather than sending them to private or voluntary institutions in distant Dublin. In contrast, at Enniscorthy, more than half the farmers accommodated at over £20 were Protestant. Richmond also tended to cater for more successful farmers although a smaller, but significant, proportion (37.5%) was maintained at £12 or less.

Farmers' acreage is another useful indicator of their socio-economic status. At Enniscorthy, Drapes sometimes recorded patients' farm acreage in his case notes on patients admitted in the 1890s. For example, Drapes noted that Patrick D.—a single fifty-eight-year-old Catholic— lived alone on his farm of seventeen acres. At the other end of the scale, Drapes wrote that Francis R., a single fifty-three-year-old Catholic farmer, had told him he had a farm of 110 acres.[46] Drapes usually recorded land acreage for female paying patients, suggesting that this was an important factor in determining their social status and financial circumstances. In some cases, Drapes detailed the land of the spouse or sibling responsible for the woman's maintenance. For example, when Hannah N. was sent to Enniscorthy aged forty and single, Drapes noted that her two living brothers, Thomas and James, 'each has over 90 acres (pt. sup) and James a mill as well'.[47] He also recorded the acreage of patients who were farmers' wives. Among these, he wrote that Catherine S. had twenty-eight acres, Anne J. had forty-eight acres, reputedly worth £46 and Margaret Sara K. had 100 acres.[48] Marcella J.'s son had a farm of thirty acres and Marcella also sold her chickens on market day.[49] Of these examples, only Margaret Sara K. was a Protestant, mirroring the fact that Protestant landowners tended to retain the larger estates. However, Johanna F., a Catholic, was reportedly the niece of a man from New Ross who owned a farm of 200 or 300 acres.[50] Likewise, the

Table 4.10 Relationship between land acreage and maintenance fees charged for paying patients admitted to Enniscorthy district asylum, 1868–1900

Fee per annum	Holding size
£8	20 acres of a farm
£12 (later reduced to £8)	28 acres
£13	30 acres free
£15	48 acres valued at £46

Compiled from Clinical Record Volumes No. 3, 4 & 6 (WCC, St Senan's Hospital, Enniscorthy); Enniscorthy minute books and admissions registers

examples of the male patients above demonstrate that Catholic farmers in Wexford could occupy both ends of the social scale.

Finally, in four cases, both the amount of land owned and the maintenance fees for Enniscorthy paying patients were recorded. As Table 4.10 demonstrates, acreage was roughly proportionate to the fees charged, indicating landholding size was a determining factor for maintenance fees. As this table reveals, even the lowest grade of paying patient at Enniscorthy (£8) could possess twenty acres, placing them well above the defining lower limit of small farmer (five acres). If these values are taken as representative, several paying patients from the farming classes could be termed part of the rising Catholic middle classes.

Those under the heading 'other occupation' comprise a medley of professions that defy any systematic classification. Predictably, several of the 'other occupations' pursued by men admitted to voluntary and private asylum tended to be professionals rather than tradesmen. Among them were white-collar workers like engineers, stockbrokers, bank managers, architects, bookkeepers and accountants. Together with clerks, members of these professions made up a large proportion of admissions to voluntary and private asylums and were usually members of the Church of Ireland.[51] This conforms to Daly's assertion that Protestants numbered disproportionately among the 'middle-class occupations' of professional and public service and the white-collar clerical and banking jobs in this era.[52] However, it is important to bear in mind that, with the exception of St John of God's, the voluntary and private asylums in this study were primarily populated by Protestants.

The proportion of men recorded as having 'no occupation' varied widely from one asylum to the next, reflecting discrepancies in record keeping. The highest numbers of male first admissions in this category were in district asylums (11%) and at Hampstead (12.3%), while 'unemployment' was lowest among men sent to Stewarts (2.3%) and St John of God's (6.4%). For Stewarts' patients, explanation for the low proportion described as having 'no occupation' might lie in the tendency to enumerate patients' social class rather than occupation; almost one-quarter of male first admissions were described as 'gentlemen'. However, 9.6% of men admitted to Hampstead were also described in terms of their social class (mostly gentlemen), suggesting that an even larger proportion of admissions to that asylum were without a particular occupation. The category of 'no occupation' therefore encompassed a wide range of social groups from the unemployed to those with independent means and maintenance fees for this group ranged from £6 to £213 per annum. Those kept at the highest rates were probably wealthy gentlemen. Certainly, in 1857, the lunacy inspectors surmised that the large proportion of private asylum patients recorded as having no occupation were mainly comprised of 'persons of independent fortune'.[53] In addition, it is plausible that at least some of this cohort would have been landlords.[54]

A final group worthy of mention is those in the army. Although not well represented in the voluntary and private asylums, soldiers were the second largest category committed to the district asylums as paying patients. This is mostly due to Richmond, where 28.3% of male paying patients admitted were soldiers. A small but notable proportion of soldiers were sent to Bloomfield (5.6%) and Hampstead (7.8%). Unsurprisingly, soldiers sent to Bloomfield and particularly Hampstead were from the higher ranks of the army, such as captains or lieutenants, while those committed to Richmond were more often described as privates or simply soldiers, in addition to a handful of army pensioners. The high proportion of soldiers admitted to Belfast (10.6%) and Richmond stems from these asylums' proximity to prominent army barracks.

The Richmond case notes provide insight into the committal and discharge of soldiers at that asylum. The military authorities took responsibility for the committal, maintenance charges and discharge of these soldiers. Accordingly, the authority of the asylum medical officer or superintendent was lessened, even in cases where they suspected a patient was not mentally ill. In several cases, the reporting physician noted his suspicion that a soldier patient was malingering in the hope of being discharged from service. By 1901, suspicions of malingering at Richmond had even spread to the patient population and a female paying patient remarked that 'Dr. Rambant [Richmond medical officer] has a lot of military fellows on getting what the patients should get. Talks of someone (the military fellows I suppose) humbugging the doctors behind their backs.'[55] In earlier case notes, the medical officers were conscious that at least some of the soldiers admitted were apparently in good mental health, although they did not state this explicitly. The first instance occurred in 1890, when Robert B. was admitted. Dr. M.J. Nolan, the Senior Assistant Medical Officer to the Richmond Asylum, reported:

> He seems anxious to attract attention of the medical officers by his conduct – when they are not present he is reported to be quiet and orderly ... Is anxious to know whether he has altogether severed his connection with the army ... Says he is very anxious to know what is to become of him – whether he is to be sent home to England or left here. He says he cannot endure the conduct of the patients.[56]

The following year, another soldier, Charles H.R., was 'closely watched ... day and night for malingering'. Although Nolan was 'satisfied that he is not insane', he noted:

> He is determined to secure his discharge from the service and is capable of enduring much discomfort in his effort to appear insane. He has today been handed over to the military authorities. Discharged 12 March 1891.[57]

When Francis B. was asked 'if he is tired of being a soldier he smiles and says he is'. Although the Army Medical Board examined him on 25 June 1891 and discharged him from service, it was not until 31 August that he was handed over to the military authorities and discharged from the asylum relieved. In the interim, Francis reportedly became 'depressed and seems disappointed that no notice has come from the military authorities concerning his removal'. When Nolan attempted to cheer him up, informing him that 'he may now be sent to England any day he only sighs, says all is over with him, that he is dead and that we mean to cut him up'.[58] It is conceivable that the military authorities were eager to make an example of malingering comrades by forcing Francis to remain wrongfully confined in the asylum.

In the case of Thomas H., a different medical officer was vigilant in his attempt to ascertain if the patient was insane.[59] Although they were unable to detect malingering, the medical officer ordered the attendants to 'take special note of his behaviour but according to them he has not at any time altered in his manner'. The medical officer then decided to launch an investigation of his own:

> Last night I awoke him and asked him how long he had been asleep. His manner of speaking and acting was brighter and more intelligent for the first few moments, though when he realised where he was he seemed to relapse into his usual dull stupid state.[60]

When the Army Medical Board examined Thomas a week later, they decided he should remain in Richmond for another month. Nolan reported that the board could not 'satisfy themselves as to his mental state'. He also noted that 'during examination he affected a dull dogged manner quite unlike his usual state'.[61] In this instance, while Nolan and his fellow medical officer were clearly certain of their patient's sanity, the Army Medical Board had the final say, thus diminishing the authority of the asylum medical officers. According to Nolan, some soldier patients went to great lengths to attempt to convince asylum staff and the Army Medical Board they were unfit for duty. Nolan claimed that Thomas H. became so 'dirty' and 'untidy in his habits' that the attendants became 'satisfied he is insane'.[62]

While the precise reasons for these soldiers' attempts to be discharged from service remain largely obscure, asylum life was clearly a preferred alternative to the army in these cases. For example, when Leo S., a Russian Jewish soldier, was admitted in 1893 and noted as being epileptic, he quickly 'admitted that he was malingering' to escape his comrades' racial insults. He explained to Nolan that he had bought '4*d.* worth of salts of sorrel' to bring on the symptoms of epilepsy and that he:

> shammed epilepsy because he was so miserable in the army; his comrades used to insult and bully him; chiefly on the sub [sic] of his nationality ... he had been much annoyed by the manner his comrades looked on him that he felt he 'was not wanted' ... In consequence of this he became depressed and gave way to drink and at the time he took the sorrel he was under sentence to the cells for absence from duty and it was partly to avoid this punishment he sought to make himself ill.[63]

Leo's frank confession to Nolan suggests his awareness that asylum staff had little say over his discharge from either the army or the asylum. By this point, Nolan seemed resigned to his diminished authority over soldier patients and following this he often simply noted 'insanity very doubtful. A soldier anxious to leave the army'.[64]

The outcome for most of these soldiers following discharge is unknown. In the case of an Irish soldier named Edward D., it is possible to conjecture. Edward informed the medical officer that 'he enlisted when drunk – that he has got a good job waiting for him if he could get out of the army but that he has no special wish to leave the service'. A month later, however, Edward changed his mind, 'says he would like to get home to his father where a good job awaits him. He has no wish to return to the Army.' Less than a month later, the patient was discharged from both the asylum and the army. He returned home where he presumably began working at the 'good job' he had mentioned to his doctor.[65]

Compared with male patients, the former occupations of female paying patients provide less clear-cut indications of their socio-economic background. In this regard, the recording process varied widely in the selected asylums, reflecting the difficulties inherent in attempting to reconstruct the occupational profile of women in the nineteenth century. Women's occupations have also tended to be under-recorded in Irish censuses because work in farming and industry was often combined with family duties. The 1871 census is a notable exception; it identified farmers' wives as part of the agricultural force and wives who contributed to family businesses as being employed in them.[66] As Daly has argued, census enumerators tended 'to assign women to the domestic or unoccupied class', reflecting 'society's belief that this was their appropriate place'.[67] In a similar vein, Melling has shown that Victorian women were often deprived of an occupational status in the English census because their labour was not recognised as valuable in its own right.[68] However, as discussed above, those filling in admissions registers for female paying patients were more concerned with ascertaining their spending power.[69]

Table 4.11 provides a crude breakdown of the principal occupational categories for female paying patients admitted to the selected asylums. Overall, more than three-quarters had no recorded occupation, though this varied significantly between regions and institutions. A disproportionately high percentage of 'unemployed' women were sent to Richmond and to a lesser extent, Belfast. In contrast, almost two-thirds of female paying patients committed to Ennis and a third of those to Enniscorthy were listed under a relatives' occupation: 'wife of', 'daughter of', and so on. The appellation 'wife of' was not peculiar to paying patients. Pamela Michael has found that female asylum patients in nineteenth-century Wales were often listed under their husband's occupation, although after marriage many may have continued to engage in paid employment that was important to family survival.[70]

The large proportion of 'unemployed' women committed to Bloomfield and Highfield is expected, given that Irish middle-class women and even some in skilled working-class families tended not to work outside the home.[71] Stewarts' female patients were far less often described as having 'no occupation' but, instead, just over half were labelled in terms of their social status. Of these, most (47% of total female admissions) were termed a 'lady', compared with only 9.8% of the women committed to the more expensive Bloomfield. At Bloomfield, 'ladies' were maintained at between £100 and £180 per annum, while at Stewarts more than three-fifths were maintained at less than £50 and some as low as £20. Those described as 'lower order', 'mid class' or 'middle' were also maintained at less than £50. These discrepancies highlight the fluidity of labels like 'lady' and 'middle class' and demonstrate the pitfalls of blindly interpreting them as representative of social class or spending power.

Women committed to Belfast, Richmond and Stewarts asylums were most often assigned designated occupations in the admissions registers. This reflects urban trends. Despite a national decline in female employment in the Irish labour force from 1861, particularly in Connaught and parts of Leinster, the highest proportions of working women were in Counties Antrim, Armagh and Down and urban areas such as Dublin City and its suburbs.[72] During the nineteenth century, the north-east rivalled areas such as Lancashire in terms of the high proportion of women working in factories.[73] Nonetheless, with the exception of two dressmakers, one upholsterer and one weaver, there is little evidence of Belfast paying patients' participation in Ulster's strong textile and clothing sectors.[74] Likewise, although dressmaking was the most popular occupation among female industrial workers in Dublin,[75] Richmond admitted only one court dressmaker, draper, dressmaker and embroiderer as paying patients. While it is possible that some of these women were engaged in factory work, it is equally, if not more, likely that they carried out these occupations in the home.

Table 4.11　Former occupations of female first admissions to the case studies, 1868–1900

Former occupation	Belfast	(%)	Ennis	(%)	Enniscorthy	(%)	Richmond	(%)	Stewarts	(%)	Bloomfield	(%)	Highfield	(%)	All	(%)
No occupation	12	31.6	5	7.2	5	14.3	95	69.9	12	4.5	131	80.4	83	76.9	343	42.2
Class specified	0	0.0	3	4.3	0	0.0	1	0.7	133	50.4	16	9.8	0	0.0	153	18.8
Designated occupation	9	23.7	5	7.2	4	11.4	17	12.5	62	23.5	13	8.0	5	4.6	115	14.1
Farming	2	5.3	12	17.4	13	37.1	3	2.2	16	6.1	0	0.0	0	0.0	46	5.7
Domestic	10	26.3	1	1.4	1	2.9	4	2.9	5	1.9	3	1.8	0	0.0	24	3.0
Wife/Widow Of[a]	0	0.0	21	30.4	10	28.6	5	3.7	27	10.2	0	0.0	0	0.0	63	7.7
Daughter/Sister of[b]	1	2.6	22	31.9	1	2.9	0	0.0	7	2.7	0	0.0	0	0.0	31	3.8
Mother of[c]	0	0.0	0	0.0	1	2.9	0	0.0	0	0.0	0	0.0	0	0.0	1	0.1
Not recorded	4	10.5	0	0.0	0	0.0	11	8.1	2	0.8	0	0.0	19	17.6	36	4.4
Student	0	0.0	0	0.0	0	0.0	0	0.0	0	0.0	0	0.0	1	0.9	1	0.1
Total	38	100.0	69	100.0	35	100.0	136	100.0	264	100.0	163	100.0	108	100.0	813	100.0

Compiled from Belfast, Ennis, Enniscorthy, Richmond, Stewarts, Bloomfield and Highfield admissions registers
[a]Includes wife/widow of farmer
[b]Includes daughter/sister of farmer
[c]Includes mother of farmer

Table 4.12 Female first admissions to the case studies associated with farming, 1868–1900

Occupation	Belfast	(%)	Ennis	(%)	Enniscorthy	(%)	Richmond	(%)	Stewarts	(%)	All	(%)
Agriculture	0	0.0	0	0.0	0	0.0	0	0.0	1	0.4		0.1
Farmer	2	5.3	2	2.9	12	34.3	2	1.5	13	4.9		4.0
Farmer & Hotel keeper	0	0.0	0	0.0	0	0.0	1	0.7	0	0.0		0.1
Farming	0	0.0	1	1.4	0	0.0	0	0.0	1	0.4		0.3
Farming class	0	0.0	9	13.0	1	2.9	0	0.0	1	0.4		1.4
Farmer's widow	0	0.0	2	2.9	0	0.0	0	0.0	0	0.0		0.3
Farmer's wife	0	0.0	10	14.5	7	20.0	3	2.2	1	0.4		2.7
Wife of gent farmer	0	0.0	0	0.0	0	0.0	0	0.0	1	0.4		0.1
Farmer's daughter	1	2.6	16	23.2	1	2.9	0	0.0	3	1.1		2.7
Grazier's daughter	0	0.0	0	0.0	0	0.0	0	0.0	1	0.4		0.1
Farmer's mother	0	0.0	0	0.0	1	2.9	0	0.0	0	0.0		0.1
Total	3	7.9	40	57.9	22	63.0	6	4.4	22	8.4		11.9

Compiled from Belfast, Ennis, Enniscorthy, Richmond and Stewarts admissions registers

As Daly has argued, aside from a small number of female professionals and commercial clerks, women with recorded occupations in the
census were poor.[76] Yet, in this study, women assigned occupations in
the admissions registers were not necessarily maintained at low rates,
suggesting that their relatives had at least a degree of spending power.
Some were accommodated at as much as £160 per annum. Designated
occupations included nuns, teachers, governesses, shopkeepers, shop
assistants and shop girls, servants, grocers, nurses and those who worked
with textiles. This list is indicative of women's rising opportunities in the
workplace towards the end of the nineteenth century. Shop assistants, in
particular, were perceived by contemporaries as representative of 'wom-
en's altered role in the public sphere' and this group was by no means
among the poor. From the mid-nineteenth century, shop assistants had
been 'manoeuvring towards membership of the Irish petit bourgeoisie'
and, by the twentieth century, female shop assistants, drapers and draper's assistants clearly enjoyed a new brand of economic independence.[77]
The recording of occupations for female paying patients in this study
therefore does not necessarily indicate poverty.

For several women in lower paid professions, poverty, particularly following the onset of mental illness, was more likely. As Melling has found
in his study of governesses and female schoolteachers admitted to three
Devon asylums, while their domestic means could be modest, it was vital
for this social cohort to avoid the publicity of their committal. Melling
demonstrates that 'many private teachers relied on connections with the
"best circles"' and 'were understandably anxious to maintain some proximity to the privileged world of their employers'.[78] Melling also argues
that relatives and friends often strove to avoid committing governesses
to pauper institutions and struggled to finance their accommodation at
private asylums such as Wonford House.[79] These findings might account
for the presence of governesses, schoolteachers and even domestic servants in the voluntary asylums in this study. However, this study suggests
that employers, rather than relatives, paid for their maintenance, a privilege they also extended to domestic servants. In Bloomfield, an unidentified source contributed £150 per annum for a 'housekeeper and ladies'
maid'. Several other unnamed individuals paid between £50 and £150
per annum to accommodate governesses there. Non-relatives paid for the
maintenance of several women committed to Stewarts. These included
three servants, a governess, a laundress, a stitcher and a teacher, though
these were at lower rates (approx. £50 per annum). For example, a Mrs.

Jameson, Mrs. Moore and Dr. Leet paid £50, £40 and £30 respectively for the maintenance of a laundress, a servant and a governess. These individuals are among the few in the financial accounts whose relationship to the patient was not specified, implying these individuals were, in fact, employers, rather than relatives or friends. This highlights the high value placed on servants and employees in Irish households and suggests that even outside traditional family settings, friends or employers were willing to invest in voluntary asylum care for women.

While designated occupations were relatively less common amongst female paying patients from rural areas, farming was more common. The percentage connected to farming either directly, through marriage or by birth is shown in Table 4.12. Notably, none of the women admitted to Bloomfield or Highfield was in this category, while more than half of female admissions to Ennis (57.9%) and Enniscorthy (63%) were linked to farming. One major difference arises between the two rural samples. At Ennis, a large proportion of farming women were listed as relatives of farmers but at Enniscorthy over one-third were identified simply as 'farmer'. This mirrors national trends. In Leinster, middle-aged or elderly widows were often reluctant to pass their family farm to a son. In the West of Ireland, 'the transmission of farms between the generations appears to have been accomplished more smoothly' and women farmers were less common.[80] Despite their engagement in most kinds of agricultural work, women were not described as farmers either in the census or by themselves unless they were the heads of households.[81] This would appear to hold true for paying patients admitted to Enniscorthy. For example, Ellen McC, who was admitted in 1898, aged fifty-three and single, lived with her 'married nephew, but house and place are hers. Has a big farm, over 100 acres.'[82] Maria C., a forty-year-old widow admitted in 1897, had overseen her twenty acres and her brother described her as a 'good business woman on farm'.

CONCLUSIONS

Elizabeth Malcolm has provided what she terms a 'superficial' profile of patients in Armagh, Belfast, Omagh and Sligo district asylums at the turn of the twentieth century. Her findings suggest that the typical Irish asylum patient was a male labourer, from a labouring or small farming family, Catholic and single.[83] Adopting this methodology, between 1868 and 1900, the 'typical' paying patient committed to the district asylums was also a male farmer. He too was Catholic, unless he was committed to Belfast, and single. This remarkably similar profile reveals that paying patients admitted to district asylums differed little from the total populations of these asylums. In contrast, the 'typical' voluntary asylum patient was a Church of Ireland (or Quaker in Bloomfield) single woman with no former occupation. Given wide variations between the types of patient committed to the private asylums, it is necessary to provide separate 'superficial profiles' for each. The 'typical' admission to St John of God's was a single Catholic man in trade, that to Hampstead was a single Church of Ireland man with an 'other occupation', usually a white-collar profession, and that to Highfield a married Church of Ireland woman with no occupation.

These profiles reveal a great deal about the socio-economic background of the individuals and families who used these asylums. Unlike district asylums, Bloomfield and Stewarts admitted more women than men. Other asylums such as St Vincent's voluntary asylum (see Chap. 2) and Highfield private asylum had a policy of admitting only women. This complicates Oonagh Walsh's assumption that non-pauper women in Ireland were more often accommodated in the home.[84] Although both MacKenzie and Walsh have argued that families were more willing to pay for male patients' asylum care because of their 'greater economic importance',[85] this study has revealed that in the Irish context, relatives and friends were willing to invest large sums of money in women's care and treatment. While this might suggest a greater determination to 'dump' unwanted female relatives, there is no concrete evidence to support this.

The occupational profile of patients in this study provides some clues as to the sort of people confined in different kinds of institutions. The underrepresentation of those in the most prominent trades of the period suggests that their families could not afford to pay for their care. White-collar professionals such as lawyers, doctors and accountants were most often found in voluntary and particularly private asylums. Men and women described as farmers were from a variety of social backgrounds, with significant inter- and intra-regional variation and could be anything from a smallholder to a relatively wealthy landowner. The religious profile of their cohort also points towards the Catholic middle classes emerging steadily in rural Ireland. However, members of the Church of Ireland were over-represented in voluntary asylums and in Hampstead and Highfield, demonstrating that the Catholic middle classes were seeking accommodation elsewhere. Voluntary and private patients' occupational profile corroborates this statement; the occupations listed tended to be dominated by Protestants in this era. While a large proportion of women in this study were described as having had no previous occupation, admissions register entries were concerned with demarcating the economic profile of these individuals and thus demonstrate a wide range of female occupations. A relatively small proportion of women in this study were assigned designated occupations. While work outside the home for women has tended to be aligned with financial necessity or even desperation, those engaged in non-domestic work in this study were usually connected to more 'respectable' forms of employment: shop girls, drapers, nurses and nuns. Sources such as these may thus add to our understanding of women and work in nineteenth-century Ireland.

NOTES

1. Report into the State of Lunatic Asylums, Part II, p. 36.
2. As has been shown, the 1875 Act attempted to address this concern in guiding boards of governors in their negotiation of appropriate maintenance fees.
3. First Report of the Inspectors General on the General State of Prisons of Ireland (342), H.C. 1823, x, 291, p. 9; 57 Geo. III, c. 106; 'Editorial Article 2,' *Irish Times*, 12 June 1860.
4. Melling and Forsythe (2006, p. 163).
5. O. Walsh (2004, pp. 73–74).
6. Malcolm (1989, p. 205).
7. Showalter (1986).
8. Busfield (1994, p. 268).
9. Showalter (1981, p. 164).
10. MacKenzie (1992, pp. 129, 135–136).
11. O. Walsh (2004, pp. 73–74).
12. Vaughan and Fitzpatrick (1978, p. 3).
13. Finnane (1981, p. 130), Cox (2012, p. 135), O. Walsh (2004, p. 73).
14. MacKenzie (1992, pp. 129, 135–136), O. Walsh (2004, pp. 73–74).
15. O. Walsh (2004, pp. 73–74).
16. Digby (1985, p. 175).
17. Cox (2012, p. 140), Malcolm (1999, p. 180). For more on marriage patterns in nineteenth-century Ireland, see Guinnane (1997, pp. 193–240), Connell (1962).
18. MacKenzie (1992, p. 169), Melling and Forsythe (2006, p. 116).
19. Digby (1985, p. 176); see Showalter (1981, p. 325).
20. Patient Accounts, 1858–1900 (Stewarts, Patient Records).

21. Cox has also found the existence of 'affective' familial bonds in her study of district asylum patients. See Cox (2012, pp. 108–109).
22. O. Walsh (2004, pp. 73–74), MacKenzie (1992, pp. 135–136).
23. Patient Accounts, 1858–1900 (Stewarts, Patient Records); Patient Accounts, 1896–1900 (Highfield Hospital Group, Hampstead and Highfield Records); Patient Accounts, 1812–1900 (FHL, Bloomfield Records).
24. Ibid.
25. Cox (2012, p. 150).
26. 'Census of Ireland 1901,' accessed 6 January 2012, http://www.census.nationalarchives.ie. Twenty-nine out of the 166 patients discharged from Ennis, Enniscorthy, Richmond, Stewarts, Bloomfield, Hampstead and Highfield between 1898 and 1900 were identified in the 1901 Census. This identification was not possible for St John of God's because restricted access to the records dictated that patients' surnames could not be included on the database. Belfast was also omitted because patients' addresses were too vague to allow for definitive linkage between asylum and census records.
27. Female Case Book, 1898–1899 (GM, Richmond District Lunatic Asylum, pp. 469–471).
28. This is contrary to the arguments put forward in Scull (1982).
29. L. Walsh (2004, p. 265).
30. Ibid.
31. Admissions and Receptions Registers, 1841–1900 (PRONI, Purdysburn Hospital, HOS/28/1/3); Admissions-Refusals, 1868–1900 (CCA, Our Lady's Hospital, OL3/1.3); Admissions Registers, 1868–1900 (WCC, St Senan's Hospital, Enniscorthy); Admissions Registers, 1870–1900 (GM, Richmond District Lunatic Asylum); Admissions Registers, 1858–1900 (Stewarts, Patient Records); Admissions Registers, 1812–1900 (FHL, Bloomfield Records); Admissions Registers, 1885–1900 (SJOGH, Patient Records); Admissions Registers, 1826–1900 (Highfield Hospital Group, Hampstead and Highfield Records).
32. MacKenzie (1992, p. 130).
33. Religious affiliation was recorded systematically in the admissions registers for the four district asylums studied. It was recorded for 100% of first admissions to Belfast and Enniscorthy, 88.1% for Ennis and 97.4% for Richmond. Religious persuasion was not recorded in the admissions registers for Bloomfield, Stewarts, St John of God's, Hampstead or Highfield. However, through nominal linkage with surviving case notes, religious persuasion has been identified for 38.8% of Stewarts', 11.1% of Bloomfield's, 16.5% of St John of Gods' and 26.9% of Hampstead and Highfield's first admissions.

34. The headings used are taken from the lunacy inspectors' annual reports in their categorisation of private asylum patients' former occupations. Preference was given to this classification system over contemporary census headings because, like this study, the lunacy inspectors were dealing exclusively with asylum populations and working with data drawn from admissions registers. The additional headings of 'clerk', 'labourer' and 'police' have been added to the lunacy inspector's model to highlight the prominence or otherwise of these occupations within certain asylum populations. 'Son of', 'pensioner' and 'social class specified' were also added to circumvent the difficulties in accurately classifying these groups.

35. This umbrella term includes merchants, grocers, shopkeepers, drapers, bakers, carpenters, butchers and commercial travellers. For more on nineteenth-century Irish industry, see Bielenberg (2009).

36. For more on industry in the North of Ireland and particularly Belfast, see Gribbon (1989, pp. 298–309).

37. Daly (1984, pp. 23–30).

38. Ibid., pp. 32, 40–41.

39. Guinnane (1997, p. 39).

40. Ibid., pp. 41–43.

41. Jones (1995, p. ix, 1).

42. Guinnane (1997, p. 41).

43. Cited in Bell and Watson (2009, p. 18).

44. See Guinnane (1997, pp. 44–47).

45. See MacDonagh (1977), Ó Gráda (1989, 1994), Comerford (1989); W.E. Vaughan (1994), Hoppen (1998). For an overview of the Irish Land Wars, see Clark (1979).

46. Clinical Record Volume No. 4 (WCC, St Senan's Hospital, Enniscorthy, pp. 373–374; 317–378, 118).

47. Clinical Record Volume No. 5 (WCC, St Senan's Hospital, Enniscorthy, p. 197).

48. Clinical Record Volume No. 4 (WCC, St Senan's Hospital, Enniscorthy, p. 239; 359); Clinical Record Volume No. 6 (WCC, St Senan's Hospital, Enniscorthy, p. 215).

49. Clinical Record Volume No. 4 (WCC, St Senan's Hospital, Enniscorthy, pp. 231, 14).

50. Clinical Record Volume No. 3 (WCC, St Senan's Hospital, Enniscorthy, p. 211).

51. Admissions Registers, 1858–1900 (Stewarts, Patient Records); Admissions Registers, 1812–1900 (FHL, Bloomfield Records); Admissions Registers, 1885–1900 (SJOGH, Patient Records); Admissions Registers, 1826–1900 (Highfield Hospital Group, Hampstead and Highfield Records).

52. Daly (1984, pp. 124–126).
53. Seventh Report on the District, Criminal, and Private Lunatic Asylums in Ireland [1981], H.C. 1854–1855, xvi, 137, p. 22.
54. Landlords usually let their land to 'intermediate landlords, commonly called middlemen, who sublet their holdings to smaller tenants and cottiers', meaning that they were not technically 'occupied' by their livelihood. See Donnelly (1989, p. 332).
55. Female Case Book, 1857–1887 (GM, Richmond District Lunatic Asylum, pp. 453, 108, 12).
56. Male Case Book, 1890–1891 (GM, Richmond District Lunatic Asylum, pp. 1–2).
57. Ibid., pp. 754–756.
58. Male Case Book, 1891–1892 (GM, Richmond District Lunatic Asylum, p. 58).
59. This medical officer's identity is unknown because he did not sign his case notes.
60. Male Case Book, 1891–1892 (GM, Richmond District Lunatic Asylum, pp. 146–147).
61. Ibid., pp. 146–147.
62. Ibid., p. 147.
63. Male Case Book, 1893–1894 (G.M, Richmond District Lunatic Asylum, pp. 433–435).
64. For example, Male Case Book, 1894–1895 (G.M, Richmond District Lunatic Asylum, pp. 53–54); Male Case Book, 1894–1895 (G.M, Richmond District Lunatic Asylum, pp. 49–50).
65. Male Case Book,1892–1893 (G.M, Richmond District Lunatic Asylum, pp. 737–739).
66. Daly (1997, pp. 2–3).
67. Ibid., p. 3.
68. Melling (2004, p. 192).
69. L. Walsh (2004, p. 265).
70. Michael (2004, p. 103).
71. Daly (1997, p. 32).
72. Ibid., p. 19. This has been attributed alternately to the economic boom experienced in rural Ireland which enabled women to 'opt out of paid employment in favour of unpaid domestic work within the family' and the collapse of domestic spinning during the post-Famine period. See Bourke (1993).
73. Daly (1997, p. 7).
74. Ibid., p. 8.
75. Daly (1984, p. 41).
76. Daly (1997, p. 32).

77. Rains (2010, pp. 152, 199–200).
78. Melling (2004, p. 192).
79. Ibid., p. 199.
80. Daly (1997, pp. 19–22). For more on farming families in the West of Ireland, see Fitzpatrick (1980).
81. *Census of Ireland*, 1861–1911, Occupational Tables.
82. Clinical Record Volume No. 6 (WCC, St Senan's Hospital, Enniscorthy, pp. 175–176).
83. Malcolm (1999, p. 182).
84. O. Walsh (2004, pp. 73–74).
85. MacKenzie (1992, pp. 129, 135–136), O. Walsh (2004, pp. 73–74).

References

Bell, Jonathan and Watson, Mervyn. *A History of Irish Farming 1750–1950*. Dublin: Four Courts Press, 2009.

Bielenberg, Andy. *Ireland and the Industrial Revolution: The Impact of the Industrial Revolution on Irish Industry, 1809–1822*. London and New York: Routledge, 2009.

Bourke, Joanna. *Husbandry to Housewifery: Women, Economic Change and Housework in Ireland, 1890–1914*. Oxford: Clarendon Press, 1993.

Busfield, Joan. 'The Female Malady? Men, Women and Madness in Nineteenth-Century Britain.' In *Sociology* 27, no. 1 (1994): 259–277.

Clark, Samuel. *Social Origins of the Irish Land War*. Princeton: Princeton University Press, 1979.

Comerford, R.V. 'Ireland 1850–70: Post-Famine and Mid-Victorian.' In *A New History of Ireland V: Ireland Under the Union, I, 1801–70*, edited by W.E. Vaughan, 371–385. Oxford: Oxford University Press, 1989.

Connell, K.H. 'Peasant Marriage in Ireland: Its Structure and Development since the Famine.' *Economic History Review* 14, no. 3 (1962): 502–523.

Cox, Catherine. *Negotiating Insanity in the Southeast of Ireland 1830–1900*. Manchester: Manchester University Press, 2012.

Daly, Mary E. *Dublin, The Deposed Capital: A Social and Economic History, 1860–1914*. Cork: Cork University Press, 1984.

Daly, Mary E. *Women and Work in Ireland*. Dundalk: Dundalgan Press, 1997.

Digby, Anne. *Madness, Morality and Medicine: A Study of the York Retreat, 1796–1914*. Cambridge: Cambridge University Press, 1985.

Donnelly, James S. 'Landlords and Tenants.' In *A New History of Ireland V: Ireland Under the Union, I, 1801–1870*, edited by W.E. Vaughan, 332–349. Oxford: Oxford University Press, 1989.

Finnane, Mark. *Insanity and the Insane in Post-Famine Ireland*. London: Croom Helm, 1981.

Fitzpatrick, David. 'Irish Farming Families before the First World War.' *Comparative Studies in History and Society* 25 (1980): pp. 339–384.

Gribbon, H.D. 'Economic and Social History, 1850–1921.' In *A New History of Ireland VI: Ireland Under Union, 1870–1921*, edited by W.E. Vaughan, 260–356. Oxford: Oxford University Press, 1989.

Guinnane, Timothy. *The Vanishing Irish: Households, Migration, and the Rural Economy in Ireland, 1850–1914.* Princeton: Princeton University Press, 1997.

Hoppen, K. Theodore. *The Mid-Victorian Generation, 1846–1886.* Oxford: Oxford University Press, 1998.

Jones, David Seth. *Graziers, Land Reform, and Political Conflict in Ireland.* Washington, DC: Catholic University of America Press, 1995.

MacDonagh, Oliver. *Ireland: The Union and Its Aftermath.* London: Allen and Unwin, 1977.

MacKenzie, Charlotte. *Psychiatry for the Rich: A History of the Private Madhouse at Ticehurst in Sussex, 1792–1917.* London: Routledge, 1992.

Malcolm, Elizabeth. *Swift's Hospital: A History of St. Patrick's Hospital, Dublin, 1746–1989.* Dublin: Gill and Macmillan, 1989.

Malcolm, Elizabeth. 'The House of Strident Shadows: The Asylum, the Family and Emigration in Post-Famine Rural Ireland.' In *Medicine, Disease and the State in Ireland 1650–1940*, edited by Elizabeth Malcolm and Greta Jones, 177–195. Cork: Cork University Press, 1999.

Melling, Joseph. 'Sex and Sensibility in Cultural History: The English Governess and the Lunatic Asylum, 1845–1914.' In *Sex and Seclusion, Class and Custody: Perspectives on Gender and Class in the History of British Psychiatry*, edited by Jonathan Andrews and Anne Digby, 177–221. Amsterdam and New York: Rodopi, 2004.

Melling, Joseph and Bill Forsythe. *The Politics of Madness: The State, Insanity and Society in England, 1845–1914.* London and New York: Routledge, 2006.

Michael, Pamela. 'Class, Gender and Insanity in Nineteenth-Century Wales.' In *Sex and Seclusion, Class and Custody: Perspective in Gender and Class in the History of British and Irish Psychiatry* edited by Jonathan Andrews and Anne Digby, 95–122. Amsterdam and New York: Rodopi, 2004.

Ó Gráda, Cormac. 'Poverty, Population, and Agriculture, 1801–1845.' In *A New History of Ireland V: Ireland Under the Union, I, 1801–1870*, edited by W.E. Vaughan, 108–136. Oxford: Oxford University Press, 1989.

Ó Gráda, Cormac. *Ireland: A New Economic History, 1780–1939.* Oxford: Oxford University Press, 1994.

Rains, Stephanie. *Commodity, Culture and Social Class in Dublin 1850–1916.* Dublin and Portland: Irish Academic Press, 2010.

Scull, Andrew. *Museums of Madness: The Social Organisation of Insanity in Nineteenth-Century England.* Harmondsworth: Penguin, 1982.

Showalter, Elaine. 'Victorian Women and Insanity.' In *Madhouses, Mad-Doctors and Madmen: The Social History of Psychiatry in the Victorian Era*, edited by Andrew Scull, 157–181. Philadelphia: University of Pennsylvania Press, 1981.

Showalter, Elaine. *The Female Malady: Women Madness and Culture in England, 1830–1980*. New York, Pantheon Book, 1986.

Vaughan, W.E. *Landlords and Tenants in Mid-Victorian Ireland*. New York: Oxford University Press, 1994.

Vaughan, W.E. and A.J. Fitzpatrick (eds.). *Irish Historical Statistics, Population, 1821–1971*. Dublin: Royal Irish Academy, 1978.

Walsh, Lorraine. 'A Class Apart? Admissions to the Dundee Royal Lunatic Asylum, 1890–1910.' In *Sex and Seclusion, Class and Custody: Perspectives on Gender and Class in the History of British and Irish Psychiatry*, edited by Jonathan Andrews and Anne Digby, 249–269. Amsterdam and New York: Rodopi, 2004.

Walsh, Oonagh. 'Gender and Insanity in Nineteenth-Century Ireland.' In *Sex and Seclusion, Class and Custody: Perspectives on Gender and Class in the History of British Psychiatry*, edited by Jonathan Andrews and Anne Digby, 69–93. Amsterdam and New York: Rodopi, 2004.

CHAPTER 5

'The Evil Effects of Mental Strain and Overwork': Employment, Gender and Insanity

In 1875, an article penned by eminent Irish asylum doctor, Dr. Frederick Maccabe, appeared in the *Journal of Mental Science*.[1] In this piece, Maccabe considered the rising levels of mental strain young men were suffering due to overwork. He claimed that in this period, more than any other, young men were compelled to study more rigorously for examinations, following which they met with greater competition and pressures in their chosen professions. Among those most at risk he counted the commercial, official, professional and literary classes. Maccabe was writing in a period of relative prosperity in Ireland. Had he conceived of his article just a few years later, he might have emphasised the mental strain produced by an economic depression that began in 1879 and endured until the mid-1890s. By then, esteemed medical commentators including Daniel Hack Tuke and Thomas Drapes both linked the extreme poverty of the Irish population to high levels of mental illness.[2] As this chapter argues, while fear of poverty afflicted the rural poor during this era, anxieties about employment and the state of the economy were seen to affect other social groups.

Drapes and Tuke were not alone in relating economic factors to insanity. Labouring men committed to the Hanwell asylum in Middlesex between 1845 and 1850 were considered anxious about their economic future, suffering intense fears of poverty.[3] These patients' fears were not emphasised in social commentary or psychiatric literature but rather by their families who named them as major causes for their insanity.[4] Following the Great Famine, Irish psychiatric thought had clearly begun

© The Author(s) 2018
A. Mauger, *The Cost of Insanity in Nineteenth-Century Ireland*, Mental Health in Historical Perspective, https://doi.org/10.1007/978-3-319-65244-3_5

149

to embrace these lay associations. In the south-east of Ireland, certifying medical officers for district asylum patients often cited fear of poverty, anxiety caused by unemployment and changed circumstances as causes of mental illness, based on evidence that family members had supplied to them. Fears such as these were thought to have a detrimental impact on patients' minds.[5]

Yet, historians of psychiatry have been curiously reluctant to emphasise medically recognised links between employment and illness in fee-paying asylum patients. In her comparison of the causes doctors assigned to York Retreat patients between 1796 and 1823 and 1874 and 1892, Digby found a tenfold rise in 'overwork' or 'over study' and a concurrent rise in 'business and money anxiety'. Despite these stark indicators of a growing reliance on work-related aetiologies, Digby has cautioned against the temptation to interpret this rise as reflecting the shift from the romantic age to the 'competitive problems associated with living in a mature capitalist economy afflicted with economic depression'. Instead, she infers that her 'fragile data' indicate 'a greater readiness to specify immediately observable features' in everyday life.[6] In contrast, this chapter argues that asylum doctors' recognition of certain life events and circumstances as causal factors of mental illness reveals much about contemporary psychiatric associations between employment, economic shifts and mental illness. Digby's findings might therefore be reinterpreted to reflect an increasing movement towards more 'psychological' understandings of mental illness.

In a similar vein, MacKenzie, in her study of Ticehurst private asylum, has argued that, between 1845 and 1915, asylum doctors assigned the causes of anxiety and overwork as 'sympathetic alternatives' to alcohol, based on her observation that some patients attributed these causes were heavy drinkers. According to MacKenzie, the reasoning behind this rested in the Ticehurst proprietors' sensitivity to families' perceptions of what had caused the mental disorder, which they largely echoed.[7] The frequent identification of alcohol as a cause of mental illness in Ireland reveals that asylum doctors there did not mirror this approach. Moreover, neither Digby nor MacKenzie have apparently made room for the possibility that families, and even patients, cited work-related or financial anxieties because they believed they had directly precipitated illness. In fact, patients and their families often reported that the pressures of employment and other economic factors were to blame. Professional opinion could outweigh these lay considerations, however, and this study has yielded no evidence that relatives dictated to the doctors who assigned causes and diagnoses.

Importantly, both medical and lay commentators tended to link employment and mental illness primarily for male patients, with medical officers characterising male anxieties as a failure to fulfil gendered economic roles.[8] However, working-class women were not immune to being assigned financial or work-related strain. In early Victorian England, employment was central to the identities of poor women and lack of work was sometimes attributed to their mental illness, by medical practitioners and patients alike.[9] In Ireland, women's anxieties about poverty were also aligned with 'maintaining appropriate standards of female respectability'.[10] As Chap. 4 discussed, a high proportion of the women in this study did not work outside the home—a trend which increased in proportion to social status or wealth. Yet, women who remained at home played an important role in contributing to the family economy.[11] Moreover, a smaller section of women in this study did engage in paid work, while others were property owners. In spite of this, medical aetiologies of wealthier women's illnesses did not tend to hinge on their economic functions in any obvious way. Instead, they focused on domestic circumstances. While the illness of wealthier women in British asylums was also unlikely to be attributed to work-related or financial concerns, several scholars have emphasised the links drawn between women's reproductive functions and mental breakdown in contemporary psychiatric literature.[12] As Suzuki has argued, 'Victorian middle-class women had hysteria as the disease that symbolised their place in the separate spheres'.[13] As will be shown, in Ireland, female non-pauper insanity was attributed to a myriad of factors, the majority of which did not hinge on their biological functions.

This chapter explores the causes assigned to paying patients in the selected asylums. 'Cause of insanity' was recorded in the admissions registers for all the asylums studied except Hampstead and Highfield. Analysis of these returns is supplemented by a survey of asylum doctors' casebooks, which cast further light on psychiatric definitions. Lay interpretations are also present in the case notes, where medical personnel recorded information supplied by families, friends and patients.[14] In addition, letters written by patients' friends and relatives provide indications of lay understandings.

MEDICAL AETIOLOGIES

It is often challenging to separate lay and medical definitions of mental illness. As we have seen, paying patients committed to asylums required two medical certificates. These forms allowed certifying doctors to record causes of illness and were later transcribed into admissions registers and casebooks, where asylum doctors could choose to confirm or alter the causes assigned.[15] Medical rather than lay authorities therefore usually had the final say over what was recorded.

Late nineteenth-century asylum doctors distinguished between moral and physical causes of insanity. Moral causes encompassed a range of 'psychological' factors such as grief, bereavement, business or money anxieties, religion and 'domestic trouble', and reveal much about perceptions of the life events or circumstances leading to mental illness. Physical causes, including accidents and injuries, physical illnesses, 'hereditary' and 'alcohol' are less instructive. Physical causes were accorded a pivotal space in the psychiatric discourse of this era, emulating widely held medical theories about the physical nature of mental illness. Asylum doctors in Ireland frequently cited alcohol and 'hereditary' as pathologies closely associated with theories of degeneration.[16] This bias towards commonly accepted causes obscures, to some extent, psychiatry's recognition of the 'psychological' causes of mental illness. It is therefore important to explore both explanations to gain a full understanding of the various frameworks embraced.[17]

As shown in Table 5.1, physical causes were more frequently reported for patients in this study. Among them 'hereditary' and 'alcohol' were

Table 5.1 Supposed cause of illness of first admissions to the case studies, 1868–1900

	Female						Male					
Asylum	Both	(%)	Moral	(%)	Physical	(%)	Both	(%)	Moral	(%)	Physical	(%)
District asylums	8	4.0	48	24.2	142	71.7	7	2.4	48	16.8	231	80.8
Bloomfield	0	0.0	4	30.8	9	69.2	0	0.0	4	50.0	4	50.0
Stewarts	5	3.9	11	8.6	112	87.5	0	0.0	9	9.6	85	90.4
St John of God's	N/A	N/A	N/A	N/A	N/A	N/A	5	1.9	72	26.7	193	71.5
Total	13	3.8	63	18.9	263	77.3	12	1.8	133	20.2	513	78.0

Compiled from Belfast, Ennis, Enniscorthy, Richmond, Stewarts, Bloomfield and St John of God's admissions registers the most often named (Table 5.2). For those assigned physical causes, 'alcohol' accounted for 43% of men and 11.2% of women admitted. This high rate of alcohol-related admissions differs from Britain. While alcohol was recognised as a factor in the admission of private patients to Dundee Royal Hospital in Scotland, it was usually associated with the working classes.[18] Alcohol abuse was also less often identified as a symptom in English private asylum patients.[19] In contrast, of the paying patients assigned physical causes in this study, those committed to private asylums were actually more likely (54.8%) than those sent to voluntary (17.7%) or district (19%) asylums to be assigned alcohol. This suggests that alcohol had especially 'Irish' associations. Certainly, during the nine-teenth century, the Irish reputation for drunkenness was publicised by English caricaturists to the extent that, according to Malcolm, 'in the English eyes, the Irish became violent, cruel and drunken'.[20] While Irish spirit consumption rose in the late 1860s and early 1870s, from 1850 temperance activities resulted in more censorious attitudes towards drunkenness, restricted opportunities for heavy drinking, and more facili-ties for sober recreation and entertainment.[21]

The influx of alcohol-related admissions to Irish asylums provoked comment from medical superintendents who observed and contem-plated the nature of their patients' inebriety. In England, the decline in alcohol consumption between the 1820s and 1870s has been attributed to several factors including the medical community's increased hostility towards drink and their reluctance to prescribe it as a medicine.[22] It is

Table 5.2 Physical and moral causes by gender most commonly assigned to first admissions to the case studies, 1868–1900[a]

	Male	Male (%)	Female	Female (%)
(%) Physical				
Alcohol	226	43.0	31	11.2
Hereditary	148	28.2	145	52.5
Biological	0	0	35	12.7
(%) Moral				
Work/Finance	64	44.1	5	6.6
Domestic	11	7.6	17	22.4
Religion	8	5.5	6	7.9
Bereavement/Grief	7	4.8	13	17.1

Compiled from Belfast, Ennis, Enniscorthy, Richmond, Stewarts, Bloomfield and St John of God's admissions registers ([a]In cases where patients were assigned multiple causes, both are included in this analysis in order to illustrate their statistical significance)

plausible that the Irish psychiatric profession shared their English colleagues' hostility.[23] Certainly, in 1904 Drapes expressed his frustration at the repeated readmission of habitual drunkards to Enniscorthy district asylum, going so far as to blame excessive drunkenness in Wexford for an increase in insanity there.[24] While Drapes was probably commenting on his pauper patients, he evidently did not regard paying patients as being above reproach. This is seen in the case studies. Contrary to Drapes' statement concerning repeat admissions, only thirty-eight patients readmitted to the asylums studied were assigned the cause of alcohol. As Finnane has contended, 'since the insanity of a drunkard was questionable, his or her state when not drunk rarely justified long detention'.[25] For those assigned 'alcohol' whose length of stay is known, almost three-quarters remained in the asylum for less than one year. Notably, among those assigned physical causes, alcohol was most commonly attributed to Enniscorthy paying patients (24.5%) compared with those in Ennis (12.1%) and Belfast (6.8%). This implies that Drapes was particularly inclined towards this framework, which is unsurprising given his keen interest in temperance activities.[26] Nevertheless, there is little doubt that accommodating the 'drunken' was very much a role for all types of Irish asylums by the late nineteenth century.

Cox and Finnane have identified alcohol's prominence in the aetiologies of district asylum patients in Ireland. For example, between 1832 and 1922 drink accounted for the illness of 12.7% of patients admitted to the Carlow asylum.[27] Both historians have highlighted the absence of inebriate reformatories or retreats in the nineteenth century, suggesting that, in their stead, district asylums became the principal receptacle for this group.[28] This argument would go some way towards explaining the high proportion of drink-related admissions among paying patients in district asylums. It does not, however, account for the even greater percentage admitted to voluntary and private asylums. One explanation lies in class-specific, medical conceptions of 'drunkenness'. In 1875, the lunacy inspectors, discussing the feasibility of establishing 'receptacles for dipsomaniacs', argued that drunkenness among the 'lower orders without social position or means' was treated as an offence or misdemeanour, while among the 'better and richer classes' it tended to be perceived as an 'incipient malady'.[29] For the rich, then, a tendency to overindulge in drink may have been treated more as an illness than an offence.

As historians of British psychiatry have observed, certifying physicians were more reluctant to assign 'hereditary' as a cause of illness to 'upper-class and aristocratic patients'.[30] This hesitancy is also visible in this study. 'Hereditary' accounted for only 7.2% of assigned physical causes for St John of God's patients and 0.3% for Bloomfield patients, compared with 53.9% for paying patients sent to district asylums and 38.6% to Stewarts. This hints at the influence of patients' social status. Degeneracy was largely characterised as a working-class problem, bound up in the belief that the labour value of future workers would be jeopardised by the reproduction and amplification of the degenerative effects of the urban, industrial life over the generations.[31] By the late nineteenth century, commentators were emphasising the impending social uselessness of the poor and destitute.[32] An institution's religious ethos also had implications for the cause of illness attributed. The exceptionally low proportion of Bloomfield patients assigned 'hereditary' is in keeping with Digby's contention that the managers of the York Retreat were particularly sensitive to this label because of high rates of inter-marriage between members of the Society of Friends.[33] Patients' gender, too, was a determinant. 'Hereditary' was cited in 52.5% of women assigned a physical cause compared with only 28.2% of men.

Naturally, causes related to the reproductive cycle, here termed 'biological', were assigned exclusively to women in this study. These causes included 'menstrual', 'child birth', 'puerperal' and 'menopause'. In the British context, Digby has argued that both lay and medical interpretations of Victorian middle-class women's mental illness centred on biological models.[34] However, Levine-Clark has suggested that biological symptoms and diagnoses were more often applied to middle-class women, while working-class and pauper women were assigned alternative causative factors.[35] Yet, in this study, biological causes were not necessarily assigned to women considered higher in social ranking. For instance, while 11.4% of physical symptoms assigned to women admitted to Stewarts were biological, one-fifth of female paying patients in the Belfast district asylum were similarly described. Furthermore, none of the physical causes attributed to Bloomfield's middle- and upper-class female patients concerned their reproductive system, suggesting that some certifying physicians accepted biological aetiologies more than others did.

The high proportion of paying patients assigned physical causes reveals that Irish asylum doctors framed much of the illness they observed in these terms. However, subtle differences between aetiological trends for Irish and British non-pauper patients suggest that these causes were not routinely class- or gender-specific. Although the Irish psychiatric profession had strong professional ties with its British counterpart, including several Irish members of the Medico-Psychological Association[36] and Irish participation in the *Journal of Mental Science*, Irish asylum doctors did deviate from the frameworks of their British colleagues. While, as Cox has demonstrated, Irish asylum doctors' explanations for the alleged increase of insanity in Ireland were mostly in line with the British and European intellectual climate, they clearly also drew upon their own personal and cultural understandings of their patient populations.[37] These cultural influences are evident in a heavier reliance on alcohol-related aetiologies in the Irish context. They are also particularly visible in the moral causes assigned, revealing that asylum doctors recognised not only the commonly held physical explanations of insanity, but also the complex socio-economic and personal circumstances which could affect mental health.

Table 5.2 details the most common moral causes assigned to patients in this study. For men, 44.1% of moral causes were work/finance-related. This category covered wide-ranging factors including overwork and over-study, business worry, anxiety, disappointment and trouble, business and money losses and want of employment, and were more often assigned in urban case studies. While, to some extent, the high proportion of work/finance-related causes might reflect a bias in the case studies in that the majority were Dublin-based asylums, as Chap. 4 discussed, half of the patients admitted to the voluntary and private asylums were not from Dublin. Nonetheless, among male patients in this study, all of the assigned moral causes at Bloomfield were work/finance-related ones, compared with only 12.5% in Enniscorthy and 30% in Ennis. Belfast was also particularly high at 64.3%, followed by Stewarts at 55.6%, revealing that business and finance-related aetiologies were seen to affect a wide socio-economic spectrum, particularly for those in urban contexts.

Women were far more frequently assigned 'domestic' causes, rather than work/finance related ones. These included domestic trouble, domestic trials, family affairs, family trouble and private trouble and situated woman snugly within the confines of the domestic sphere. Related causes were grief or bereavement of a family member which had reportedly affected women (17.1% of moral causes) more than men (4.8% of moral causes). The higher proportion of women assigned 'domestic' aetiologies (22.4% of moral causes) compared with men (7.6% of moral causes) reveals that these causes were gendered. Notably, almost one-third of these women were either farmers or had a designated occupation recorded. As will be shown, even when women exhibited anxieties about their businesses or financial concerns, these were rarely attributed as causes of their illness.

To what extent, then, did patients' socio-economic background shape the identification of their illness? Robert A. Houston has argued that social position was an important determinant and this argument holds equally true for Ireland.[38] Patients' former occupation also influenced the causes attributed to their mental illness, particularly for male patients. Of those assigned moral causes, students were most often assigned 'over study' (80%), while more than three-fifths of those in trade, law or medicine were assigned work/finance-related causes. Among physical causes, alcohol was most commonly assigned to policemen (59.1%), clergymen (56.7%) and those in trade (55.4%). Alcohol was also believed to have caused the illness of six out of the seven publicans in this study, in keeping with Finnane's contention that a publican's occupation was perceived as a constant source of temptation.[39]

While we have seen that a myriad of medical and socio-cultural factors, including attitudes towards alcohol consumption, degeneration, gender and social class, influenced asylum doctors attributing causes, the opinions of patients and their relatives are obscured. The following sections explore medical case notes and the correspondence of patients' relatives and friends to gain a more nuanced appreciation of the lay and medical explanations of mental illness. These sections also examine the interactions between patients and their relatives and friends in accounting for the onset of their illness.

URBAN ECONOMIES

During the 1840s, the proprietor of Hampstead House, Dr. John Eustace II, kept a casebook on patients admitted to his private asylum. Although his notetaking coincided with the Great Famine, Eustace did not refer to this cataclysmic event nor to any financial hardship afflicting the patients he described.[40] The most plausible reason for this omission is that Hampstead patients tended to be comfortable or wealthy Dubliners, for whom the consequences of the Famine were less devastating than for other social groups. Eustace's case notes do, however, set the stage for several other themes which emerge strongly in later casebooks for Enniscorthy, Richmond, Stewarts, Bloomfield, St John of

God's, Hampstead and Highfield. These themes include overwork for men and domestic trouble for women.

Eustace's notes on his male patients are comparable, in some respects, to those compiled by asylum doctors writing in the 1890s. For instance, he wrote of one patient, a John H., that he had 'held a situation in a Brewery where his business required him to remain up all night' resulting in insanity.[41] By the 1890s, medical and lay associations between work and mental illness were more pronounced. Suzuki has found that clerks sent to Hanwell in the mid-nineteenth century suffered from fears of losing their positions.[42] In this study, between 1868 and 1900 the illness of eight out of the nineteen clerks assigned moral causes was ascribed in the admissions registers to similar anxieties. However, case notes compiled about clerks in the 1890s indicate that several more than this number cited work-related and financial anxieties. In addition to fearing loss of their position, some clerks also reportedly suffered from overwork, a cause that Suzuki has argued was usually monopolised by middle-class men and women in mid-nineteenth-century psychiatric discourses.[43]

Reporting physicians at Richmond were particularly inclined to associate clerks' working life with their illness during the 1890s. Admitted in 1900, James L., a bookkeeper and clerk, was diagnosed with acute melancholia and the assigned cause was unknown. The case notes, however, attributed his illness to 'hard work and study. Little games or amusement of any kind'. James also cited overwork as a cause, believing that 'he let himself get run down and work too hard' and blamed himself: 'thinks that if he had taken a holiday and rest he might have recovered without coming to the Asylum'. The pressures to excel in his profession had clearly taken their toll: 'I had regrets that I had not got on as well as I might have done—as I had intended to get on'. As a result, James feared the loss of his rank and respectability, stating that 'he had an idea that he was going to turn into a low class character and lose his situation—also feared that he might take to drink (though never drank in his life)'.[44] Although not a clerk, Thomas B., a melancholic army sergeant, also supposedly fell ill due to clerical responsibilities:

a large amount of work, of an exceptionally worrying and responsible nature, including manipulation of stock to the value of £7000. For two months past this played on his mind, he made errors of calculation; unduly forgot things which he had just done, was very much worried by this, feeling that his mind was breaking down, contemplated suicide very frequently.[45]

Financial worries continued to trouble Thomas, who later told the medical officer that 'the prospect of his return to his family with only his pension for support, and his inability to increase the monies by any effort of his causes great depression'.[46]

These cases mirror the arguments put forward by MacCabe in his 1875 article:

In the competition of the present day the struggle of life is in itself a sufficient strain; and when we remember that, notwithstanding hard work, such a degree of success as would insure freedom from pecuniary care rarely comes to the young professional man, it is highly probable that the *res angusta domi* of the present, combined with the feeling of uncertainty as to the future, favours other conditions constituting a minor form of mental strain.[47]

MacCabe did not just cite competition as a cause of mental strain, but the nature of work itself:

Sometimes, even with moderate success, if the work imposed is very constant, men of scrupulous temperament suffer from a feeling of morbid anxiety as to the proper discharge of their duties; they take their work too much to heart, and a distressing feeling of being unequal to their responsibilities is very liable to supervene, and to pass into a form of strain that is particularly difficult to deal with, and that occasionally deepens into a state of mind but little removed from melancholia.[48]

Both James L. and Thomas B. were apparently plagued with anxieties about their ability to discharge their duties properly. While the case notes suggest that asylum physicians often defined patients' identity in relation to their former occupation, they also imply that relatives and patients placed immense importance on the capacity to work.

Other work-related factors were also said to take their toll. Suzuki has found that patients and relatives expressed resentment or anger towards their employers. He ties this to a working-class 'resentment of aristocratic frivolity' as labouring men were seen to be overworked with little regard for their physical or mental health.[49] Richmond paying patients also became embittered with their former employers, although these instances resulted from job loss rather than perceived exploitation, most likely reflecting better working conditions for the social cohorts examined in this study. Joseph Patrick O'B., admitted to Richmond in 1891, had worked as an Inland Revenue clerk in London and then Donegal. Following four consecutive periods of three months' leave, he was dismissed permanently, an episode which:

> affected him a good deal: At home he is always 'abstracted', will do nothing and has turned against every member of his own family: full of delusions of conspiracy against him on the part of the Inland Revenue Board, his family and 'others' whose identity appears to be indefinite.

Joseph Patrick's disillusionment with the Inland Revenue was so marked that he apparently refused to accept the pension he was offered 'as he said he had a right to stay on in the office'. Whether this pension was applied to his maintenance is impossible to ascertain, although his fees were £20, suggesting that either Joseph Patrick or his relatives had some source of disposable income.[50] Edward S., who had previously worked as a commercial traveller, was also committed to Richmond in 1891. Edward had allegedly been 'an industrious, anxious man generally sober but now and again indulging in "spirits"'. In consequence, Edward's employer had been obliged to dismiss him on more than one occasion but repeatedly reinstated him in periods of recovery due to his 'business capacity'. Ultimately, Edward was dismissed and:

> this affected his spirits, and the depression this set off was markedly increased when he failed to get any employment. He then developed such active symptoms that he was confined in Dr Patton's private asylum [Farnham House].

Edward's eventual transfer to Richmond from a more expensive private asylum implies a descent down the social scale. While in Richmond, Edward was maintained at £27 per annum, though he died in the asylum six months after admission.[51]

The Richmond case notes also record the anxieties of those who had failed to excel in a professional capacity. Edward K., the son of an architect, was committed in 1892. Prior to admission, he had secured employment as solicitor's clerk. However:

his constant mistakes... led to his discharge after about 2 years, and he was then without employment for a considerable time. When he again took work, this time in another solicitor's office – he failed to give satisfaction, and left his occupation after a row with his employer. Since this time, about 12 months ago – he has been without work, nor has he sought any.[52]

A more bizarre manifestation of professional failure was David Charles S., who was admitted to Richmond in 1898. As a student, David Charles had been removed from his university due to his 'dislike of the hats of the professors. Whenever he found one lying about he would hide it'. Following this, David was appointed as clerk in the Railway Office. However, after about two years he was discharged for 'irregularity in his work'. This apparently constituted doing 'anything other clerks told him to do such as standing on his head or going on foolishly'.[53]

White-collar professionals in voluntary asylums were also identified as having fallen ill due to their working conditions. In 1891, Joseph McC, a railway clerk, was noted on admission to Bloomfield to have had 'long hours and irregular meals'. After just four months, Joseph was discharged 'cured' and clearly deemed capable of resuming his occupation: 'left and is to return to business. Is quite well'.[54] An inability to work was an important determinant for a patient's admission. As Houston has found, the alleged incapable were judged according to their ability to carry out the tasks required of their occupation or their station in life.[55] The same can be said for patients in this study, for whom such incapacity was perceived as evidence of mental illness. For example, Stewarts patient and former office clerk, Thomas McD B., was admitted in 1889 after he 'became listless and would not occupy himself and was dismissed'.[56] In 1896, another clerk, George J., was admitted to Stewarts after he 'became "odd" in manner, fearful of having made mistakes in his books'.[57]

In addition to those recorded as being unable to work properly, during the last decade of the nineteenth century, several Stewarts patients were admitted expressing business anxieties. Richard M., a tailor, had reportedly been 'brooding over business affairs, cannot settle his mind to any employment although heretofore was a very busy man doing a large trade'.[58] Grocer, Charles Alfred M's mental illness was 'said to be induced by adversity in business'.[59] Finally, Eli S., a single, Jewish, dental mechanic was admitted to Stewarts suffering from mania. The 'supposed cause' in the admissions register was business disappointment and, in the case notes, business worry. Eli had reportedly been 'bad for about 10 weeks' having 'taken into business with another man in Limerick as dentist and as the partnership turned out a failure he lost all the money he had'.[60]

In their discussion of work and recreation in the Norfolk Lunatic Asylum, Steven Cherry and Roger Munting have emphasised the importance placed on rehabilitation and self-reliance in the outside world.[61] In the Irish context, Cox has found that capacity or willingness to work could predicate a patient's discharge from the asylum.[62] In this study, ability to return to work was generally seen as a sign of recovery. The progress of Joshua L.W., a twenty-two-year-old clerk admitted to Bloomfield in 1895 was clearly measured against his ability to resume employment: 'says he is not well enough to think of leaving or doing any business. Mopes about most of the day'.[63] Similarly, Frederick James H. was first admitted to Stewarts in June 1899, at which point his occupation was recorded as being a mercantile clerk and the cause of his disorder as 'alcohol'. While at Stewarts, Frederick James was eager to return to work. One evening he informed the medical superintendent, Frederick E Rainsford, 'he was off as he had to do stock taking' and the following day urged the doctor to consider that 'Findlater & Co. could not get on without him'. The following month he was allowed home on thirty days' leave of absence, after which he was discharged recovered in October 1899.[64] However, in February 1900, Stewarts readmitted Frederick James, now recorded as a bookkeeper. Rainsford wrote that 'since his discharge has kept well and able to attend to business. Says that he was at work up to Monday Feb 19th but he was latterly making mistakes in his books & could not put them right so that on that date his master sent him home'. Frederick James' inability to perform his job seemingly upset him and his difficulties continued at home. The case notes continued:

> He is now apparently in a state of active melancholia. Laments his fate. Trembles and weeps. Says he will never be well again and that he is greatly to be pitied. Says his wife treated him badly and that he has not seen her for months.[65]

Frederick was again discharged cured after just two months in Stewarts.[66]

There is no record that either private asylum patients or their relatives cited economic failure as a cause of illness. Nevertheless, employment was seen as an important part of their identity and many allegedly evinced an eagerness to resume employment. For instance, Thomas M., a priest admitted to St John of God's in 1899, reportedly 'never ceases to be highly indignant at his enforced detention here, claiming he is still perfectly well able to earn his living if only granted his liberty'.[67] The reporting physician, P.O'Connell, placed emphasis on patients' desire or ability to resume employment. In 1885, he wrote of one patient: 'he is now 20 years away from business and evinces no anxiety to return to business. Does this indicate weak-mindedness?'[68] Securing employment after discharge, meanwhile, was viewed as a justification for discharge.[69] In 1900, O'Connell wrote of another patient: 'he is well recovered. A situation has been secured for him'.[70]

Hampstead patients were less inclined to cite work or financial pressures as a cause of illness, or to be attributed these causes. This complicates Houston's findings concerning wealthy madmen in eighteenth-century Scotland, whose mental health was judged according to their capacity to conduct their affairs.[71] One exception to this was George C., a married grocer admitted to Hampstead in 1892, who repeatedly spoke to John Neilson Eustace about his business anxieties:

He began to refuse food, said he was 'the ruin of his family' 'had ruined the business', was 'bankrupt'. He threatened suicide but said he had 'not sufficient courage' 'shd have performed the act long ago' 'was not half a man' & c. 'His people would all soon' be dead & c ... Refers chiefly to financial affairs 'that he is bankrupt', 'has destroyed or will destroy thousands of people', he 'has been an awful fool & sh. have killed himself long ago & c'.[72]

George's characterisation of his business failures highlights his anxieties about his status as a breadwinner and, in turn, his masculinity. Suzuki has identified similar anxieties among mid-nineteenth-century London labourers, where male heads of households crumbled under the pressure to provide a stable income for their families. Cox has corroborated Suzuki's findings that 'medical officers attributed male anxiety at failing to fulfil gendered economic roles as causes of insanity' such as being able to provide for their families. However, while Suzuki has argued that new working-class notions of manhood were a factor behind 'anxiety-driven cases of madness' and both Cox and Suzuki have focused primarily on pauper asylum populations,[73] it is clear that conditions of employment could also trouble wealthier business owners. In his case notes, Eustace recorded the cause of George's illness as 'business and domestic trouble', suggesting that he too believed these factors were responsible for George's breakdown. Although in this study there is little record of wealthier businessmen overtly citing failure to provide for their families as a source of anxiety, these sentiments may have been generally understood or accepted. Certainly, while anxieties concerning the pressure to remain economically productive were evident among the poor, MacCabe highlighted these anxieties among the wealthier classes in language couched in social Darwinism:

> It is true that in this contest for civil employment and professional pre-eminence the 'survival of the fittest' may possibly result; but the struggle itself is, I believe, attended with such serious risk to the mental integrity of the competitors that it occurs to me as not inopportune for this [Medico-Psychological] Association to raise a warning voice against the evil effects of mental strain and overwork.[74]

At least for male urban populations, evidence exists that there was a very real danger of mental breakdown resulting in committal when an individual could no longer function in an occupational capacity. The comparatively predominant discussions of work and finance in the Richmond and Stewarts case notes suggests that these anxieties were greater, or at least perceived by asylum physicians as being so, for those lower down the social scale. Patients maintained at lower rates of maintenance were more likely to have experienced financial difficulties. It is also plausible that Stewarts' 'middle-class' patient population and white-collar workers in district asylums, anxious to assert their respectability, drew their identity at least in part from their occupations and financial prowess. Reporting physicians from similar social backgrounds to these patients probably shared these sentiments. As Suzuki has pointed out, middle-class doctors sympathised with their social peers in their characterisation of them as 'too sincere followers of a rigorous work ethic'.[75] MacCabe's emphasis on the wealthy suggests the existence of comparable sympathies in the Irish context.

Rural Economies

Fears about livelihood and economic productivity were by no means exclusive to urban communities. In rural populations, tensions existed between familial loyalty, marriage and business interests. Many Irish paying patients came from apparently loving familial and spousal relationships. However, these relationships often eroded when land and property interests were at stake. This conforms to commonly held representations of rural Ireland.[76] Although historians have emphasised the detrimental impact of issues such as the consolidation of landholdings, emigration, land hunger and Famine memories on emotional familial bonds, which produced families that were 'devoid of emotional gratification', Cox has identified a 'range of familial emotional contexts' among those committed to Enniscorthy and Carlow asylums. This broadly corresponds with Guinnane's contention that rural Irish families shared a strong sense of familial obligation, which extended to encompass celibate farmers.[77] Likewise, Oonagh Walsh has demonstrated that at Ballinasloe, families sent letters, querying treatment, offering advice and enclosing food and money for patients.[78] In the English context, Melling and Forsythe have noted that the families of pauper patients in Devon frequently visited and demonstrated intense anxiety about their treatment, while MacKenzie has provided a comparable characterisation of the relatives of upper-class and aristocratic patients admitted to Ticehurst.[79]

The complexity of rural familial relations is particularly visible among the property and business owners in the Enniscorthy asylum. Despite the disproportionate number of single and widowed paying patients, the themes of love and marriage remain dominant in the case notes, providing insight into contemporary concerns regarding courtship and marriage among the non-pauper mentally ill. Intimately linked with these concerns are issues of property and financial gain, which also played a decisive role in family relationships and the experience of mental illness. The case of John D. is exemplary. Aged seventy-seven, John was admitted to Enniscorthy in 1891 with 'senile insanity'. Reportedly a 'healthy old man', his personal history was provided by his two sons. The first symptoms noticed were that he 'wanted to marry a girl of 20, who was a servant to him':

> Says if he doesn't marry her his soul is lost and that he'll burn in hell ... he is very supple and has often tried to take away across the country to get to

> this girl ... Son says he won't allow bedclothes to be changed or bed made since the girl left, as he says no one can make it but her.[80]

While in the asylum, the girl visited John in the guise of his niece. Following this, the patient's sons instructed the medical superintendent to prevent any further communication between the girl and their father. They were very much against John's planned marriage, stating that 'she and her family are a designing lot and that they all encourage her to get him to marry her'. One son informed Drapes that 'it is his opinion that his father would have married "anything in petticoats" for the past two years or so'. Allegedly, the girls he proposed to were 'not at all suitable, and "streelish" in appearance and habits'.[81]

Underlying this narrative were anxieties about John's property. A farmer and a shopkeeper, John certainly had some degree of wealth. His maintenance was £18 per annum and, while in the asylum, he presented Drapes with a further £16 'to keep for him'. On one visit, John's son stated that 'latterly he was not capable of properly doing business in his shop' and elaborated with a description of the confusion this caused among the customers. This portrayal is in keeping with that of the urban professionals and white-collar workers, outlined above. It also supports Houston's findings concerning the social construction of madness in eighteenth-century Scotland.[82] John's sons' motivations for having him committed, however, became apparent when the patient later informed Drapes that 'he gave his sons up his land, but wished to retain his shop himself and get a wife to mind it for him'. John also provided what Drapes termed a 'rational explanation' regarding his romance with the servant girl:

> the girl had been so spoken of in connection with him that her character had suffered, and that if he did not make her the only reparation he could by marrying her, he would suffer in the next world.[83]

Just two months after his committal, John was discharged. Drapes noted that this was 'greatly against the wishes of his sons, but I have not been able to find any distinct evidence of his insanity'. According to the census, by 1901, John, now aged eighty-seven, had married a woman of twenty-seven, possibly the servant girl.[84] However, ten years later his son resided at John's address with his own wife and six children, suggesting that he had ultimately inherited the property.[85] The most plausible reason for this was that John's wife had not borne his children, which would have prevented her from being entitled to property rights following his death.[86]

This case is important in two respects. Firstly, it highlights contemporary fears among the public about the wrongful confinement of asylum patients for the pecuniary gain of their relatives. That John's sons professed to have committed their father to protect their family business is clear. Whether they actually feared for his mental state is less likely. Secondly, this case demonstrates that in instances where the asylum doctor identified wrongful committal by relatives, he could and would intervene.

Notably, while this case portrays the public's anticipated behaviour of relatively comfortable landed families, far more evidence can be gleaned of familial love and emotional bonds. For example, James S., a sixty-six-year-old farmer diagnosed with recurrent mania, informed Drapes: 'I cry all night for my wife and home'.[87] Fanny K., on the other hand, 'did not cry or seem affected at all parting with husband' when she was admitted.[88] The very fact that Drapes commented on Fanny's behaviour suggests that many other spouses did display an emotional reaction at being separated from their family upon committal to the asylum. Beveridge has found similar in the Scottish context, where patients committed to the Morningside asylum exhibited feelings of despair.[89] Like other patient populations, family visits also played an important role in the lives of paying patients in Enniscorthy and, to a lesser extent, Richmond.[90] The case notes for several paying patients at Enniscorthy recorded a visit from a least one relative.[91]

Letters from concerned relatives further corroborate the care and affection they exhibited. When Margaret K. was admitted to Enniscorthy as a paying patient, her husband informed Drapes that 'he would have sent her here long ago but her mother wouldn't allow it'. While she was in the asylum, Margaret's mother Sarah wrote the following letter to Drapes:

> I write to ask you how is my child Margaret K. Would you think if she was brought home the change might do her good or cheer her up. She wrote a letter to me a few weeks ago ... The first of her trouble came on from torments this is why she got into a nervous state. I being ill at the time and not able to go to her she was left alone by herself and got into a low

state... She asked me to send for her in the letter she wrote me. I sent it to her husband when I got it [sic].[92]

The 'child', a married woman of thirty, was discharged relieved within two months of the letter's receipt

Yet, in instances where property or business interests were at stake, these factors tended to eclipse those of familial devotion. Indeed, the high numbers of paying patients who had displayed an inability to control their business or function in their profession suggests that this was a major reason for committal. Oonagh Walsh has asserted that people in the west of Ireland would go to great lengths to secure property as it became a measure both of citizenship and stability.[93] Yet, with the exception of the case of John D., this study has revealed very little evidence to support this contention. While the extent to which John D. struggled in his shop is difficult to ascertain, it is conceivable that other relatives' claims regarding patients' incapacity to work were justified. In these instances, families may have viewed committal as a last resort to protect their resources or livelihood. This is especially true of paying patients in Enniscorthy, whose relatives would have little control over the actions or interactions of a lunatic positioned behind the shop counter or at a farmers' market. As Suzuki has maintained, families in England feared for the lunatic and his or her property as they would be 'easy prey to unscrupulous wretches' in the public sphere.[94] This implies that the extent to which wrongful committals occurred may have been exaggerated in the public imagination. As Walsh has argued, many patients with a 'genuine mental illness' accused their relatives of confining them for pecuniary gain.[95]

Again, mirroring Houston's findings concerning incapacity to work,[96] several paying patients were committed to Enniscorthy following an inability to conduct their affairs. James S., the man who had cried all night for his wife and home, was committed in 1897 because he

Goes out at night and hunts his sheep by the light of a candle and insists on his wife coming with him ... He often would go out in pouring rain, and stay about until his clothes were soaked. One night he stayed out (with her) ... from 12 to 4am trying to drive sheep into a house they never were in before. Mrs S left him for a few minutes and went into the house thinking he might follow her, but he did not, and when she went out again she found him sitting in a pool of water.[97]

While in the asylum, James continually wrote to his wife enclosing small presents he had managed to appropriate in the asylum. Drapes listed the gifts he sent, which included 'a ball of yarn', 'a ball of twine', 'a broken head', 'thimbles', 'sweets' and 'tobacco'. Sadly, James was not reunited with his wife, but died in the asylum after a residence of four years, aged about seventy.[98]

Laurence D. was admitted in 1896 with chronic mania. The first symptoms noticed were 'sleeplessness' and 'no ability to manage his business'. Like James, Laurence had been 'a good business man in the first part of his career, but since he began to drink 6 years ago, has failed in capacity for doing any'. Laurence was a family man who clearly had affection for his children. In a letter to a neighbour, Laurence wrote, 'I wish you to inform me how my two dear children are'.[99] While in the asylum, Laurence repeatedly insisted upon his sanity and often asked Drapes to re-examine him. Laurence's incapacity, however, appeared to be legitimate:

> He had a mania for ordering goods far more than he wanted, then couldn't pay for them, so had to get brother's assistance and in this way was induced to sign this deed ... Was very unmanageable at times: used to shut shop door and turn his family out in the street ... Memory has been failing: often gave directions twice over, and would mark things in shop over again at prices below what they cost, and would go to customers and tell them they had been overcharged by his wife and brother ... he accused [his wife] of 'stealing' goods out of the shop during his absence from home, at the time that his brother William was managing the business ... Whereas wife states that she had a perfect right to take anything she required (clothes &c) for her own, or her children's use: and what he referred to was a piece of cashmere, some tablecloths and woollen and cotton goods which she took for that purpose.[100]

Laurence had managed his business up to three years before he was committed to Enniscorthy. Despite the alleged difficulties and even threats Laurence posed to the family business, it is striking that his relatives cared for him for three years prior to committal. When his family decided he was no longer capable of handling his affairs, a deed was drawn up handing management over to his brother, William. Following this, Laurence visited several solicitors in Dublin but failed to break the deed. When his brother died, his wife, Ellen, took up management of the business and, at the time of Laurence's committal, had been running the shop for six months. Laurence took especial offence to this, complaining to Drapes that his business had been taken out of his hands and misman-aged by his wife. It is unlikely that Ellen would have adopted a man-agerial position had it not been for her husband's absence, in keeping with Cox's finding that mental illness could 'disrupt gendered domestic roles and boundaries' and place women in a position of authority in the household.[101]

In this case, Drapes favoured Laurence's family, and especially his wife. On admission, he was stated to have 'violently assaulted wife on several occasions'. However, Laurence 'denied having ever hurt his wife, but says he did strike her lightly with his foot across her legs, which he had every right legal or divine to do if she did wrong and that he consid-ered she had acted very badly'. Based on his observation of an interview held in the asylum between Laurence, his wife and her brother, Drapes noted that the patient's manner toward her was 'nasty and overbear-ing, all through adopting the style of a cross-examining lawyer'. Drapes appeared shocked by his patient's behaviour:

> At commencement of interview his demeanour towards [brother-in-law] was similar to that towards wife, and in fact he began by ordering him out of the room peremptorily (probably thinking he could bully his wife more easily). This I did not allow. [The brother-in-law] impressed me as an honest, straightforward fellow, patient and good tempered and to have certainly not the slightest hostile feeling towards D: and before the inter-view was over (after wife had left the room, not feeling well) – D, although knowing that she has been subject to some internal painful affect, in speak-ing of it as 'that convenient pain that she gets' – the two men were con-versing in a quite friendly manner, D calling him Willie and even joking and laughing.

Laurence was discharged on probation after just over a year's residence in the asylum. He was sent in the charge of an attendant to his family home as his wife 'would not send for him, and refused to be responsible for him'. Drapes noted that he had 'conducted himself sensibly here' and the Board ordered his discharge on probation 'on condition that he was not to touch drink, and not meddle with the business'. Drapes' interest in the case continued after discharge, noting four months later: 'heard he went to America and was found dead in his bed at an hotel: Death believed to be due to an overdose of whiskey'.[102] This appendage is particularly grim, given the man's affectionate references to his daughters while in the asylum and it suggests that, although discharged, the former patient failed to put down roots following emigration. Four years later, Laurence's widow Ellen was listed in the census as a draper and 'head of family', living with one daughter and a draper's assistant, apprentice and manager. By 1911, Ellen had retired and lived with her two daughters who had both become governesses.[103]

In addition to tradesmen, several farmers admitted to Enniscorthy referred to the unfavourable state of their financial affairs. The first symptoms of illness noticed in Martin B, a cattle dealer, shopkeeper and farmer, were that he 'got notice to leave his home, took this to heart thinking he wouldn't get another'.[104] Fear of eviction or the state of one's farm reportedly dominated some patients' thoughts. Like female patients in Enniscorthy and neighbouring Carlow,[105] Marcella J. expressed severe anxieties regarding her status as a paying patient, becoming 'rather agitated now as a rule: thinks all her money is gone: that we are running up a big bill against her here which she will never be able to pay'. A few days later she got 'depressed and agitated: has no money: no use my writing a bill against her' until finally she became 'very agitated: keeps crying out: "I can't I can't: I've no money, no money at all"'. The primary cause for Marcella's apprehensions might be that, on admission, she had delusions that 'the cattle on the land have been burned'.[106] In the case of Francis R., who owned a farm of 110 acres, the economic hardships he experienced were attributed to his mental breakdown:

> He has been farming for past 10 years or so, but did not know very much about it as he lived at home up till then (father was sessional crown solicitor ... now retired) ... Found it hard enough ... that it did not pay and added that was what sent him in here.[107]

It is therefore plausible that, for some, the impact of the agricultural hardship which continued into the early 1890s may have contributed to or been exacerbated by mental illness. Even later in the century, these issues were referred to. As late as 1899, 'the only cause' of illness that the sister of paying patient, Kate K., could give Drapes was that 'they lost a grass farm and this appeared to prey on her mind'.[108]

For landlords, excessive spending or even charity were viewed as indications of illness. John Neilson Eustace wrote of Henry O.B.:

His philanthropy is excessive, some beggars in the village have their rents paid by him, all the children look to him for pence, a pedlar used to receive 2/6 a visit & was told by him not to come more than once a month. Needless to say, during the man's lifetime he came as often as he sd. An att who married & left for Australia asked for some money & was lent £80 & given £10. This appeared at the time & has since found (I believe) to be an exceedingly bad investment.[109]

Similarly, 'gentleman' patient, George Leslie K reportedly:

gave away a great deal of property to his tenants & on the Lord Chancellor taking care of his estates he extorted money to the extent of £600 from his wife in order 'to buy more property for the poor tenants'. The money was kept in his trousers pocket & he always slept with this garment under his pillow.[110]

These narratives, most likely supplied by relatives, once again highlight the importance placed on land in rural communities. Like the paying patients admitted to Enniscorthy, failure to properly conduct property or business interests eclipsed family ties resulting in committal.

The influx of paying patients with property and business interests into district asylums like Enniscorthy supplied asylum doctors with new challenges. In many ways, the doctor was cast in the role of judge or mediator between family members, as they attempted to uncover the motivations behind individual committals.[111] Drapes appeared to embrace this role as he endeavoured to get to the bottom of complex familial conflicts. This could work in favour of the patient or the committing party, depending on the facts he accumulated, and did not appear to be gender-based. While many families exhibited affection and care for their mentally ill relatives, the outcome for patients who had ceased to conduct the family business efficiently was usually bleak.

POLICEMEN, VIOLENCE AND ALCOHOL

Like white-collar workers, another group whose conditions of employment were seen to affect their mental health negatively was members of the police force. The private lives of Royal Irish Constabulary (RIC) men were often subject to intense scrutiny, due to the wide-ranging codes of regulations imposed on them. When a policeman married, he was forbidden from serving in his wife's native county, meaning that marriage was a major cause of transfer within the RIC.[112] Several policemen admitted to Enniscorthy as paying patients had been forced to live separately from their wives. In February 1895, William H., aged 36, married Margaret in Tipperary. Margaret remained there for five months before her husband asked her to join him in Enniscorthy. Their cohabitation was cut short just eleven days later when William's station was changed and 'he said there was no accommodation for her'. Enforced separation from a spouse was also assigned as a cause of illness, implying that at least a degree of spousal affection had existed. Bernard C., an RIC constable and paying patient at Enniscorthy had moved '2 years ago from Ballywilliam where his wife resides: felt this separation a good deal and attributes this state of his mind to this'.[113]

The pressures of a position in the RIC also affected the wives of policemen. When Anne McC. was admitted to Richmond in 1892, she said she had not seen her husband, a detective inspector in the RIC, for about ten years. Prior to this, she had travelled around with him before being committed to Stewarts asylum and eventually transferred to Richmond. Anne stated she did 'not know exactly who sent her here [Richmond], if her children, they must have been instigated to do so by the constabulary or the Lord Lieutenant'. She later reiterated that 'the constabulary must be the cause of all her suffering'.[114]

The personal histories of paying patients from the police force, sometimes admitted as dangerous lunatics, are characterised by violence and make for vibrant, although at times disturbing, accounts of the lives of mentally ill Irish policemen. During their short time together, William H. exhibited numerous signs of violence towards his new wife. On admission, it is recorded that he threatened to shoot her and 'once took a knife and made the movement of sharpening it, and when she asked him what he was doing that for he said, "oh, for business"'.[115] Perhaps more harrowing, however, is the case of Sergeant K. The sergeant, a forty-four-year-old married policeman, was admitted to Enniscorthy as a dangerous lunatic in April 1897, before being named a paying patient. The warrant stated that he had attempted 'to locate a revolver' with the intention of killing a bird 'that was annoying him', as well as threatening to shoot the head constable. When his wife, Mary Jane, a ladies' nurse in Dublin, came to visit him, he 'received her affectionately', kissed her and they walked in the grounds together. However, Mary Jane informed

Drapes of her husband's history of violence, from which he compiled the following:

> They are 17 years married. Was only 4 days married when he threatened to kill her. Before he was married he beat her when in drink. About 3 years ago wife spoke to him about the company he was keeping, and he tried to kill her with a hatchet ... tried to smother wife 2 years ago in the night and she got up and left him finally ... She has often to rush out of the house in her night-dress.[116]

Just four months after his admission, Sergeant K. was discharged 'recovered'. Yet, the family's relationship with the asylum and Drapes did not end there. A newspaper clipping from an unidentified source was appended to the case notes, detailing the man's disappearance. Sergeant K.'s whereabouts was eventually detected and his wife wrote to Drapes in desperation:

> Dear Sir,
>
> The old trouble has come to me again. What I am to do with my husband I do not know ... On discharge he disappeared and for ages I knew nothing of him. Now he comes to the house and swears he will murder me ... I dare not sleep at night fearing my life, the hatchet as his constant companion.[117]

In Richmond, policemen were frequently associated with violence. John K. reportedly 'took up a poker to his daughter', while the warrant for Edward B., a pensioner from the Dublin Metropolitan Police, stated that he 'did assault his wife'.[118] So apparently ingrained was violence among the police force, that police constable Peter C., who was not violent, believed he would never be fit to return to duty 'as any fighting or drunken row affects his nerves very much and "makes him all a tremor"'.[119]

The ties between policemen and violence are especially significant, given their role in law enforcement. However, the high social status afforded to this group was undermined by their unruly behaviour, causing public scandals and spectacles. Mary Jane K. was shocked by the erosion of her husband's social values and struggled to come to terms with her plight. The remainder of her letter to Drapes read: 'I gave him a good home and he had not anything to do except keep respectable, live honestly and off he has gone ... Pardon my troubling you so much. Yours, Nurse K.'

Recognition by asylum doctors of the high levels of violence these men displayed towards their wives complicates McCarthy's contention that 'male violence against women and children was hidden and condoned' by the state and that female victims of domestic violence were often committed to Enniscorthy in the early twentieth century.[120] In addition to violence, 'excess of alcohol' was frequently given as a cause of insanity for policemen in this study, as outlined above. Like other patients assigned this cause, policemen stayed for a relatively short period of time in the asylum; almost 70% were discharged before six months and 84.6% before twelve months. The case of Michael D., a thirty-five-year-old, single, RIC constable who was admitted to Enniscorthy in 1897 with *mania a potu* was typical:

Seems always nervous, hands trembling and voice hesitating. Denied that he drank much, says the police are mostly blackguards and told lies of him ... Admits he has a bad record in the police, but attributes it to false charges against him, and his nervous manner being attributed to drink.[121]

Michael was discharged recovered after just one month in the asylum. Seeing as several of the policemen who were dismissed from the force were allowed to re-join,[122] it is conceivable that patients in this study might be permitted to do so following recovery. Certainly, Sergeant K., who had been in the police force for twenty-five years when committed, told Drapes he was 'once punished for drink when he had been 8 years in the force but never since'.[123]

WOMEN, WORK AND DOMESTICITY

Links between conditions of employment and mental illness were far more tenuous for female patients in this study. Eustace II's notes on women admitted to Hampstead in the 1840s reveal an early medical alignment of women's mental illness with failure to fulfil domestic duties.[124] Anna Maria D. was admitted to Hampstead in 1845, after she 'became gloomy and reserved and neglected her husband and children, desiring to be alone'.[125] This behaviour continued while Anna Maria was at Hampstead and Eustace recorded: 'some of her family have called to see her, their visits have not improved her. She received them unkindly'.[126] In the same year, Helen B., who railed 'very much against her husband & threatens him very much', was admitted with 'habitual intoxication'. Her husband informed Eustace that 'in consequence of her conduct to him he has not slept with her for two years'.[127] While commentary on a woman's failure to fulfil conjugal duties was obviously confined to married women, single women were expected to behave appropriately towards family members, especially when they relied on them for financial support. Refusal to do so was also viewed as a sign of illness. In 1846, Eustace II reported that Florinda C.'s monomania was 'manifested in the most violent dislike to her brother where kindness to her had been for years her almost sole support'.[128] Almost half a century later, Drapes wrote of Catherine S., a paying patient in Enniscorthy: 'husband states that her mind began to be affected about ? months. Has done no work in the house since then (except a little knitting)'.[129]

As Chap. 3 discussed, the relatives of Ennis patients who were called upon to contribute towards maintenance frequently referred to their straitened circumstances. Family friends, writing in support of these claims, also blamed female 'domestic trouble' for mental illness. In 1889, James Frost JP wrote to Gelston concerning the financial condition of a potential patient's husband:

> A neighbour of mine, Mrs G[-] of Ballymorris has become insane and she must be placed in the Lunatic Asylum. As to the capacity of her husband to pay for her while she remains an inmate, I would say it is very slight. He holds about thirty acres of land, and has a few cows, but he is up to his ears in debt. He owes two years rent, and I do not see him to possess any adequate means to meet the payment of it. For a long time past, he was not even able to pay the wages of a maid servant and his poor wife had to do all the work of the house besides taking care of the children.[130]

Richard Studdert, a governor of Ennis asylum, also wrote to Gelston concerning Mrs. G.:

> she seems to have been respectably brought up and educated and was doing well until a sad succession of misfortune came upon her – 5 of her 9 children having died within a few weeks, also her father in law at the same time a hitherto comfortable man became quite otherwise from reduced circumstances. All resulted in her going out of her mind.[131]

These representations succeeded in convincing the Ennis asylum board to admit Mrs. G. as a pauper patient.[132] Ten year later, a parish priest, James Cahir, wrote to Gelston about the financial affairs of another female patient, Mrs. K. According to Cahir, twenty-three years earlier, Mrs. K.'s husband:

> owing to money difficulties left his family and went to America where I believe he is still living although he never writes home. When he left, his stock was reduced to one cow and his poor wife in struggling to maintain herself and three young children was so worried by difficulties that she lost her senses and had to be sent to the Asylum leaving only one cow on the farm and rent in arrears.[133]

In this case payment was also 'remitted'.

These letters reveal lay interpretations of factors which precipitated female mental illness. Those writing in support of patients' families pin-pointed financial decline resulting in increased housework, childcare, farming duties and family bereavement as the cause of their illness. These lay opinions differed from those asserted by Eustace II in the 1840s and Drapes in the 1890s; while failure to perform domestic duties was viewed as a *symptom* of mental illness by medical observers, increased domestic duties and 'domestic trouble' were characterised as a *cause* of illness in lay explanations.

'Domestic trouble' also reportedly featured for women in paid work. Several female patients admitted to Stewarts exhibited fears about their financial condition and their family businesses. Ann Elizabeth Ellen M. had allegedly 'suffered great domestic trouble thro' bankruptcy of her husband' and the cause of her illness was attributed to adverse circumstances.[134] Jane D., whose husband was a butcher with a shop on Moore Street in Dublin City, 'was associated with her husband ... in business and as such was kept a good deal indoors ... got very silent and fretted a good deal about business wh. was then dull. Slept badly'. The 'supposed cause' of Jane's illness was not 'business worry' but 'domestic bereavement', suggesting her role in the business was considered domestic rather than commercial. This was reflected in the admissions register, where her occupation was recorded as 'butcher's wife'. When she recovered, Jane's husband clearly appreciated that she needed a rest from the butcher's shop and took her home 'with a view to sending her to the seaside'.[135] Even when female patients had a designated occupation, such as Eliza Jane K., a single woman and shopkeeper who was 'greatly concerned about money matters', or Elizabeth Jane M., a married draper, who had 'had great business anxiety thro' boycotting', business worry was not cited as a cause of their illness.[136] Instead, Eliza Jane was assigned no cause and Elizabeth Jane was assigned 'hereditary'. Disparities between male and female aetiologies most likely stem from contemporary attitudes towards women's work. From the mid-nineteenth century, official interpretations of productive labour shifted and influenced how women's occupations were enumerated in the census returns. By 1871, married women who worked with their husbands and single women who engaged with the family business were classified as being in domestic occupation.[137] It is plausible that asylum physicians were likewise inclined to characterise female business concerns as domestic rather than commercial.

Although not engaged in commercial work, women in wealthier households played a significant role in maintaining the household budget, deciding where to shop and seeking credit.[138] Accordingly, women committed to Highfield were sometimes measured against these functions. Like men who were deemed fit to resume employment, female paying patients who demonstrated an ability to resume domestic roles were seen as improved. John Neilson Eustace wrote of Margaret W., a sixty-year-old widow with no recorded occupation, 'she is a capable business woman & frequently goes into town shopping'.[139] Eustace clearly viewed Margaret's ability to shop as a sign of improvement. On the other hand, an inability to manage one's financial affairs could be viewed as evidence of insanity. Emily H., who was maintained at Stewarts at £50 per annum, was 'said to have had grandiose ideas and that she went into Arnotts [department store] and bought £40 worth of goods'.[140]

CONCLUSIONS

Historians have been curiously reluctant to emphasise the importance asylum doctors placed on patients' working life prior to committal and the potential this had to cause mental illness.[141] This chapter has argued that greater historiographical significance should be accorded to factors such as alcohol, employment, and financial and domestic troubles in the aetiologies attributed to fee-paying patients. In this study, both lay and medical commentators commonly recognised these factors as having triggered mental illness in paying patients. Like labouring men in

Victorian London,[142] urban life reportedly held challenges for Irishmen who fell prey to the anxieties generated by employment within the commercial sector. The working life of certain occupational groups, including clerks, was often identified as precipitating insanity. Policemen were another group whose working conditions attracted psychiatric attention. Subjected to an extremely regimented lifestyle, RIC men suffered marital problems and displayed a tendency towards alcohol abuse and violence, resulting in committal. This association between working life and insanity speaks volumes about contemporary society's interpretations. In relation to social status, those unable to maintain their position within a given occupation were defined in terms of this failure.

Both Cox and Oonagh Walsh have emphasised the presence of familial bonds in the rural south-east and west of Ireland respectively.[143] This chapter has revealed that, among paying patients, land disputes and an inability to manage one's affairs threatened to shatter these bonds, often resulting in committal. Discussion of women's reproductive functions did not tend to occupy lay or medical narratives of female insanity in this study. Instead, patients, their relatives and their doctors discussed the mental strain of domestic circumstances, which could even include business anxieties. That domestic causes were often applied to female mental illness in place of work/finance is to be expected, given contemporary understandings of productive employment and female occupations. Nonetheless, lay explanations of female illness indicate awareness and even appreciation of the potential strain—both domestic and economic—of women's work in late nineteenth-century Ireland.

Notes

1. MacCabe was the resident physician to the State Criminal Asylum at Dundrum in Dublin and honourable secretary to the Medico-Psychological Association and had previously been resident medical superintendent at the Waterford district asylum.
2. Cox (2012, pp. 56, 62–64). Tuke was the editor of the *Journal of Mental Science* for seventeen years during the economic depression and published several articles in it on the alleged increase of insanity in Britain and Ireland. Drapes was a 'notable Irish asylum physician'. Educated at Trinity College Dublin, he was a licentiate of the Royal College of Surgeons in Ireland, member of the British Medical Association, editor of the *Journal of Mental Science* during World War I

and one of the few Irish asylum superintendents who published on the causes of mental illness in Ireland. See Cox (2010, pp. 281–282). For more on Drapes' career, see Kelly (2016, pp. 93–96).

3. Suzuki (2007, p. 118).
4. Ibid.
5. Cox (2012, pp. 59, 121).
6. Digby (1985, p. 212).
7. MacKenzie (1992, p. 152).
8. Suzuki (2007, p. 121).
9. Levine-Clark (2004, p. 123).
10. Cox (2012, pp. 121–122) and Cronin (2010).
11. See Bourke (1993) and Luddy (2000).
12. Digby (1989) and Oppenheim (1991, pp. 181–232).
13. Suzuki (2007, p. 118).
14. The reporting physician, at times, openly refuted these lay narratives. For example, Clinical Record Volume No. 3 (WCC, St Senan's Hospital, Enniscorthy, p. 264); Clinical Record Volume No. 4 (WCC, St Senan's Hospital, Enniscorthy, p. 208).
15. Cox (2012, p. 220).
16. Ibid., pp. 60, 220.
17. In cases where patients were assigned both physical and moral causes, both are included to illustrate their statistical significance.
18. Walsh (2004, p. 262).
19. MacKenzie (1992, p. 152).
20. Malcolm (1986, p. 332).
21. Ibid., pp. 328, 331.
22. Harrison (1971 pp. 298–347).
23. Malcolm (1986, p. 326).
24. Finnane (1981, p. 147).
25. Ibid.
26. Kelly (2016, p. 95).
27. Cox (2012, p. 221).
28. Finnane, pp. 146–150, Cox (2012, pp. 60–61, 221–222).
29. The Twenty-Forth Report on the District, Criminal, and Private Lunatic Asylums in Ireland, H.C. 1875 [319] xxxiii, p. 18.
30. MacKenzie (1992, p. 151). See also Digby (1985, pp. 208–209).
31. Pick (1989, p. 197).
32. Ibid.
33. Digby (1985, pp. 208–209).
34. Digby (1989, pp. 192–220). For the American context, see Theriot (1993, pp. 1–31).
35. Levine-Clark (2004, pp. 123–148).

36. Healy (1996, pp. 314–320).
37. Cox (2012, p. 65). See also Kelly (2016, pp. 96–100). See Rosenberg (1992, p. xvi).
38. Houston (2004, p. 59).
39. Finnane (1981, p. 150).
40. Notably, after the Famine, doctors at the Carlow district asylum reported fear of subsequent famines and destitution as causes of illness in some patients, see Cox (2012, p. 121). These fears were not reported to affect paying patients in this study.
41. Hampstead Casebook 1840s (Highfield Hospital Group, Hampstead and Highfield Records, p. 11).
42. Suzuki (2007, p. 124).
43. Ibid., p. 123.
44. Male Case Book 1900–1901 (GM, Richmond District Lunatic Asylum, pp. 333–335).
45. Male Case Book 1892–1893 (GM, Richmond District Lunatic Asylum, p. 438).
46. Ibid., pp. 438–439.
47. MacCabe (1875), p. 397.
48. Ibid.
49. Suzuki (2007, pp. 123–124).
50. Male Case Book 1891–1892 (GM, Richmond District Lunatic Asylum, pp. 409–411).
51. Ibid., p. 258.
52. Ibid., pp. 897–898.
53. Male Case Book 1898 (GM, Richmond District Lunatic Asylum, pp. 275–276).
54. Bloomfield Case Book (FHL, Bloomfield Records, p. 1).
55. Houston (2004, pp. 55–56).
56. Case Book 1889–1900 (Stewarts, Patient Records, p. 6).
57. Ibid., p. 85.
58. Ibid., p. 126.
59. Ibid., p. 17.
60. Ibid., p. 175.
61. Cherry and Munting (2005, p. 45). See also Melling and Forsythe (2006, p. 192).
62. Cox (2012, pp. 156, 160).
63. Case Book (FHL, Bloomfield Records, p. 61).
64. Case Book 1889–1900 (Stewarts, Patient Records, p. 156).
65. Ibid., p. 166.
66. Ibid., p. 166.
67. Casebook Two (SJOGH, Patient Records, p. 59).

68. Ibid., p. 1.
69. Cherry and Munting 2005, p. 45; Cox 2012, p. 160.
70. Casebook Two (SJOGH, Patient Records, p. 73).
71. Houston (2004, pp. 54–58).
72. Hampstead Casebook 1890s (Highfield Hospital Group, Hampstead and Highfield Records, p. 26).
73. Suzuki (2007, pp. 121, 127–128) and Cox (2012, p. 121).
74. MacCabe (1875, pp. 391–392).
75. Suzuki (2007, p. 123).
76. Fitzpatrick (1985) and Guinnane (1997).
77. Cox (2012, pp. 108–109) and Guinnane (1997, pp. 142–143, 230–235).
78. Walsh (2001, p. 145).
79. Melling and Forsythe (2006, p. 100) and MacKenzie (1992, p. 215).
80. Clinical Record Volume No. 3 (WCC, St Senan's Hospital, Enniscorthy, p. 264).
81. Ibid.
82. Houston (2004).
83. Clinical Record Volume No. 3 (WCC, St Senan's Hospital, Enniscorthy, p. 264).
84. 'Census of Ireland 1901,' accessed 10 July 2012, http://www.census.nationalarchives.ie.
85. Ibid.; Clinical Record Volume No. 3 (WCC, St Senan's Hospital, Enniscorthy, p. 264).
86. See Bourke (1993, p. 272).
87. Clinical Record Volume No. 6 (WCC, St Senan's Hospital, Enniscorthy, p. 408).
88. Clinical Record Volume No. 4 (WCC, St Senan's Hospital, Enniscorthy, p. 198).
89. Beveridge (1998, p. 437).
90. See, for example, Cox (2012, pp. 108–109, 157) and Melling and Forsythe (2006, p. 100) and MacKenzie (1992, p. 215).
91. See, for example, Clinical Record Volume No. 3 (WCC, St Senan's Hospital, Enniscorthy, pp. 3, 166, 264); Clinical Record Volume No. 4 (WCC, St Senan's Hospital, pp. 208, 240); Clinical Record Volume No. 5 (WCC, St Senan's Hospital, p. 16); Clinical Record Volume No. 6 (WCC, St Senan's Hospital, pp. 112, 128, 407); Clinical Record Volume No. 7 (WCC, St Senan's Hospital, pp. 392, 356).
92. Clinical Record Volume No. 6 (WCC, St Senan's Hospital, p. 216).
93. Walsh (2001, p. 141).
94. Suzuki (2001, pp. 120–121).
95. Walsh (2001, p. 141).

96. Houston (2004, pp. 55–56).
97. Clinical Record Volume No. 6 (WCC, St Senan's Hospital, pp. 120, 407).
98. Ibid. For another example see Clinical Record Volume No. 5 (WCC, St Senan's Hospital, pp. 93–94).
99. Clinical Record Volume No. 5 (WCC, St Senan's Hospital, p. 390).
100. Ibid., p. 190, 389–390.
101. Cox (2012, p. 150).
102. Clinical Record Volume No. 5 (WCC, St Senan's Hospital, pp. 189–90, 389–90, 392, 411).
103. 'Census of Ireland 1901,' accessed 6 January 2012, http://www.census. nationalarchives.ie.
104. Clinical Record Volume No. 3 (WCC, St Senan's Hospital, p. 297).
105. Cox (2012, pp. 121–122).
106. Clinical Record Volume No. 4 (WCC, St Senan's Hospital, p. 231).
107. Ibid., pp. 317–318, 118.
108. Clinical Record Volume No. 7 (WCC, St Senan's Hospital, p. 122).
109. Hampstead Casebook 1890s (Highfield Hospital Group, Hampstead and Highfield Records, p. 16).
110. Ibid., p. 20.
111. See also Finnane (1985).
112. Griffin (1997, p. 168).
113. Clinical Record Volume No. 3 (WCC, St Senan's Hospital, p. 196).
114. Female Case Book 1892–1893 (GM, Richmond District Lunatic Asylum, pp.126–127).
115. Clinical Record Volume No. 5 (WCC, St Senan's Hospital, pp. 311–312).
116. Clinical Record Volume No. 6 (WCC, St Senan's Hospital, pp. 46, 359).
117. Ibid., p. 359.
118. Male Case Book 1890–1891 (GM, Richmond District Lunatic Asylum, p. 384); Male Case Book 1894–1895 (GM, Richmond District Lunatic Asylum, p. 65).
119. Male Case Book 1894–1895 (GM, Richmond District Lunatic Asylum, p. 436).
120. McCarthy (2004, p. 123, 135).
121. Clinical Record Volume No. 6 (WCC, St Senan's Hospital, p. 128).
122. Griffin (1997, p. 170).
123. Clinical Record Volume No. 6 (WCC, St Senan's Hospital, p. 46).
124. For the twentieth century, see McCarthy (2004, p. 134).
125. Early Hampstead Casebook 1840s (Highfield Hospital Group, Hampstead and Highfield Records, p. 16).
126. Ibid., p. 17.

127. Ibid., p. 14. For more on violence and women in Victorian England, see Marland (2004).
128. Early Hampstead Casebook 1840s (Highfield Hospital Group, Hampstead and Highfield Records, p. 18).
129. Clinical Record Volume No. 4 (WCC, St Senan's Hospital, p. 240).
130. James Frost J. P. to R.P. Gelston, 10 Jun. 1889 (CCA, Our Lady's Hospital, OL1/7 Letter 1577).
131. Richard Studdert to R.P. Gelston, date unknown (CCA, Our Lady's Hospital, OL1/7 Letter 1577b).
132. Minute Book, 1888–1891 (CCA, Our Lady's Hospital, OL1/5, p. 183).
133. James Cahir P P to R.P. Gelston, 7 Apr. 1899 (CCA, Our Lady's Hospital, OL1/7 Letter 2606).
134. Case Book 1889–1900 (Stewarts, Patient Records, p. 154).
135. Ibid., p. 168.
136. Ibid., pp. 90, 41.
137. Luddy (2000, p. 45). See also Daly, (1997) and Bourke, 1993.
138. Luddy (2000, p. 55).
139. Highfield Casebook (Highfield Hospital Group, Hampstead and Highfield Records, p. 11).
140. Case Book 1889–1900 (Stewarts, Patient Records, p. 163).
141. Digby (1985, p. 212) and MacKenzie (1992, p. 152).
142. Suzuki (2007).
143. Walsh (2001, p. 145); Cox, (2012, p. xviii, 108–9, 148–149).

REFERENCES

Beveridge, Allan. 'Life in the Asylum: Patient's Letters from Morningside, 1873–1908.' *History of Psychiatry* 9 (1998): 431–469.

Bourke, Joanna. *Husbandry to Housewifery: Women, Economic Change and Housework in Ireland, 1890–1914.* Oxford: Clarendon Press, 1993.

Cherry, Steven and Munting, Roger. '"Exercise is the Thing"? Sport and the Asylum c. 1850–1950.' *The International Journal of the History of Sport* 22, no. 1 (2005): 42–58.

Cox, Catherine. 'Health and Welfare in Enniscorthy, 1850–1920.' In *Enniscorthy: A History*, edited by Colm Tóibín, 265–287. Wexford: Wexford County Council Public Library Service, 2010.

Cox, Catherine. *Negotiating Insanity in the Southeast of Ireland 1830–1900.* Manchester: Manchester University Press, 2012.

Cronin, Maura. '"You'd be Disgraced!": Middle-Class Women and Respectability in Post-Famine Ireland.' In *Politics, Society and Middle Class in Modern Ireland*, edited by Fintan Lane, 107–129. Basingstoke: Palgrave MacMillan, 2010.

Daly, Mary E. *Women and Work in Ireland*. Dundalk: Dundalgan Press, 1997.

Digby, Anne. *Madness, Morality and Medicine: A Study of the York Retreat, 1796–1914*. Cambridge: Cambridge University Press, 1985.

Digby, Anne. 'Women's Biological Straitjacket.' In *Sexuality and Subordination: Interdisciplinary Studies of Gender in the Nineteenth Century*, edited by Susan Mendes and Jane Rendall, 192–220. London and New York: Routledge, 1989.

Finnane, Mark. *Insanity and the Insane in Post-Famine Ireland*. London: Croom Helm, 1981.

Finnane, Mark. 'Asylums, Families and the State.' *History Workshop Journal* 20, no. 1 (1985): 134–148.

Fitzpatrick, David. 'Marriage in Post-Famine Ireland.' In *Marriage in Ireland*, edited by Art Cosgrove, 116–131. Dublin: College Press, 1985.

Griffin, Brian. 'The Irish Police: Love Sex and Marriage in the Nineteenth and Early Twentieth Centuries.' In *Gender Perspectives in Nineteenth-Century Ireland: Public and Private Spheres*, edited by Margaret Kelleher and James H. Murphy, 168–178. Dublin: Irish Academic Press, 1997.

Guinnane, Timothy. *The Vanishing Irish: Households, Migration, and the Rural Economy in Ireland, 1850–1914*. Princeton: Princeton University Press, 1997.

Harrison, Brian. *Drink and the Victorians: The Temperance Question in England, 1815–72*. London: Faber, 1971.

Healy, David. 'Irish Psychiatry. Part 2: Use of the Medico-Psychological Association by its Irish Members – Plus ça Change!' In *150 Years of British Psychiatry*, edited by Hugh Freeman and German E. Berrios, 314–320. London: Athlone Press, 1996.

Houston, Robert A. 'Class, Gender and Madness in Eighteenth-Century Scotland.' In *Sex and Seclusion, Class and Custody: Perspectives on Gender and Class in the History of British and Irish Psychiatry*, edited by Jonathan Andrews and Anne Digby, 45–68. Amsterdam and New York: Rodopi, 2004.

Kelly, Brendan. *Hearing Voices: The History of Psychiatry in Ireland*. Newbridge: Irish Academic Press, 2016.

Levine-Clark, Marjorie. '"Embarrassed Circumstances": Gender, Poverty and Insanity in the West Riding of England in the Early Victorian Years.' In *Sex and Seclusion, Class and Custody: Perspectives on Gender and Class in the History of British and Irish Psychiatry*, edited by Jonathan Andrews and Anne Digby, 123–148. Amsterdam and New York: Rodopi, 2004.

Luddy, Maria. 'Women and Work in Nineteenth- and Early Twentieth-Century Ireland: An Overview.' In *Women and Paid Work in Ireland, 1500–1930*, edited by Bernadette Whelan, 44–56. Dublin: Four Courts Press, 2000.

MacCabe, Frederick. 'On Mental Strain and Overwork.' *Journal of Mental Science* 21 (Oct., 1875): 388–402.

MacKenzie, Charlotte. *Psychiatry for the Rich: A History of the Private Madhouse at Ticehurst in Sussex, 1792–1917.* London: Routledge, 1992.

Malcolm, Elizabeth. *Ireland Sober, Ireland Free: Drink and Temperance in Nineteenth-Century Ireland.* Dublin: Gill and Macmillan, 1986.

Marland, Hilary. *Dangerous Motherhood: Insanity and Childbirth in Victorian Britain.* Basingstoke: Palgrave Macmillan, 2004.

McCarthy, Áine. 'Hearths, Bodies and Minds: Gender Ideology and Women's Committal to Enniscorthy Lunatic Asylum, 1916–25.' In *Irish Women's History*, edited by Alan Hayes and Diane Urquhart, 115–136. Dublin: Irish Academic Press, 2004.

Melling, Joseph and Bill Forsythe. *The Politics of Madness: The State, Insanity and Society in England, 1845–14.* London and New York: Routledge, 2006.

Oppenheim, Janet. *'Shattered Nerves': Doctors, Patients and Depression in Victorian England.* New York and Oxford: Oxford University Press, 1991.

Pick, Daniel. *Faces of Degeneration: A European Disorder, c. 1848–1918.* Cambridge: Cambridge University Press, 1989.

Rosenberg, Charles E. 'Framing Disease: Illness, Society and History.' In *Framing Disease: Studies in Cultural History*, edited by Charles E. Rosenbery and Janet Golden, xiii–xxvi. New Brunswick and New Jersey: Rutgers University Press, 1992.

Suzuki, Akihito. 'Enclosing and Disclosing Lunatics within the Family Walls: Domestic Psychiatric Regime and the Public Sphere in Early Nineteenth-Century England.' In *Outside the Walls of the Asylum: The History of Care in the Community, 1750–2000*, edited by Peter Bartlett and David Wright, 115–132. London: Athlone Press, 2001.

Suzuki, Akihito. 'Lunacy and Labouring Men: Narratives of Male Vulnerability in Mid-Victorian London.' In *Medicine, Madness and Social History: Essays in Honour of Roy Porter*, edited by Roberta Bivins and John V. Pickstone, 118–128. Basingstoke: Palgrave Macmillan, 2007.

Theriot, Nancy M. 'Women's Voices in Nineteenth-Century Medical Discourse: A Step towards Deconstructing Science.' *Signs: Journal of Women in Culture and Society* 29 (1993): 1–31.

Walsh, Lorraine. 'A Class Apart? Admissions to the Dundee Royal Lunatic Asylum, 1890–1910.' In *Sex and Seclusion, Class and Custody: Perspectives on Gender and Class in the History of British and Irish Psychiatry*, edited by Jonathan Andrews and Anne Digby, 249–269. Amsterdam and New York: Rodopi, 2004.

Walsh, Oonagh. 'Lunatic and Criminal Alliances in Nineteenth-Century Ireland.' In *Outside the Walls of the Asylum: The History of Care in the Community 1750–2000*, edited by Peter Bartlett and David Wright, 132–152. London: Athlone Press, 2001.

CHAPTER 6

'A Great Source of Amusement': Work Therapy and Recreation

Psychiatry's emphasis on employment went beyond assigning causes of illness to encompass treatment. Work therapy was a key facet of moral treatment, which remained a dominant form of therapy in nineteenth-century asylums. Asylum doctors stressed the usefulness of work therapy for patients, including distraction from their malady, rehabilitation and their eventual resocialisation following discharge.[1] However, by the 1860s, asylum doctors' optimism about moral treatment was gradually replaced by a therapeutic pessimism.[2] The benefits of moral therapy were most famously expounded by Samuel Tuke, in his *Description of the Retreat* published in 1813.[3] These included the distraction of patients from painful or disturbing thoughts through providing them with occupations and pastimes. The York Retreat's therapists believed that the proper regulation of the mind was connected with disease prevention and. stemming from this, work therapy was intended to 'encourage the growth of mental abilities and especially the power of concentration'.[4] This reflected the influence of the Society of Friends' discipline on the Retreat's therapists, which aimed to inculcate habits of Christian self-denial, moderation and uprightness of character in its youngest members.[5] In the absence of these habits, patients were provided with a domestic setting, in the form of the York Retreat, where they could be resocialised.[6]

Unsurprisingly, for women in this study, work therapy was exclusively confined to domestic occupations, further underscoring a gender bias in Irish non-pauper asylum care. In voluntary and private asylums, doctors counteracted the difficulties they faced in delivering appropriate work therapy for wealthier patients by offering more varied and stimulating recreations.

© The Author(s) 2018
A. Mauger, *The Cost of Insanity in Nineteenth-Century Ireland*, Mental Health in Historical Perspective,
https://doi.org/10.1007/978-3-319-65244-3_6

189

PRODUCTIVE EMPLOYMENT

In Irish district asylums, as elsewhere, work was considered essential as a therapeutic regime and fundamental to Victorian concepts of respectability. In Ireland, asylum medical staff perceived patients' failure to work as a 'refusal to join the ranks of the "respectable" poor'.[7] A number of the doctors in this study clearly subscribed to the therapeutic benefits of occupation and recreation. However, they often struggled to find suitable employment for their wealthier patients. This was not a uniquely Irish problem. Digby has noted the difficulty in employing private patients at the York Retreat, contending that resistance to manual labour stemmed from a perception that it was menial and degrading. She has also highlighted the problem of 'matching possible work to previous life habits' for this social cohort, a pursuit which was vital to the provision of moral treatment.[8] Nevertheless, asylums could provide outlets for skilled and semi-skilled workers. For instance, at Staffordshire asylum in England, male paying patients who were tailors and shoemakers occupied themselves at these trades.[9] In Irish district asylums, employment was as much part of asylum life for paying patients as their pauper counterparts and many were given work that was related to their former occupation. The degree to which individual paying patients were willing to engage in work varied a great deal. Some reportedly did no work, a point which was frequently noted by the reporting physician. However, there is no evidence that paying patients who refused to work in district asylums did so due to a sense of social superiority.

Physical labour was considered an especially appropriate tenet of moral treatment in Ireland due to the large numbers of agricultural labourers in the asylum population,[10] and several paying patients who were previously farmers worked on the asylum farm. Other patients deemed physically fit, such as soldiers, were sent to work on the farm in Richmond. In Britain, work therapy has been attributed to an ethos of political economy in asylums, making savings on maintenance costs and staffing, especially where asylums were understaffed, to accomplish a degree of institutional self-sufficiency.[11] At the Norfolk asylum, food was produced directly, using patients' labour on the gardens and farm.[12]

Paying patients in this study often contributed to the economy of the asylum, performing tasks at which they were skilled. For example, at Enniscorthy, Harvey Henry M., a boot and shoe shopkeeper, was reportedly 'very fond of polishing boots' and asked the attendants to allow him to polish theirs.[13] When William Henry P., previously a carpenter, broke a window sash while trying to escape, he was employed at fixing it 'and being a carpenter he had no difficulty in mending window'. Following this, William Henry asked Drapes to allow him to work and was sent to the carpenter's shop where he 'worked steadily'.[14] Ellen W., who had been '6 years in America as waitress in a hotel', was sent to work in the kitchen, and Teresa C., a tailor's wife, did 'a little needle-work'.[15] John B., a painter suffering from acquired epilepsy, was 'put to work at painting during this month and he kept fairly well at it, but has to stop at times if he has had a fit'.[16] At Richmond, Francis F., a porter, was 'retained as a ward worker in hospital'.[17] Christopher O'K., a painter, was employed at painting and 'working with the farm gang', while Thomas G., a civil service pensioner, worked as a clerk.[18] These examples clearly illustrate that paying patients, a number of whom were skilled, could be employed advantageously by the asylum, which benefited from the influx of skilled workers, capable of painting, mending and crafting as the authorities desired. Furthermore, working in familiar areas could be considered therapeutic and even rehabilitative for patients, putting them on a road to recovery and fostering self-reliance outside the asylum.[19]

Work therapy was manifestly seen as rehabilitative at St John of God's, where its medical superintendent, O'Connell, noted frequently when patients performed tasks linked to their former occupations. For instance, O'Connell recorded that patient Daniel C., a priest, 'read at least part of the divine office' almost daily. However, he 'still absents himself from chapel' and was 'at times, cranky and quarrelsome as well as insulting to his fellow priests ... he has been somewhat more disagreeable to his fellow priests, in their special sitting-room, during the winter'.[20] Eventually he was 'left much to himself in the priests' sitting-room where he has no one with whom to quarrel' until ultimately the priests' sitting room was described as 'the special room formerly set apart for priests'.[21] James C., a lay brother, was more devout: 'he frequents the chapel as usual ... never forgets to go to chapel privately, every day after dinner'.[22] Another priest, Patrick B., reportedly often attempted to give sermons, saying that he was 'a most elegant preacher'. When asked to preach, Patrick would 'say something and repeat it several times, giggling at his own words'.[23] O'Connell's motivation for recording such information can be inferred from his notes on patient Michael K., a farmer:

He takes much interest in cattle and horses of which he is a very good judge... He is easily roused from these thoughts to take him to a fair or market to buy or sell cattle is sufficient... While there is any excitement for him, as the recent Horse Show, at Ballsbridge, which he delights to visit, or a race at Leopardstown, he is in excellent spirits. He takes keen delight in farming affairs of all kinds and is thoroughly skilled at all that pertains to agriculture... If he can engage from time to time in anything pertaining to farming it acts as a great stimulus to rouse him and to keep him from thinking of himself – from interpretation... I often fancy that if he had constant mental occupation, such as his farm must give, he could take care of himself and do his business well.[24]

This extract suggests that O'Connell considered employment a worthy means of distraction for his patients. O'Connell also viewed lack of work as problematic, writing of Louis de L.V.W., who was admitted in 1885: 'no mental change except that he is rather stupid and sleepy, due, no doubt, to not being employed'.[25] This was not confined to fee-paying patients. Medical staff in district asylums found any resistance to work in the asylum particularly troubling, interpreting such refusals as symptoms of continuing poor mental condition.[26]

Although they stressed the importance of useful work, district asylum doctors did not force paying patients to stick to one form of employment, especially when they did not appear to enjoy or excel at it. James L., was therefore allowed to give up weaving 'because he disliked noise of looms' and was moved to gardening.[27] A sixteen-year-old schoolboy, Charles L., worked in several areas during his patient career including the tailor's shop, the smith's shop, the shoemaker's shop, the weaving shop, the bookshop and the farm. He was also employed at driving one of the carts.[28]

Voluntary and private asylum patients were accorded relatively few opportunities to work, as asylum staff found it hard to provide class appropriate employment. As early as the 1830s, Bloomfield's managing committee commented on the 'difficulty of finding employment or amusement as would be beneficial to the patients' and issued an appeal to the asylum's subscribers for any suggestions they might have.[29] The issue of how best to employ patients continued to daunt the committee. In the same decade, they noted that one patient had been removed to 'another asylum, where greater facilities were afforded for agricultural employments, which it was hoped might in his case be attended with advantage'.[30] In 1850, Bloomfield's managing committee was pleased to report that 'in the course of the past year the manifest benefit arising from out-door employment, and the steady improvement in the order and discipline of the house which has kept pace with the introduction of means to amuse and employ, have been very gratifying'.[31] 'Employments of an industrial character, together with suitable recreations, and an enlarged supply of newspapers, periodicals, and useful and entertaining books' were not only credited with rendering Bloomfield's patients more comfortable and having 'fostered habits of self-control and propriety of demeanour' but also with contributing to the 'improvement of their bodily health'.[32]

Predictably, the committee noted that several male patients were employed in the garden and grounds, while female patients tended to perform fancywork and needlework.[33] This is corroborated in the house steward's casebook for this period, where he documented many male patients assisting the gardener, sweeping up leaves in the shrubbery, moulding cabbages, painting and undertaking 'trellis work'. Others raked and trimmed the walks in the ladies' field, pumped water, chopped wood and helped in the laundry.[34] As with paying patients in district asylums, while those at Bloomfield were actively encouraged to engage where possible, they were not confined to one occupation and clearly had at least a measure of freedom in how they spent their time. One patient, David S., reportedly 'adopted the coachman as he own' and stated his intention to retain his services when he left the institution. In the meantime, he performed various jobs to assist the coachman. The following week he was found busy in the garden, 'with the idea that it was assisting the groom'.[35] The employment of male patients in the vegetable garden hints at the ethos of economy and self-sufficiency outlined earlier. Nonetheless, as will be seen, far more attention was paid to occupying Bloomfield patients at recreational pursuits, suggesting that distraction rather than economy was the principal regime for patients at this asylum.

Despite improvements in providing occupational therapy during this period, Bloomfield's managing committee was still concerned with how best to occupy patients. Bloomfield's visiting physician, Dr. Valentine Duke, wrote in his 1863 report of his difficulties in engaging patients in employment, which he argued were 'increased rather than diminished, as the patient occupies a higher position in the social scale'.[36] In later reports, Duke juxtaposed the industry witnessed in district asylums with the relatively poor output of Bloomfield's patients:

> In those Asylums intended specially for the accommodation of the work-ing classes, the entire range of manual and mechanical employment can be called into aid, but with us these are scarcely, if at all available: a little car-pentry, some painting and working in the garden and grounds, being all we can adopt.[37]

Duke elaborated the following year:

> For farming or other rural employment our resources are but limited, and the general sphere of life, and antecedents of the greater number of our patients, would render mere manual labour an unsuitable and inadequate occupation. We must therefore seek other resources.[38]

In fact, in that year, two patients had angrily objected to the notion that they might assist in the garden moulding cabbage plants. When Stanley asked Joseph R., to do so, Joseph retorted that 'he was not of that trade and wouldn't do anything of the kind'.[39] A month later, Stanley asked former grocer David S., to perform the same task and 'at first he declined saying his dignity would be reduced if seen in my [Stanley's] company'. However, he eventually agreed to work in the garden, albeit for 'a short time'.[40] This mirrors the behaviour of non-pauper patients at the Morningside asylum in Scotland, where a sense of social superiority was common and posed challenges for asylum authorities.[41]

By the 1890s, Stewarts' managing committee was also commenting on the complexities they faced in this regard. This committee, however, did not appear worried, reporting that 'an excellent dietary, pure air, cheerful associations, and such entertainment as can be provided … are powerful factors in bringing about recoveries'.[42] Case notes for Stewarts' patients contain few specific examples of patients actually carrying out work. As was the norm for patients in nineteenth-century asylums, those who did work were employed largely in line with traditional gender roles.[43] Reports of female employment detailed needlework, sewing and 'household work',[44] though these occupations might equally be deemed as recreational activities for wealthier female patients. For example, at Staffordshire asylum in England, first-class women 'knitted and sewed for pleasure' rather than work.[45] Stewarts' medical superintendent, Frederick

E. Rainsford, stressed the gendered divisions of patient labour when he wrote of Eliza Edith A., making 'senseless requests such as being allowed to work on the farm'.[46] Like patients in Enniscorthy and Carlow,[47] Stewarts' patients also engaged in housework.[48] However, male patients employed indoors tended to undertake 'masculine' activities such as working with the carpenter, in the engine room at 'various mechanical works' or raking gravel. Notably, patients carrying out these jobs were paying lower fees of £50 or £60 per annum, suggesting that those who paid higher rates were not expected to carry out manual labour.[49] It is highly unlikely that wealthier patients who did not work in civilian life were employed in asylums.[50]

This is corroborated by an exploration of the case notes for Hampstead and Highfield patients. There is no record whatsoever of Hampstead's exclusively male patients carrying out any work. Similarly, Highfield's all-female patient population seemed to engage in very little housework. While Lucy D., 'did some serving', she reportedly showed 'very little enthusiasm for her work'.[51] Another patient, Kate L., 'did some needlework' and was 'useful in the house and garden' but she also 'read steadily' and was able 'to play a good game of whist'.[52] Yet, at the less expensive St John of God's, patients were strongly encouraged to work. Several worked in the laundry, the poultry yard, the linen room, peeled fruit and vegetables in the kitchen, cleaned and dusted the 'cells', the refectory and the 'agitated division' and one patient polished his boots, a task which he reportedly insisted on doing himself.[53] Michael D. was said to be outstandingly helpful and assisted in looking after his fellow patients:

> is always most willing to do light jobs of work and to assist old and feeble patients... he always dusts the furniture in the day-room after the floor has been swept... He makes himself useful especially in leading Mr G to and from the refectory etc... He also goes to the agitated division at times to play the piano for the patients in it.[54]

These accounts suggest that the patients in St John of God's were willing to assist in the running of the asylum. One patient, Joseph H., was 'perpetually insisting on looking for work and will steal away to some part of the House and fuss there. When not given work to do, he will go out in the garden and fist up grass blades growing in the walks'.[55] The relatively industrious characters of Richmond and Enniscorthy district asylums and

St John of God's, compared with Bloomfield, Hampstead and Highfield, suggest that work therapy was very much an occupation for less wealthy asylum patients.

RECREATIONAL ACTIVITIES

Given the strong emphasis on productive occupation in the district asylums, it is, perhaps, unsurprising that paying patients there had less time to engage in amusements. Recreational pursuits in district asylums were often limited as overcrowding resulted in the conversion of dayrooms and exercise yards into dormitories.[56] In relation to recreational activities, there are very few accounts of district asylum paying patients doing anything more than reading or playing cards.[57] At Richmond, there is an isolated reference to one female paying patient playing the piano.[58] While another patient, Frances N., would 'do no work of any kind', when she informed a medical officer that she had won prizes for some of her paintings at various exhibitions, she was 'supplied with paints & c but she is unable to fix her attention so as to produce a picture. What she paints one day she spoils it the next'.[59] In addition, the hospital grounds at Richmond were open to patients every day and sports, picnics and entertainments were sometimes organised.

In more expensive asylums, patients were encouraged to occupy themselves in a wide range of amusements and entertainments. Comparably wide-ranging activities were on offer to patients at the Crichton Royal Asylum in Dumfries, where the superintendent, William Alexander Francis Browne (1837–1857), 'devoted enormous energy and ingenuity to the moral discipline and treatment of his charges'. Browne was concerned with restoring his well-to-do patients to sanity and later confessed that activities such as these combated the monotony of asylum life.[60] Annual reports and case notes for Bloomfield and Stewarts patients abound with evidence that recreation, rather than work, was considered a vital part of the therapeutic regime in voluntary asylums. In 1863, Duke alluded to the reasoning behind this. While he highlighted the difficulties inherent in finding socially appropriate employment for Bloomfield's patients, Duke opined that:

It is not possible to compel the mind which has been educated, and accustomed to activity either to rest completely, or remain idle. Mental repose cannot be insisted on, there is no forcing the intellectual faculties to lie fallow.

Duke therefore stressed the importance of creating sufficient 'diversion of thought, and to secure a healthy interest in surrounding objects'. He counted among the most useful 'party evenings', when patients could 'enter into the spirit of the scene, enjoying the presence of strangers, performances of music, acting of characters, &c.' and pronounced himself gratified 'to think that their happiness is even temporarily prompted by inducing a forgetfulness of self'.[61] Party evenings, dances and other evening entertainments became a frequent element of voluntary and private asylum life. However, the gaiety of such evenings could be disrupted by patients, as is evidenced by the report on St John of God's patient, Richard A.P., who, at an evening entertainment, became 'quite excited' and required 'four men to remove him from the recreation hall'.[62]

From the 1880s, Pim detailed the recreations on offer at Stewarts, which were promoted in the asylum's annual report. These included the availability of daily papers, books from a lending library, books and periodicals donated 'from some of our kind friends', a billiard table which was 'a great source of amusement to those who can play' and a piano 'for the ladies, many of whom are very good performers'.[63] The woods and pleasure grounds were continuously being enlarged and additional walks were constructed by male former pupils of the imbecile branch, who were engaged in gathering fallen leaves and digging.[64] In the summer of 1898, Stewarts organised carriage drives for patients to 'places of interest'.[65] During the winter months, various forms of indoor entertainment were adopted, including 'magic lantern exhibitions, conjuring, cinematography, Punch and Judy, Concerts, & c'.[66] Stewarts' managing committee was keen to point out the benefits of the asylum's small population and attractive location. Overcrowding was guarded against, while the grounds were said to be 'fully taken advantage of for recreative [sic] purposes'.[67]

Physicians writing case notes on Stewarts' patients in the 1890s took care to note the sorts of amusements they enjoyed. Frederick James H., took an 'interest in books and reads a good deal', while Maude Frances C., could 'enjoy a dance'.[68] H.P., an architect, 'employed himself making architectural drawings and worked with neatness and precision'.[69] Several attempts were also made to occupy patient Henry Richard Q., a professor of music. In the asylum, he played his 'harmonium a little'. Sadly, however, the professor, who had been diagnosed with 'senile decay', was unable to enjoy his music:

> Tried American Organ in Dining Hall yesterday but could make very little of it owing to the weak state of his legs being unable to work the bellows ... Attends Divine Service, attempts to sing gets out of time and loses his place.[70]

During the 1890s, Bloomfield's patients were kept busy with games, outings, visits, reading and various other amusements. Among references to amusement in the case notes, Joshua L.W., was allowed to take 'tea in the parlour with his sisters', William G., 'reads the papers, plays chess, ball, croquet, and such like' and Henry Jacob H., spent 'a good deal of time painting or drawing various things about the place'.[71] Patients also went out for drives, played billiards, walked in the garden, smoked, played the piano, read books, spent a month at the seaside, sewed, knitted and played 'Haluna'.[72]

Patient amusements at St John of God's were less varied. In this asylum, patients read newspapers, played cards, chess or billiards, the violin and piano, walked in the garden, or went on country walks.[73] Some patients also pursued their own pastimes. Frederick K., was reportedly 'fond of postage stamps and ... glad to get some ... he amuses himself at times by pasting old postage stamps into an old Dublin City directory'.[74] Thomas K., was 'fond of being out of doors hunting rats or shooting', while James M., amused himself caring for a parrot.[75] Recreation was clearly important at St John of God's though. In the early twentieth century, additional arrangements were made including the establishment of a library in 1904 and a handball court a few years later.[76] At Hampstead during the 1890s, frequent references were made to recreation in the casebooks, where patients played chess, cards, draughts, billiards, croquet, tennis, walked on the farm, cycled, played handball, had long walks and 'carriage exercise', read novels and newspapers, and watched cricket, tennis and football matches.[77] It is important to note, however, that patients were not always willing to engage in recreational activities. For example, John Neilson Eustace wrote that Palms S.M., an army lieutenant, sometimes had 'to be stimulated to walk as far as the garden but the sight of the wheelbarrow to wheel him in is usually enough of a stimulus!'[78]

Given the more common characterisations of asylum life as ordered, monotonous and isolating,[79] the degree of freedom accorded to voluntary and private asylum patients was refreshingly large. In the Staffordshire asylum in England, freedom to go beyond the asylum complex 'was a prerogative of wealth' and patients visited a dairy farm, the theatre, relatives and the seaside.[80] In keeping with the practice at the York Retreat,[81] in Irish voluntary and private asylums, carriage drives and day trips were organised for those considered suitable to attend. For example, in 1864, Stanley accompanied three of the male patients to the Botanic Gardens and Glasnevin Cemetery in Dublin, where they visited Daniel O'Connell's tomb.[82] Voluntary asylum patients were also allowed to walk outside the grounds of the institution, sometimes unattended. In addition, other excursions were organised from the 1860s, including visits to 'popular exhibits, to launches, reviews, &c.'.[83] In some cases, patients chose their own entertainment. When Bloomfield patients William G., and James H., saw an advertisement for the Christy Minstrel's concert at the Rotunda Lying-In Hospital in Dublin, they sought permission from Bloomfield's superintendent, Mary Pryor, to attend, which they were granted and went in the charge of two attendants. They later told Stanley that 'they were particularly pleased that it was a rich treat and that the singing was performed with good taste and ability'.[84]

This substantial liberty was also accorded to private asylum patients. In August 1908, a party of thirty, comprised of St John of God's patients and attendants, went for a picnic to the Glen of the Downs, County Wicklow, while patients in that asylum were permitted to go on country drives, walks, excursions and picnics.[85] Highfield patient, Elizabeth B.P., attended two garden parties where she played croquet.[86] Fellow patient, Christina McF.S., went to the Gaiety theatre in Dublin 'several times since admission in company with her husband & always conducted herself in a perfectly rational manner' and was allowed home for Christmas.[87] At Hampstead, Mosley C.S., an army captain, was granted parole to attend entertainment in town accompanied by an attendant. He visited the Zoological Gardens and the Botanic Gardens in Dublin. These visits reflected Mosley's keen interest in botany; he was said to spend 'most of his days walking about observing farm and garden interests' and 'gathered and refined special garden seeds' for John Neilson Eustace.[88] Eustace also had a house in the seaside town of Killiney and patients sometimes stayed there in the summer.[89]

Just as the dangers of patients working in district asylums could bring about further disruption,[90] allowing patients to leave the asylum did not always go to plan. Robert P., a Hampstead patient diagnosed with alcoholic insanity, frequently went into town and to the theatre. On these occasions, he was accompanied by an attendant partly on account of his alcoholic tendencies and partly due to his nervousness at venturing far alone. His liberty was eventually reduced when 'it was suspected that patient has been taking some drink on his visits to Dublin'.[91] At St John of God's, O'Connell did not always support his patients' liberty. In 1905, he wrote of patient James M.:

> In the intervals between his attacks he goes about far too much. I do not understand why he is permitted to go where he pleases and when he pleases ... He has taken to motor driving during the past six months and goes out too much for his good. Motor driving is far too exciting for him and to this I attribute the frequent recurrence of his attacks. He should be kept under more restraint – confined more to the grounds.[92]

In spite of the enhanced sense of liberty among voluntary and private asylum patients, these excursions were not always dignified or enjoyable. When Maria Jane E.T., was taken along with other Stewarts' patients to a picnic in Howth, she became quite excited, 'kept screaming out "go away", "don't annoy me", when no one was near her, spitting all round her &c'.[93] When Joshua S.B., was taken to the park to see a royal visit, he 'wanted to throw stones at King's horses', believing he was ordered to.[94] These examples illustrate that, contrary to the positive tone of annual reports for voluntary asylums, which championed patients' excursions, the reality of providing recreational activities for asylum patients was often more challenging.

CONCLUSIONS

Moral therapy remained the dominant ideological framework for treating insanity throughout much of the nineteenth century. Although this framework was initially developed for patients at the York Retreat private asylum, it met with challenges both at York[95] and for asylums caring for Irish paying patients. The key issue was to find class-appropriate occupations for those who had not engaged in manual work in the outside world. While asylum doctors placed emphasis on employing paying patients, those who had not worked prior to committal were not forced to do so. Nor were patients who refused to work punished, but instead they were encouraged to distract themselves in other ways. In the asylums studied, there is evidence that asylum doctors allowed patients to engage in pursuits they enjoyed, even when these might be considered meaningless. For wealthier patients, amusements provided an alternative means of occupation. Providing patients with suitable distractions therefore overtook institutional economy or self-sufficiency as the principal regime for fee-paying patients.

NOTES

1. Digby (1985, pp. 42–49), Cherry (2003, pp. 53–81). See also Cherry and Munting (2005, pp. 42–58).
2. Digby (1985, pp. 57–104). See also Scull (1982).
3. Tuke (1813).
4. Digby (1985, pp. 34, 42).
5. Ibid.
6. Ibid.
7. Cox (2012, p. 156).
8. Digby (1983, p. 63; 1985, p. 42).
9. Wynter (2010, p. 47).
10. Finnane (1981, pp. 134–135).
11. Cherry (2003, pp. 59, 80), Andrews (1991, p. 75). See also Cherry and Munting (2005, pp. 42–58). For the Irish context, see Cox (2012, pp. 212–216).
12. Cherry (2003, pp. 59, 80).
13. Clinical Record Volume No. 5 (WCC, St Senan's Hospital, Enniscorthy, p. 369).
14. Clinical Record Volume No. 4 (WCC, St Senan's Hospital, Enniscorthy, p. 4).
15. Clinical Record Volume No. 7 (WCC, St Senan's Hospital, Enniscorthy, p. 182); Clinical Record Volume No. 5 (WCC, St Senan's Hospital, Enniscorthy, p. 186).
16. Clinical Record Volume No. 3 (WCC, St Senan's Hospital, Enniscorthy, p. 336).
17. Male Case Book, 1887–1888 (GM, Grangegorman Records, p. 142).
18. Male Case Book, 1891–1892 (GM, Grangegorman Records, pp. 181–183); Male Case Book, 1898 (GM, Grangegorman Records, p. 618).
19. Cherry (2003, p. 65); Cherry and Munting (2005, p. 45).
20. Casebook Two (SJOGH, Patient Records, p. 11).

21. Ibid., p. 348.
22. Ibid., p. 30.
23. Ibid., p. 38.
24. Ibid., p. 41.
25. Ibid., p. 2.
26. Cox (2012, p. 156). See also Melling and Forsythe (2006, p. 192).
27. Male Case Book, 1900–1901 (GM, Grangegorman Records, p. 335).
28. Male Case Book, 1898 (GM, Grangegorman Records, p. 194); Male Case Book, 1899–1900 (GM, Grangegorman Records, pp. 184, 956, 959).
29. *Annual Report of the State of the Retreat* (Dublin, 1836), p. 5.
30. *Annual Report of the State of the Retreat* (Dublin, 1839), p. 7.
31. *Annual Report of the State of the Retreat* (Dublin, 1850), p. 5.
32. *Annual Report of the State of the Retreat* (Dublin, 1852), p. 8.
33. *Annual Report of the State of the Retreat* (Dublin, 1860), p. 6.
34. Edward Hyde, Notice of Particulars (FHL, Bloomfield Records).
35. Ibid., 1 Oct. 1862, 8 Oct. 1862.
36. *Annual Report of the State of the Retreat* (Dublin, 1863), p. 9.
37. *Annual Report of the State of the Retreat* (Dublin, 1866), p. 9.
38. *Annual Report of the State of the Retreat* (Dublin, 1867), p. 8.
39. Edward Hyde, Notice of Particulars (FHL, Bloomfield Records, 28 May 1864).
40. Ibid., 29 Jun. 1864.
41. Beveridge, 1998, p. 50.
42. *The Stewart Institution and Asylum Report* (Dublin, 1897), p. 21.
43. See Showalter (1986, p. 82), Cherry (2003, pp. 61, 67), Busfield (1994, pp. 259–277). For the Irish context, see Cox (2012, p. 212), McCarthy (2004, p. 132).
44. Case Book 1889–1900 (Stewarts, Patient Records, pp. 32, 149, 97).
45. Wynter (2010, p. 47).
46. Case Book 1889–1900 (Stewarts, Patient Records, p. 71).
47. Cox (2012, p. 212).
48. Case Book 1889–1900 (Stewarts, Patient Records, pp. 57, 103).
49. Ibid., pp. 110, 64.
50. Wynter has made this argument about first and second-class women at Staffordshire: (Wynter 2010, p. 46).
51. Highfield Casebook (Highfield Hospital Group, Hampstead and Highfield Records, p. 31).
52. Ibid., p. 41.
53. Casebook Two (SJOGH, Patient Records, pp. 2, 18, 25, 28).
54. Ibid., p. 12.
55. Ibid., p. 71.
56. Cox (2012, p. 214).

57. Clinical Record Volume No. 3 (WCC, St Senan's Hospital, Enniscorthy, pp. 212, 420); Clinical Record Volume No. 6 (WCC, St Senan's Hospital, Enniscorthy, p. 407); Male Case Book, 1887–1888 (GM, Grangegorman Records, p. 202); Male Case Book, 1890–1891 (GM, Grangegorman Records, p. 158); Clinical Record Volume No. 3 (WCC, St Senan's Hospital, Enniscorthy, p. 4); Clinical Record Volume No. 5 (WCC, St Senan's Hospital, Enniscorthy, p. 190).

58. Female Case Book 1895–1897 (GM, Richmond District Lunatic Asylum, p. 168).

59. Female Case Book, 1891–1892 (GM, Grangegorman Records, p. 459).

60. Scull (1993, p. 296).

61. *Annual Report of the State of the Retreat* (Dublin 1863), pp. 9–10.

62. Casebook Two (SJOGH, Patient Records, p. 63).

63. *The Stewart Institution and Asylum Report* (Dublin, 1884), p. 20, *The Stewart Institution and Asylum Report* (Dublin, 1887), p. 22, *The Stewart Institution and Asylum Report* (Dublin, 1889), p. 21, *The Stewart Institution and Asylum Report* (Dublin, 1894), p. 25.

64. *The Stewart Institution and Asylum Report* (Dublin 1890), p. 21. *The Stewart Institution and Asylum Report* (Dublin, 1891), p. 22.

65. *The Stewart Institution and Asylum Report* (Dublin 1898), p. 25. Carriage drives were also organised for patients at St Patrick's Hospital, see Malcolm, 1989, p. 161.

66. *The Stewart Institution and Asylum Report* (Dublin 1899), p. 24.

67. *The Stewart Institution and Asylum Report* (Dublin 1894), p. 24; *The Stewart Institution and Asylum Report* (Dublin, 1900), p. 19.

68. Case Book 1889–1900 (Stewarts, Patient Records, pp. 150, 156).

69. Edward Hyde, Notice of Particulars (FHL, Bloomfield Records, 21 Dec. 1864).

70. Case Book 1889–1900 (Stewarts, Patient Records, p. 144).

71. Case Book (FHL, Bloomfield Records, pp. 9, 19, 61).

72. For example, Case Book (FHL, Bloomfield Records, pp. 7, 14, 16, 22, 31, 45).

73. Casebook Two (SJOGH, Patient Records, pp. 1, 328, 5, 7, 11, 12,42, 19, 32, 39).

74. Ibid., p. 7.

75. Ibid., pp. 27, 16.

76. Ibid., pp. 27, 29.

77. Hampstead Casebook 1890s (Highfield Hospital Group, Hampstead and Highfield Records, pp. 2, 6, 3, 10, 32, 17, 12, 13, 33, 56).

78. Ibid., p. 3.

79. See for example Reynolds (1992, p. 179), Cox (2012, pp. 195–239). For the Scottish context see Beveridge (1992), pp. 438, 440–441.

80. Wynter (2010, p. 46).
81. Digby (1985, p. 46).
82. Edward Hyde, Notice of Particulars (FHL, Bloomfield Records, 16 May 1864).
83. *Annual Report of the State of the Retreat* (Dublin 1867), p. 14.
84. Edward Hyde, Notice of Particulars (FHL, Bloomfield Records, 23 Nov. 1864). In the English context, Rob Ellis has argued that local townspeople displayed hostility at Epsom county asylum patients' excursions. Ellis (2013).
85. Casebook Two (SJOGH, Patient Records, pp. 25, 53, 19).
86. Highfield Casebook (Highfield Hospital Group, Hampstead and Highfield Records, p. 51).
87. Ibid., p. 21.
88. Hampstead Casebook 1890s (Highfield Hospital Group, Hampstead and Highfield Records, p. 6).
89. Ibid., pp. 3, 10.
90. Cox (2012, p. 213).
91. Hampstead Casebook 1890s (Highfield Hospital Group, Hampstead and Highfield Records, p. 8).
92. Casebook Two (SJOGH, Patient Records, p. 3).
93. Case Book 1889–1900 (Stewarts, Patient Records, p. 38).
94. Ibid., p. 25.
95. Digby (1983, pp. 63, 1985, 42).

REFERENCES

Andrews, Jonathan. 'Hardly a Hospital, But Charity for Pauper Lunatics?' In *Medicine and Charity before the Welfare State*, edited by Jonathan Barry and Colin Jones, 63–81. London: Routledge, 1991.

Beveridge, Allan. 'Life in the Asylum: Patient's Letters from Morningside, 1873–1908.' *History of Psychiatry* 9 (1998): 431–469.

Busfield, Joan. 'The Female Malady? Men, Women and Madness in Nineteenth-Century Britain.' In *Sociology* 27, no. 1 (1994): 259–277.

Cherry, Steven. *Mental Healthcare in Modern England: The Norfolk Lunatic Asylum/St Andrew's Hospital circa 1810–1998*. Suffolk: The Boydell Press, 2003.

Cherry, Steven and Munting, Roger. '"Exercise is the Thing"? Sport and the Asylum c. 1850–1950.' *The International Journal of the History of Sport* 22, no. 1 (2005): 42–58.

Cox, Catherine. *Negotiating Insanity in the Southeast of Ireland 1830–1900*. Manchester: Manchester University Press, 2012.

Digby, Anne. 'Moral Treatment at the Retreat 1796–1846.' In *The Anatomy of Madness: Essays in The History of Psychiatry Vol. II: Institutions and Society*, edited by W. F. Bynum, Roy Porter and Michael Shepherd, 52–72. London and New York: Tavistock, 1983.

Digby, Anne. *Madness, Morality and Medicine: A Study of the York Retreat, 1796–1914*. Cambridge: Cambridge University Press, 1985.

Ellis, Rob. '"A constant irritation to the townspeople"?: Local, Regional and National Politics and London's County Asylums at Epsom.' *Social History of Medicine* 26, no. 4 (2013): 653–667.

Finnane, Mark. *Insanity and the Insane in Post-Famine Ireland*. London: Croom Helm, 1981.

McCarthy, Áine. 'Hearths, Bodies and Minds: Gender Ideology and Women's Committal to Enniscorthy Lunatic Asylum, 1916–1925.' In *Irish Women's History*, edited by Alan Hayes and Diane Urquhart, 115–136. Dublin: Irish Academic Press, 2004.

Melling, Joseph and Bill Forsythe. *The Politics of Madness: The State, Insanity and Society in England, 1845–14*. London and New York: Routledge, 2006.

Reynolds, Joseph. *Grangegorman: Psychiatric Care in Dublin Since 1815*. Dublin: Institute of Public Administration, 1992.

Scull, Andrew. *Museums of Madness: The Social Organisation of Insanity in Nineteenth-Century England*. Harmondsworth: Penguin, 1982.

Scull, Andrew. *The Most Solitary of Afflictions: Madness and Society in Britain, 1700–1900*. New Haven: Yale University Press, 1993.

Showalter, Elaine. *The Female Malady: Women Madness and Culture in England, 1830–1980*. New York, Pantheon Book, 1986.

Tuke, Samuel. *Description of the Retreat: An Institution near York for Insane Persons of the Society of Friends*. York: W. Alexander, 1813.

Wynter, Rebecca. 'Good in all Respects: Appearance and Dress at Staffordshire County Lunatic Asylum, 1818–1854.' *History of Psychiatry* 22, no. 1 (2010): 40–57.

CHAPTER 7

Respect and Respectability: The Treatment and Expectations of Fee-Paying Patients

In addition to providing class- and gender-appropriate occupations and amusements, proponents of moral therapy preached the benefits of maintaining harmonious surroundings. Yet, rising patient numbers and the consequent need for expanded facilities could greatly disrupt moral therapy.[1] While moral therapy was used in Irish district asylums, the late nineteenth century has been characterised as an era of therapeutic pessimism for asylum doctors, due to the ever-rising and accumulating numbers of chronic or 'incurable' patients in the system.[2] In modest-sized and large district asylums, financial and management problems impacted negatively on patient care.[3]

As a counterpoint, this chapter considers whether smaller, sometimes underfilled voluntary and private asylums were better equipped to provide moral therapy into the late nineteenth century, exploring the treatment and expectations of paying patients in the public, voluntary and private sectors. In her discussion of district asylums, Cox has argued that the language of social class and difference partly constructed the space between patients and staff.[4] In the Scottish context, Beveridge has found that social class created tensions between patients and staff and between patients themselves.[5] This chapter engages with these findings, by exploring the extent to which paying patients' expectations of asylum care were informed by their social status and class identity.

As Chap. 2 discussed, district asylum doctors and the lunacy inspectors were apprehensive about mixing paying and pauper patients in district asylums. Despite the Privy Council's decision to restrict paying patients to the same rules, regulations and treatment as the pauper

© The Author(s) 2018
A. Mauger, *The Cost of Insanity in Nineteenth-Century Ireland*, Mental Health in Historical Perspective,
https://doi.org/10.1007/978-3-319-65244-3_7

patients, there was clearly an expectation of more class-appropriate care based on their social standing. This included receiving food to which they were accustomed and privacy from the pauper patients with whom they were compelled to reside. Despite concerns to limit jealousies between paying and pauper patients, differences in social class and status resulted in tensions. Many paying patients, anxious to reassert their respectability, expressed unease about their pauper cohabitants' social origins.[6] Moreover, the social and political upheaval in Ireland resulted in religious and political divisions between patients. In contrast, the payment of higher maintenance fees at voluntary and private asylums translated into more class-appropriate accommodation and treatment, while the wealthiest patients could expect separate lodgings and special attendants. In these institutions, problems surrounding class, religion and politics were far less common, probably due to the segregation of patients from different social backgrounds.

As this chapter argues, while wealthier patients expected to be treated with 'respect', their carers anticipated certain standards of 'respectable' behaviour in return. This is evidenced in the case notes, where asylum doctors frequently commented on patients' violent behaviour, manners, dress and appearance. These considerations were influenced by not only the doctrines of moral therapy but also the physician's own understanding of class identity and social status. Notably, although voluntary and private asylums provided care tailored to social class, in line with other asylum populations, social decorum in these institutions was compromised by a surprisingly high level of violence among their more privileged clientele.[7]

EXPECTATIONS OF CARE

To assess patients' expectations of institutionalisation effectively, it is first necessary to contextualise their treatment. Studies of the treatment employed in Irish district asylums trace the decline of moral therapy throughout the nineteenth century and the eventual gloom that replaced this ideal towards the century's close. Resulting from the growing involvement of the medical community in district asylums, from the 1830s more 'medical' systems of treatment were adopted.[8] Of the asylums studied here, Bloomfield had the strongest association with moral treatment because it was modelled on the York Retreat. From the outset, the committee which established Bloomfield 'solicited direct assistance' from the founder of the York Retreat, William Tuke, who was consulted on the construction of an addition to the existing premises and even asked to interview a candidate for superintendent.[9] Although physical treatments, including leeching and the administering of emetics, were very much a part of Bloomfield's early regime of care, moral therapy came to play an increasing role.[10] Relatively little is known of the early therapeutic regimes at Hampstead, although it is plausible that the asylum's founders, all medical men, shared similar optimism about the potential of medicine to 'cure' insanity, at least initially. This contrasts with the first district asylums, which were inspired by the ideology of moral treatment and managed by laymen who fashioned themselves as 'moral governors'.[11]

By the late nineteenth century, some resident medical superintendents, including Richmond's Lalor (superintendent, 1857–1883) and his successor, Norman (superintendent, 1886–1908), took steps to reinforce the provision of moral treatment. By the 1890s, Norman, who unsuccessfully advocated the 'boarding out' of patients in the community, also increased occupational activity for patients and opened workshops for them.[12] As we have seen, the grounds at Richmond were open to patients every day where sports, picnics and entertainments were organised.[13] These principles in many ways reflected what had long been the norm in voluntary asylums like Bloomfield and Stewarts, or private asylums such as Hampstead House and Highfield House. Contrary to the overcrowded and unsanitary conditions in late nineteenth-century Richmond, smaller voluntary and private asylums benefited from lower patient numbers and more spacious arrangements. Obviously aware of this, Bloomfield's visiting physician, Dr. Valentine Duke, stated in 1862, that the advantages of moral treatment:

> can be better experienced in a well conducted asylum of moderate extent, partaking in the domestic arrangements a good deal of a private family, than in some of those very large public establishments which number their patients by hundreds.[14]

Stewarts, meanwhile, was sometimes underfilled and reported space to accommodate more patients. In 1881, the asylum, which could accommodate up to 120 patients, contained only eighty-two.[15]

During the 1860s, Duke also made numerous recommendations for improved medical treatments, including the erection of a Turkish bath and procurement of seaside lodgings. Duke framed his suggestions with the medical benefits they would bestow, demonstrating a growing emphasis on physical rather than moral treatment.[16] In this era, small tensions arose between the asylum's non-medical and medical staff over the most effective forms of treatment. When the visiting surgeon applied leeches to a patient's head, Bloomfield's house steward, Stanley wrote: 'the leeching made it appears to me, no improvement whatever in him'.[17] The following day, when Duke gave 'four powders' to the patient and produced blisters on his temples, Stanley again protested 'but all have proved useless and he appears to be beyond the reach of human skill'.[18] Stanley had his own views on what constituted useful therapies for male patients. He was a keen proponent of outdoor exercise and introduced 'football recreation', which he actively participated in almost every afternoon.[19] Stanley also frequently remonstrated with elderly patients in a bid to encourage them to go out in the fresh air. Despite any tensions between Stanley and Duke, Bloomfield's managing committee took Duke's recommendations seriously. Stanley later reported that three of the male patients had taken Turkish baths, that 'they seem to have enjoyed them' and that one patient 'thinks they may likely benefit his health'.[20] Meanwhile, lodgings were taken in the summer at the seaside town of Bray for some female patients 'whose state of health indicated the want of such a change'. The committee were impressed by these outcomes, reporting that 'the salutary result has satisfied us of its advantage', and patients continued to be sent to Bray throughout the nineteenth century.[21]

The blending of moral and physical principles of treatment at Bloomfield demonstrates the complexities of therapeutic programmes for the insane. Just as individual district asylums were influenced by the ideologies and character of the physicians who presided over them,[22] voluntary and private asylum doctors had the authority to promote a change of regime. Overall, however, ever-rising patient numbers in district asylums such as Richmond frustrated the attempts of even the most innovative asylum physician, who was often powerless to treat anything more than physical illnesses.[23]

Treatment was also influenced by the amounts spent on care. In voluntary and private asylums, patients kept at the highest sums could expect larger, even separate, living quarters, higher quality clothing and a special attendant. As such, voluntary and private asylums tailored accommodation to suit patients from wealthy backgrounds. In the

1890s, Stewarts patient, Isabella McE, a fifty-two-year-old widow who had previously been a patient at the Derry district asylum, was initially maintained at £50 per annum. While at Stewarts, she accused the RMS, Rainsford, 'daily of robbing her. Says I get millions sent for her, that hampers of wine and game come for her every morning which matron and I appropriate, that her food is poisoned &c'. She was later 'much pleased' when her maintenance fees were raised and she was transferred to her own separate bedroom.[24] In contrast, Beatrice Katherine Q., who accused Rainsford of 'having stolen her money and spent it on women', was removed to an ordinary room after her fees were reduced from £100 to £60 per annum, presumably after a shift in her financial circumstances.[25] After John Charles B. became a Chancery patient, he was moved to a separate bedroom and dined in the 'better dining room'.[26]

The same applied at Bloomfield. In the 1890s, when William R. began to masturbate publicly, he was repeatedly restrained in a straitjacket. Several attempts were made 'to do without his jacket' including the application of 'a lighter jacket with straps round arms' but this did not restrain him from masturbating and a few months later he began 'taking his clothes off on the grounds and exposing his person'. The following year he was still wearing the jacket when in the garden. On another trial without it, he began to throw stones over the garden wall and 'annoyed the neighbours'. A month later, the reporting physician commented:

> He has been wearing his jacket while in the garden lately. Unless a man were constantly to stand by him it is not possible to check him suddenly exposing his person, or throwing stones ... over the wall and as he only pays a small sum per annum, we cannot give him a special attendant.

This suggests that had William been maintained at a higher sum, he might have been under the care of a special attendant rather than in restraints. William, who had been admitted to Bloomfield in 1850, was then maintained at £31 per annum. There is no record of his maintenance fee being raised but, by the 1890s, the 'small sum' paid towards his maintenance probably put him at the lower end of the fee scale at Bloomfield.[27]

In district asylums, paying patients' experiences were shaped by the Privy Council rules as they were subject to the same treatment as pauper patients. This meant that the amount paid towards patients' maintenance had very little impact on their treatment. Nonetheless, some paying patients and their relatives and friends expected superior treatment, particularly at Richmond. According to one medical officer, Thomas D., a pensioner patient from the Dublin Metropolitan Police was 'constantly asking for special extras ... there is a general tendency to the expression of a sense of superiority'.[28] Families and friends could also intervene. When Daniel McK's son, who contributed £26 per annum for his father's maintenance, wrote to the board of governors 'requesting that he may be allowed to wear his own clothes', the board refused, insisting that Daniel should 'wear clothes of institution'.[29] A family friend of another paying patient, Daniel N., stressed that the patient was 'respectably connected' and requested 'that he be separated from ordinary lunatics and no expense spared for his benefit'.[30]

Notwithstanding these expectations, the lunacy inspectors strictly upheld the Privy Council's guidelines. In 1891, the Office of Lunatic Asylums wrote to Ennis asylum:

> Referring to a passage in the Auditors report in which he states that there are three patients in the asylum whose friends contribute in excess of the average cost, and receive for such payment more indulgences as to Food and clothing than other cases – I am directed by the Inspectors to request you will report the facts of these cases to them.[31]

While the asylum board's response is not documented, a subsequent letter from the Office drew the board's attention to the Privy Council rules and to the auditor's report that had identified the problem.[32] These letters indicate that the Office sought to guard against the preferential treatment of paying patients and did not tolerate it.

Dietary became a key area of difficulty in the treatment of paying patients in district asylums. In the nineteenth century, this was an important element of asylum therapeutics and for most patients, the aim was to improve nutritional intake.[33] Good feeding was considered essential for the recovery of mental health to a physically healthy body.[34] This emulated the beliefs of the physician superintendent at the Royal Edinburgh Asylum, Dr. Thomas Clouston (1873–1908), that stoutness was conducive to mental health and his development of a 'Gospel of Fatness' which involved the feeding up of patients.[35] In Ireland, the lunacy inspectors were keen that asylum dietaries resemble those of the patients outside the asylum, hoping that it would help them to acclimatise to asylum life.[36] However, in keeping with the concerns expressed by a number of medical superintendents at the 1857–1858 commission, and later criticisms of the Trench commission (see Chap. 2), several paying patients, especially those from more affluent backgrounds and accustomed to a better standard of living, were given an inferior diet to what they ate at home. In fact, there is no record that paying patients in this study were given food other than the standard asylum dietary. The only extra reportedly supplied to paying patients was alcohol. Although often used for medicinal purposes, in Enniscorthy the prescription of alcohol appeared in a few cases to be more of a small indulgence on the part of the RMS. Anne J. would not eat but said she would drink some 'alter wine'. In an attempt to compromise, the RMS procured some port wine, but Anne refused to take it. Later on, it was noted that Anne 'likes a drop of punch' and she was given whiskey and later poitín.[37] Similarly, when Teresa C. wished 'for a little bitter in evening', she was given '3 oz of bitter extra'.[38]

Although some paying patients, such as Mary E. at Richmond, complimented the diet they were given—'says ... she gets a beautiful dinner every day'—most paying patients' responses to their food were negative.[39] Suggesting their unease at being given a pauper patient's dietary, paying patients complained about both the quality and quantity of the food they received. This is in direct contrast to patients at the Royal Edinburgh asylum, for whom the emphasis on hearty eating was a focus of resentment.[40] At Richmond, Mary B., whose relatives paid over £29 per annum for her maintenance, was 'very dissatisfied with her dinner' and was later discharged to a private asylum.[41] Frances N., whose maintenance was over £24 per annum, had previously been a patient at St Patrick's. While at Richmond, Frances was 'continually asking to be sent home, and complains bitterly of the arrangements, feeding ect [sic] in this place and compares her life now to the life of luxury she had before she came in'.[42] John H., meanwhile, said that 'he is happy that his appetite is good but he does not get enough to eat'.[43] At Enniscorthy, Anne J. had delusions that 'those around her mean to starve her'.[44]

Those who complained about the quantity of their meals were often characterised by the medical staff as greedy or having abnormally large appetites. At Richmond, Catherine C., who was contributing highly at £24 per annum, complained that:

they don't give her potatoes as a right but of rice (she is greedy and grumbling at meals) … Asked if she gets enough to eat says she sometimes only gets one cut of bread '& that's not enough for Catherine C'! Says she ought to get two cups of tea, and one cup of milk.

The nurse reported that 'she has a terrible appetite and is always fighting about her food'. When Catherine informed a medical officer that 'they forgot to give her dinner yesterday, she got a piece of rotten plum pudding', he noted in brackets that 'she got meat as well'.[45] Although most of these complaints came from patients contributing high sums for their maintenance, this was not exclusively the case. Mary W.P., whose relatives contributed a moderate £12, also 'grumbles against the attendants for not giving enough to eat' and it was noted that she 'seems to have a very large appetite'.[46]

Some paying patients in Richmond requested additional food articles such as mutton and eggs.[47] Edwina Matilda D. wrote to a relative, Pauline, imploring her to bring food:

It is dreadful – please bring clothes to me I am in great affliction. I am hungry for want of a chicken and grapes in much need of sympathy come as soon as you can I am as cold as a stone nearly … come at once as I am cold and want to see you Pauline. I never was in such trouble in my life.[48]

In late nineteenth-century Dublin, articles like beef or mutton were a rare luxury for the poor and were generally reserved for the family breadwinner, while eggs were considered a luxury, because of their commercial value. Grapes and chicken were also less common delicacies and certainly did not feature at the tables of the impoverished.[49] Paying patients in Richmond were therefore openly contesting the provision of more run-of-the-mill foodstuffs. Whether as an assertion of their social standing or simply a longing for the more rich and varied mealtimes they had previously enjoyed, paying patients were clearly unimpressed with the dietary on offer. Little wonder, perhaps, that Enniscorthy paying patient, Francis R., literally dreamt of a more varied dietary; at eleven o'clock one morning, he imagined that he had already eaten a dinner 'of salt herrings and potatoes'.[50]

At Enniscorthy, Drapes took account of the types of food paying patients consumed at home, suggesting he was mindful of the disparities in dietary customs. In 1897, Drapes noted that Maria C. 'took no breakfast but eat [sic] her dinner: would not take porridge though brother told me she eat [sic] it at home'.[51] The following year, when Margaret Sara K. refused her food and had to be tube fed, the nurse suggested that she was 'particular about her food and thinks she might get her to take some if she cooked it for her in division'. Drapes allowed this and the following week it was recorded she was 'taking her food better'.[52] Because the provision of dietary fell within the realm of medical treatment, resident medical superintendents retained control over whether relatives could supply additional food articles. Although not explicitly prohibited by the Privy Council rules, at Enniscorthy, relatives were not allowed to provide luxuries. In 1877, the RMS, Edmundson, wrote to one paying patient's daughter asking that she 'might please not bring Beef tea &c. to your father as he is supplied with everything we deem fit for him here'.[53] At Richmond, relatives could supply extras. Hesta W's mother and friends brought her food, although she refused to accept it, believing it was poison.[54] Patrick C. refused 'very nearly all the food supplied by the asylum, but takes freely whatever his brothers bring or send him'. In this case, the patient declined to say why he refused the institution's food.[55]

The centrality of food within the case notes examined indicates the medical emphasis on good feeding as a facet of treatment. The frequency and similarity of patients' complaints recorded in the case notes, however, suggests that diet was one area where district asylum care did not meet paying patients' expectations. At Richmond, some campaigned for improved dietary standards. Walter J.H., formerly a staff sergeant in the army, wrote a letter to Norman after two of the other medical officers allegedly consented to his 'making some suggestions for the improvement of the management of this establishment'. He pointed out that:

the food as supplied to sick patients is not what it should be – Before I can draw up a good plan, I should require to see what facilities you have for cooking purposes – what arrangements are made to ensure cleanliness & what is done to prevent waste of unconsumed food. It appears to me that under the present regime waste is inevitable. If Dr Reddington's invitation to me to attend a Board Meeting could be carried out, I am sure that you would profit by my presence.[56]

The validity of Walter's supposed invitation is questionable and there is no record of Walter actually attending board meetings. Nonetheless,

Walter's letter suggests that some paying patients perceived themselves as being especially positioned to improve asylum management.

Another paying patient, Michael C., was more concerned with improving conditions for himself. Prior to becoming a paying patient in Richmond in 1892, Michael had been in the North Dublin Union infirmary ward. While there, he reportedly felt that a nurse had taken 'a dislike to him'. He therefore decided to refuse his food, hoping to be moved to another ward, and was 'very well satisfied with the result of his experiment'. While in Richmond, Michael was described as a:

> quarrelsome old man who insists on having his own way in everything. If he has not his own way, he begins to refuse food, knowing well that he will be fed with the tube in hospital. He has taken food from tube for long periods.

Food refusal became an important weapon for Michael. His reasons for doing so varied depending on his latest grievance. On one occasion, he complained that an attendant would not supply him with his full amount of 'stimulants'. On another, he stated that he refused food because he had not been given his morning paper. His ultimate demand, however, was to be allowed to eat his meals in the open air. As illustrated in Fig. 7.1, Michael's wish to eat out of doors was eventually granted and he was photographed having finished one such meal, the crockery lying on the grass beside him in a spacious green area.

Michael was not the only patient who successfully managed to eat meals alone. When Frances N. exhibited 'a curious reluctance to go down to dinner', she was allowed to dine in a separate division.[57] Nevertheless, paying patients were not generally accorded separate eating quarters from pauper patients. In one instance, a paying patient at Enniscorthy 'attacked a patient … and flung his tin of tea over him at breakfast'.[58] The victim of this incident was a pauper patient, indicating that the two were dining in the same quarters.

Michael C., used artificial feeding as leverage so often that he became accomplished at feeding himself with the apparatus: '[He] has even held the bowl while the tube was passed and has even passed the tube himself'. Later, it was reported that the patient 'will feed himself passing the nasal tube with a certain amount of pride'. The asylum authorities, in this instance, were clearly willing to give into the patient's demands, effectively shifting the balance of power from staff to patient. This

Fig. 7.1 Photograph of Michael C., male paying patient, Richmond district asylum, 20 May 1900. Appended to 'Male Case Book 1892–1893', (GM, Richmond District Lunatic Asylum, attached to p. 339)

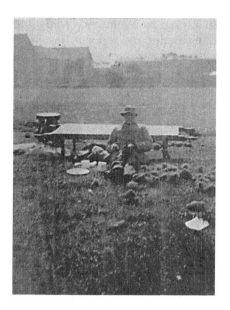

may have stemmed from the fact that Michael was a paying patient. As Andrews has argued, asylum records are often 'prejudiced in favour of the wealthy, educated, articulate or extrovert patient', as these individuals were regarded as more interesting, and received more attention than their less privileged counterparts.[59] While there is little evidence that paying patients received vastly preferential treatment to pauper patients in the asylums studied, it is conceivable that some were allowed small indulgences. For Michael C., eating outdoors became a regular ritual and it was noted that 'he insists on sitting out in the grounds in all weathers, summer and winter, wet or fine. He says he has no appetite for his meals unless when out in the open air'.[60] Of course, asylum staff may have preferred this course of action to continually force-feeding the patient.

The main problem with paying patients' diet in district asylums was that it simply had not been designed for this social cohort. Outside the asylum by the post-Famine period, while the staples of Irish diet—potatoes and milk—were beginning to be supplemented with additional foodstuffs including tea, bread, butter, bacon and flesh meat, these changes did not take place in asylums and the lunacy inspectors' main criticism of district asylum dietary was lack of variety.[61] District asylum dietary was thus now falling below what patients were accustomed to eating at home. According to the lunacy inspectors in 1890, at Enniscorthy, the ordinary breakfast consisted of oatmeal, rice in stirabout and milk, tea, sugar and milk, and bread. Ordinary dinner was bread or potatoes, milk and on Sundays, Tuesdays and Thursdays female patients were given one quart of soup. Supper consisted of more bread, tea, sugar and milk and cocoa. Only those on the 'extra' diet were given meat for dinner and the hospital diet was whiskey, wine, eggs, rice, beef tea and any other articles to be 'ordered by the physicians when necessary'.[62] At Richmond, the ordinary diet was more varied. Breakfast consisted of bread and tea but for dinner, patients were given pea soup or coffee and bread two days a week, beef four days a week and pork on another day. Potatoes were provided twice a week and 'other fresh vegetables' on another three days. For supper, patients were also provided with bread and cocoa, while those on the 'extra' diet received coffee and extra bread at dinner and tea and extra bread at supper. The hospital diet at Richmond was especially varied, including beef tea, chops, eggs, wine, whiskey, brandy, rice, tea, chicken, butter, extra milk, ricemilk, arrowroot and any extras ordered by the physicians. Soup consisting of a 'liquid in which the meat is boiled, seasoned with salt, spices and celery', peas, flour and red herrings was also provided along with cocoa with sugar and milk. Richmond's dietary also provided for Lenten and other fast days for its Roman Catholic patients, consisting of coffee, sugar, milk, bread and butter.[63] While the dietaries listed in the inspectors' annual reports do not necessarily reveal what patients were given nor the quality of the articles supplied, they do offer an indication of the types of food available to patients.

Voluntary asylum diets were much more diverse. For the period 1820 to 1850, Malcolm has argued that the diet in St Patrick's was 'far more lavish than that offered in district asylums'.[64] Stewart's asylum had fortyeight acres of farmland and pleasure grounds and this provided 'a large quantity of all seasonable vegetables and potatoes, and the milk of six cows'.[65] Stewart's medical superintendent, Pim, reported that the dietary in the lunatic asylum branch consisted of bread and butter, tea, coffee or cocoa at breakfast and tea, and soup, fish, meats in variety, potatoes and an 'abundance of vegetables all of the best quality' for dinner, with an after-course almost daily. Alcoholic beverages were not allowed unless specially ordered by a medical attendant.[66] This contrasted with Bloomfield, where beer and wine were not listed under medical expenditure, suggesting that alcohol formed part of the dietary there.[67] Both the lunacy inspectors and patients appeared to approve of the diet on offer at Stewarts. After visiting the asylum during dinner in 1871, Hatchell reported that 'the food was of excellent quality, and the allowance to each was liberal'.[68]

The diet at Stewarts included a large amount of fresh produce; a garden of three statute acres reportedly 'daily supplies the house with an abundance of every ordinary vegetable in season, and during the fruit months such delicacies as gooseberries, currants, apples, pears, &c., are liberally distributed'. In addition, the asylum farm provided 'all the necessaries for such an establishment (excepting meat, bread and butter)'. Surplus produce from the farm was sold in the Dublin markets, suggesting that it was producing more than enough for the patients.[69] Similarly, at Bloomfield in the 1850s, the gardens and grounds were 'rendered highly productive by judicious cultivation'.[70] As has been shown, several male patients worked in the vegetable garden, suggesting that Bloomfield possessed a degree of self-sufficiency. Stanley was clearly protective of the vegetable garden. On one occasion, he had patient William R. confined for a few hours in the padded-room 'to prevent him plucking up the vegetables or injuring anyone by throwing stones across the walls'.[71] In 1864, Stanley recorded the purchase of two pigs from Smithfield Market, suggesting that patients were also provided with pork.[72]

While glowing committee reports concerning the diet at Stewarts should be regarded with caution, given that they were intended to bolster the institution's reputation, it is noteworthy that there were no food-related criticisms recorded in the case notes. In contrast, patients at Bloomfield did complain about their dietary. Isabella K., exhibited 'some difficulty about her food' and would eat only stirabout, milk, beef tea and bread, and later on an egg and tea. Isabella refused to speak other than to request food, suggesting that diet was an important element of her life at Bloomfield. When she eventually spoke to the reporting physician, he asked her to take some meat, but she replied, 'I was just going to ask you not to give me any more food ... I don't want to get well.'[73] Another patient, John Francis H. was 'very hard to please about his food', despite reportedly taking an 'abundance of food, such as he wishes for, e.g. bread, butter, fruit'. Like Isabella, John Francis also refused meat and eventually insisted on subsisting only on bread and water.[74] While voluntary asylum patients clearly had more say over what they ate compared with paying patients in district asylums, when they refused food, artificial feeding was resorted to.[75] When Bloomfield patient John F. 'persisted in living on bread and water' and 'seemed to suffer in health', he was artificially fed with liquids, beef tea, milk and eggs' and subsequently had 'eaten and drunk freely'.[76]

Private asylum patients also expressed anxieties about their food. St John of God's patient, Edward A.P., said to have 'a great appetite is the first and the last out of the refectory', was:

> never done grumbling that he does not get enough of meat – beef steak which he thinks he should receive three times daily ... The coffee is 'dirty water not fit for a dog'. The food 'is not what I am accustomed to: it is not fit for a priest'.

Not unlike the district asylum doctors, O'Connell interpreted these complaints as indicating the patient's greed, stating, 'I believe he would eat meat ten times a day if he got it. He complains because he does not get it for supper in addition to getting it at breakfast and dinner.'[77] Christopher C., a barrister, was also reportedly particular about his food:

> Very closely inspects any bit of food he likes, but it is not possible to please him ... If, for example, he be given fried eggs at breakfast, he says he prefers boiled eggs. If the eggs be boiled, then he wants them fried.[78]

In this instance, O'Connell attributed Christopher's behaviour to his fear 'to eat lest he or his friends cannot pay for his support. Always gives as an excuse for not eating heartily, that the food disturbs him'.[79]

These complaints in the more expensive asylums, Bloomfield and St John of God's, suggest that diet was a subjective and important element of patients' expectations. Nonetheless, it is likely that voluntary and private asylum patients were supplied with meals that more closely resembled what they had eaten at home. Paying patients in district asylums were thus at a disadvantage, as the medical principle of supplying patients with their accustomed dietary or better was eclipsed by the legal requirement to limit them to the pauper patient's dietary.

CLASS, RELIGIOUS AND POLITICAL TENSIONS

As we have seen, during the 1857–1858 commission of inquiry, the lunacy inspectors and numerous asylum doctors were worried about the intermingling of patients from various social classes, fearing jealousies would arise between them. In practice, accommodating paying patients in district asylums did create tensions, not just between patients, but with attendants and medical staff. This mostly stemmed from paying patients who disliked mixing with those from a different social background.[80]

Case notes reveal that some paying patients at Enniscorthy tended to associate with one another, perhaps forming their own sub-group within the asylum population. Many paying patients walked together. James C. walked in the grounds with James S. every day, while Bridget C, a nun, and Johanna F., a farmer, also kept company in the grounds.[81] Other paying patients disliked mixing with others. As Richmond paying patient, Elizabeth H., stated:

> I hate being here with these dirty abominable women – their dirty language at meal-times ... Says she does not like to sit at the fire, owing to the disagreeableness of the other patients. The nurses might prevent the annoyance the pts give if they like, but they don't.[82]

Several paying patients apparently looked down on other patients and servants in the asylum. For example, James S., a farmer who had previous been in St Patrick's voluntary asylum, paid £25 per annum at Enniscorthy. While in the asylum, he complained: 'this is no place to have me, they are all madmen and ruffians here.'[83] Frances N. in Richmond was eager to differentiate herself from pauper patients: 'said she was not a pauper like the others although she was wet and dirty'.[84]

Class tensions between paying patients and asylum staff also came into play. In the Morningside asylum in Scotland, many of the more affluent patients looked down on the attendants and found it undignified to take orders from those they considered their 'coarse and uncivilised' social inferiors.[85] Asylum staff in Ireland tended to be drawn from the less affluent, while the demanding nature of the job caused a high turnover in staff.[86] District asylum staff were regularly drawn from the military, because of their experience of working in disciplined roles,[87] although it is unclear whether voluntary and private asylums attracted similar attendants.

Female paying patients at Richmond were particularly vocal about their distaste for asylum attendants and physicians, possibly stemming from the large number and high turnover in this institution. Rose C. 'wrote a letter full of abuse of the doctor, attendants, patients and the asylum generally'.[88] Rebecca B. considered 'Dr. Norman the greatest scoundrel on earth', while Catherine B. was described as:

> extremely disdainful in manner. Says an heiresses' life would suit her … objects to associating with Nurse Murphy and Nurse Hagans and doctors and shadows. Says she should own this institution … Says I am taking a great liberty in speaking to her. [89]

Mary Jane A. was clearly unhappy with her life at Richmond:

> 'Oh to think I'm here' 'Oh what sort of a place is this' 'Oh what is going to be done to me at all – to think that I was born to die in some wild place like this – oh what will happen when you are all away and nobody near me – oh what will I do. What is to become of me at all?' She is too agitated for any coherent conversation. She says 'to be walking about among a lot of dead people, not near a shop or anything – is not it terrible?'[90]

On the other hand, some paying patients were apparently pleased with their accommodation and attendants. Maria F. spoke most highly ' … of this Asylum, saying we are "blessed with good attendants" and expressing the highest recommendation of our arrangements'.[91]

At Enniscorthy, James C. had a blatant distaste for servants and asylum staff. Prior to his admission, James attacked a servant in his brother's house, threatening and striking him.[92] He told Drapes that:

> his brother's house is being robbed by a servant man named Dillon, that they have stripped the house of glass and delph, also that another servant named Margaret is in on the robbery. He adds that another man named Ennis who was in his brother's employment was a damn ruffian and that he assaulted him on one occasion, giving a box in the head.

Drapes considered this tale to be 'all a delusion'. While in the asylum, James' aversion towards attendants and servants continued. He threw stones at a painter and a few days later attacked one of the attendants in the same manner, insisting both men had threatened him.[93] Eliza M. also reportedly slapped the male servants.[94] While district asylums were often witness to outbreaks of violence between patients, nurses and attendants,[95] existing tensions in the relationship between staff and patient could only have been exacerbated by social inequalities between the two parties. This is further evidenced in a note on Hampstead patient, Richard Charles Edward M., an army lieutenant:

> Last night he had been unusually noisy, restless & excited up to 2am. About an hour & a half after this he suddenly became rational, asked why the atts were holding him in bed, said his father's servants wd not be permitted to do so, that he was a gentleman & shd be treated as such.[96]

At St John of God's, staff struggled to manage patient James Edward G., a medical student:

> He remains in bed in the morning much longer than was his habit a year or two ago, and, in consequence, does not come to breakfast often till all others are finished. The attendants are afraid to make him get up earlier.[97]

According to O'Connell, former grocer, John B., also gave his attendants trouble: 'he frequently defecates in his trousers to annoy the attendant ... frequently dirties his clothes, sometimes wilfully to give annoyance'.[98] Patients' hygiene was also a subject of remark by O'Connell and some patients could not be induced to wash themselves. Of one patient, a lay brother, he reported, 'he never takes a bath—occasionally washes his feet ... Three weeks ago, he was compelled to take a bath the first I ever knew him to take'.[99] In 1903, another patient, a clerk and bookkeeper, was described as:

> Dirty, filthy, most inquisitive, abusive and [?] as usual. A troublesome, dangerous man. I wish he were out of this Asylum ... dirty and he never bathes – I have never known him take a bath. He says he took only one while in the House!![100]

O'Connell's distaste reveals the tensions between private asylum staff and their wealthy clientele. Yet, disputes could work in favour of patients. In Hampstead in the 1840s, when a servant woman allegedly provided a patient, Helen H., 'with a key to make her escape ... the servant was discharged on her accusation & on the servants own confession'.[101] Half a century later, Hampstead patient, George G., was visited by the Registrar in Lunacy to whom he complained of the 'roughness of Att. Craber'. In response, John Neilson Eustace 'gave Att. C a month's notice on the following day as I had previously cautioned him'.[102] This suggests that private asylum patients, by virtue of their high social standing, exercised greater influence over their conditions of care.

In voluntary asylums, paying patients were usually kept separate from free patients and, accordingly, class tensions between patients arose far less frequently. In addition to classification by sex and severity of illness, moral management stressed the importance of segregating patients by social class.[103] Although Bloomfield did not strictly follow this principle, additional privacy was accorded to those maintained at the highest sums. Nonetheless, some patients disliked mixing with others. A Bloomfield patient, Anna C., would 'not on any account mix with the other ladies' and as a result, the reporting physician had 'great difficulty in getting her open air exercise'.[104] Similarly, at Stewarts, patient Eli S., a dental mechanic, objected 'to having to associate with other patients says he is a gent and they are pigs, not society for him'.[105] Another patient, Adelaide Amy J., appeared to Rainsford:

> to think that she is a person of great importance and much too good to associate with anyone about the place ... She refuses as a rule to look at anyone and hides her face with her hand when speaking and suddenly runs away to some more quiet place ... Refuses to come near me and runs away when I approach her ... Says I have nothing to do with her that she has to consider her father's name.[106]

Although she was later reported 'to talk to the other patients and seems rather pleasanter and in better spirits', she subsequently 'threw a cup of tea over a gentleman who was in the dining room saying that he was robbing her of her tea'. Two months later, Adelaide developed a notion that she was in danger of becoming diseased and wrote 'to her mother demanding her removal owing to contagion'. Unfortunately, Adelaide's attempt to interact with other patients was frustrated when another patient, Mrs. B., 'ran after her when out walking with a nettle. Miss. J. much upset. Took to bed and said she had typhoid'. Following this, she declined to speak to Rainsford or any of the patients and refused to go out walking with them. She later complained that 'all around her are dressmakers &c not fit for her to associate with'.[107]

Alongside social class, religion played an integral role in patient identity. In spite of the political and religious tensions in society at large during the period studied, this was not seen to impact to any great extent on the mental health of patients in the study. Nonetheless, there is evidence of class and religious tensions between patients and sometimes staff. It is difficult to disentangle religion from class identity in this era. By the mid-nineteenth century in England, religious denomination gave a distinctive identity to particular communities and classes, the most notable being the association between the middle class and a Christian way of life.[108] Adherence to evangelical Protestant forms became an accepted part of respectability, which increasingly came to include church-going, family worship and an interest in religious literature.[109] In post-Famine Ireland, attitudes shifted towards a range of social and cultural behaviours, including a dramatic alteration in devotional routine that culminated in a more respectable, mid-Victorian Irish populace.[110]

In addition to links between religious observances and respectability, in Ireland, religion could be a marker of one's political affiliation. Both religious and political tensions ran deep in Irish society and these could permeate asylum life. Although psychiatry held mixed views about the effects of religion on mental health, religion was believed to have a potentially positive influence on the mind and the provision of religious services formed part of the therapeutic regimes in Irish asylums. Nonetheless, the provision of religious facilities intersected with anxieties about the vulnerability of institutional inmates to proselytising.[111] Frictions arose between asylum staff and local clergymen during the 1840s about the degree of access Catholic parish priests were accorded to the Carlow asylum, as there were fears it would become a 'domain of Protestant influence'.[112] There were also heated debates surrounding the appointment of chaplains in the Belfast asylum, which admitted members of seven different creeds during the 1850s and 1860s.[113] By the mid-nineteenth century, however, most medical superintendents in Britain and Ireland 'were happy to have official chaplains fulfil the role originally carried out by the lay moral manager' and in 1867, the Lord Lieutenant of Ireland was empowered to appoint chaplains to district asylums.[114] Religious tensions in district asylums continued into the twentieth century. At Ballinasloe asylum, the asylum board prohibited the establishment of a Catholic chapel within the asylum grounds, fearing a 'Catholic takeover of the institution itself' and signifying broader political concerns at a time when schools, hospitals and universities were denominational.[115]

As we have seen, paying patients in district asylums tended to be disproportionately Protestant compared with both pauper patient populations and society at large. This resulted in an increased intermingling of patients from different religious persuasions which bred religious and political tensions in the asylums. In 1901, an Enniscorthy paying patient, Edward S., was said to have an 'aversion to Protestants, all of whom he regards as Orangemen. Moore [an attendant] often hears him muttering when he passes, e.g. that if he had the chance he would do away with all "Orangemen", and Protestants'. Edward also accused a fellow Roman Catholic inmate of becoming a Protestant to 'get the privileges', which Drapes interpreted as 'being allowed to walk about on parole'. Edward's distaste towards Protestants extended beyond those in the patient population. Drapes, an active member of the Church of Ireland, also came under fire: 'told me more than once that it was my "bigotry" which was keeping me here: and that it was I who got him sent here'.[116]

The extent to which religion was essential to patient identity is further indicated in the case of another Catholic paying patient at Enniscorthy, Lawrence D. In 1896, as part of a rather extensive campaign to avenge his wife, brother-in-law and former solicitor, whom he charged with wrongful confinement and forgery, Lawrence wrote to his parish priest, David Bolger. The letter is worth quoting from at length, as it is exemplary of religious preoccupations among not only paying patients, both also the Catholic clergy in Wexford:

> I will thank you to send me here a post office order for one pound, the amount I gave for a Baptismal Fee at the Baptism of my infant son Lawrence John: I had then more money than brains, and I have now more brains than money ... You did not think it worth your while or trouble to answer my letter of the 21st June, although you could lecture me in the jail of Wexford on the 30th July 1895 and tell me that it was a shame for me to employ a Protestant solicitor ... I replied that the last solicitor I employed was not even a Christian, he is a Jew ... I know now how a Catholic solicitor served me and he is now in the hands of the police ... I will tell you how a Protestant Nobleman, Lord Maurice Fitzgerald treated me. I wrote to him on the 23rd ult. and had his reply written from Johnstown Castle on the 27th July at one o'clock on the 28th. So much for the Protestant son of Ireland's only Duke ... So much for Catholics, Protestants and Jews

... Mind don't forget sending the money as I require it for my solicitor. Lawrence D.[117]

The patient's disillusionment with the Catholic Church is evident in his demand for the return of the £1 baptismal fee, which he now judged as an ill-conceived gesture. Lawrence's disenchantment with Catholicism appears further heightened by his admission that his former Catholic solicitor is now in prison. The priest's alleged distaste for a Protestant solicitor further indicates that religion played an important role in identity in late-nineteenth century Wexford outside the asylum as much as inside.

Religious tensions were also perceptible in the Richmond asylum. For example, Ellen C., a Protestant woman who had been previously confined in Stewarts:

> Would forgive her husband anything, but putting her where the majority are Roman Catholics. Considers that her kneeling to say her prayers is made a subject of remarks. On my pointing out to her that many patients are seen kneeling in the dormitories, she replies, 'They are Roman Catholics'. Complains that Mary M talks to her about priests and nuns.[118]

Catholic paying patient Edward F. reportedly felt that he was being kept from attending mass:

> during the isolation due to Beri-beri, he suffered much annoyance by being kept from attending his church. However, he laid the whole moral responsibility off his own shoulders and on Dr. Norman's.[119]

Ellen O'C., a Catholic paying patient aged seventy-four, seemingly resisted examination on religious grounds: 'When I went to examine her she got over excited and said it was wrong and immodest of me to go near her. She kept constantly praying and asking "are you all Catholics"'.[120]

Relatively little evidence exists of religious tensions between the wealthier clientele in voluntary and private asylums. This is despite the mixing of patients from various creeds (see Chap. 4). One reason for this stemmed from the religious characters of these institutions. In the 1860s, Bloomfield provided religious services for Quaker patients.[121] However, when queried on what provision existed for the religious attendance of those of other denominations during the 1857–1858 commission, Bloomfield's superintendent, John Moss, asserted 'we are not visited by any ministers of other denominations, unless a patient requires it, or his friends'. This was arranged on admission and Moss claimed that 'we have not the least objection to the ministers of their respective religious denominations visiting them'.[122] By the 1890s, an Episcopalian clergyman also visited the house every fortnight, but no patient was considered capable of attending Divine service outside the asylum.[123] Divine services were held weekly in Stewarts for Protestant and Catholic patients and the RMS reported that attendance to both was 'very considerable'. In addition, those who were 'capable' were permitted to attend their places of worship on Sundays.[124] The lunacy inspector, E.M. Courtenay, praised Stewarts for providing religious services, stating that 'the religious wants of the patients appeared to be carefully attended to'.[125] Certainly, although Jane M., a Church of Ireland patient, became 'very excited' one afternoon when she was not allowed to attend a service, it was later noted that she was able to go to church on Sundays.[126] Meanwhile, Maude Frances C., a Catholic, attended mass at Chapelizod.[127]

The lack of religious tensions between voluntary and private asylum patients suggests the asylum authorities proactively avoided potential difficulties arising from accommodating patients of various creeds. This is reflected in Stanley's record of preparations to receive Lady R., the daughter of a Baron and a member of the Church of Ireland, in Bloomfield in 1868:

> Doctor Owen made a visit of inquiry today respecting the admission of a daughter of Baron R[-] who is insane on Religious matters – the lady it appears has a great dislike to Roman Catholics and although a special attendant is not required, she should have a Protestant Servant to attend her ... It was the intention of her Friends to have her placed in a private Family, but the Baron who came here last week with Doctor Owen on a visit of inspection liked the place and the Doctor wishes to be informed the terms with and without an Attendant and if such a Servant would be provided.[128]

The appropriation of staff of the same religion was not unusual in nineteenth-century Ireland. Church of Ireland families, in particular, tended to hire servants of their own faith.[129] Although there is no record of Lady R. being admitted to Bloomfield, her case reveals that those providing care for the wealthier classes were mindful to achieve a balance between supplying religious services for those who wanted them and negating against any religious divisions that might arise in institutions receiving patients of various, often conflicting, religious persuasions.

Inextricably linked with religious tensions and class identity in Ireland was political unrest. In her study of the Ballinasloe district asylum, Walsh has found patients discussing the various bodies of political opinion and the same can be said for paying patients in the district asylums studied here.[130] In his 1894 article on the alleged increase of insanity in Ireland, Drapes argued:

> the almost constant political agitation to which our people are sub-jected, deeply arousing, as it does, the feelings of a naturally emotional race ... Mr. Lecky says somewhere, 'Religion is the one romance of the poor.' There is another which, as a vision of the future haunts the mind of the Irish peasant. Rent abolished, his land and homestead for himself, and a Parliament in College Green, these make up the dream which fills his fancy. Disappointed often, but still not despairing, betrayed as he has often been, he still clings with a wonderful tenacity to the picture of an ideal Ireland which his imagination, aided by the eloquence of his politi-cal teachers, has fabricated. But the hopes, fears, and anxieties, the stir-ring up of emotions, some evil, some generous, engendered by this almost chronic condition of political unrest, can hardly fail to have a more or less injurious effect on a not over-stable kind of brain, and such as those who, like Gallio, care for none of these things, may find it a little difficult to realise.[131]

These assertions betray Drapes' own political and class stance and his wishes to maintain existing class and political structures.[132] Although Drapes focused on the 'Irish peasant', these events held equally distress-ing ramifications for wealthier groups and discussion of political unrest was prevalent among Richmond's paying patients. Among Catholics, Anne R. had visions of St Patrick and Daniel O'Connell and heard Charles Stewart 'Parnell's voice every day calling her bad names'.[133] John C., a soldier pensioner 'talks in a silly rambling incoherent manner about Mrs. O'Shea, priests, Parnell, bloody Fenians &c'.[134] Protestant patients were equally preoccupied with political figures. Mary A F stated 'I am Queen Victoria' and later 'I am Robert Peel's wife'.[135] Hannah Louisa F talked 'incoherently about Mrs. O'Shea', while Fanny M. referred to 'Mr. Gladstone as a "beast"'.[136] Prior to her confinement in Richmond, Mary B. had been in the Armagh Retreat private asylum.

Mary, whose mother described her as being 'of a philanthropic turn' and a 'trustee for some money for 20 poor ladies' had complained on admission, 'says the government are not giving her good value for her money and talks of leading a rebellion against the Government'.[137] After just one day at Richmond, Mary was discharged to a private asylum.

There is no record of voluntary or private asylum patients discussing politics with their doctors. Nonetheless, in her study of St Patrick's voluntary asylum, Malcolm has strongly argued that events like the 1916 rising and the civil war often had a 'significant impact on the mental health of Irish people', not just on soldiers engaged in military service, but on civilians.[138] She also cites William Saunders Hallaran's identification of the 'terror' caused by the 1798 rebellion and finds supporting evidence in the patient records for St Patrick's.[139] In this sample, there was only one reference to political upheaval. When Mary Julia G.C., was admitted to Bloomfield in the 1860s, she was reportedly 'very terrified of Fenian Mischief'.[140] In the admissions register, the cause of her mental illness was attributed to her 'living a solitary life. Bad management of her own state of health and brought to a crisis by panic from imaginary Fenians at Wicklow'. Unfortunately, there are no surviving case notes on Mary Julia, so it is not possible to learn whether she continued to speak of her political anxieties following admission. Mary's fear of 'Fenian Mischief' does, however, inform of her political views. The relative prominence of issues surrounding class, religion and politics in the case notes on district asylum paying patients says much about contemporary medical perceptions of non-pauper mental illness. Reporting physicians clearly felt it worthwhile to record patients' anxieties about their political and social status and in turn their class identity. Yet while there is evidence of class and religious tensions between patients and staff, in most cases voluntary and private asylum authorities managed to avoid these by segregation and provision of religious ministrations for all denominations.

EXPECTATIONS OF PATIENTS

Historians of Irish asylums have highlighted the high levels of violence perpetrated by patients and their carers.[141] Violence became key to lay cultural understandings of insanity to the extent that asylums became intrinsically linked with 'dangerous insanity'.[142] Interpretations of the dangerous lunatic legislation are at the centre of these discussions, as it framed an important route of admission into district asylums.[143] Individuals considered as dangerous and of unsound mind could, following 1867, be committed directly to district asylums, effectively bypassing more tedious, bureaucratic and often unsuccessful routes into the asylum.[144] Importantly, the 1867 Act pertained only to district asylums; it did not provide for dangerous lunatics being committed to private or voluntary institutions. Yet, there is little doubt that a number of the patients received there exhibited violent and even dangerous behaviour.

By the 1890s, asylum case notes contained a field marked 'dangerous to others'. Table 7.1 reveals that those committed to more expensive asylums, particularly Hampstead and Highfield, were the most frequently described as being dangerous to others. The diagnoses assigned to patients in this study also reveal medical recognition of violent symptoms among paying patients. The two primary diagnostic categories of mania and melancholia encompassed a wide range of symptoms and behaviours.[145] Of the two, mania, which was medically associated with violence and disruptiveness, was the more common diagnosis, accounting for almost half of first admissions (see Table 7.2). Melancholics were the next largest group, constituting over one-fifth of first admissions. Aside from these two classic diagnoses, a much smaller proportion of paying patients were diagnosed with dementia, general paralysis, epilepsy or other far less common conditions such as paranoia, imbecility and congenital mental deficiency. Paying patients in rural asylums, Ennis (65.8%) and Enniscorthy (73.1%), were particularly prone to mania diagnoses. This contrasts with the neighbouring Carlow asylum, where only 39% of diagnosed patients (pauper and paying) were identified as suffering from mania,[146] and implies that paying patients were perceived as being especially violent. Male (46.4%) and female (46.5%) paying patients had almost equal chances of being diagnosed with mania, suggesting that women were considered just as capable of violent acts as their male counterparts. Certainly, violence was a distinctive feature of asylum life and perpetrated by paying patients of both sexes. The disruptive behaviour which characterised mania posed challenges to the moral therapy regimes.[147]

Voluntary and private asylum patients were reportedly particularly violent. At Bloomfield, patient John P.I. was 'liable to outbursts of violence and has assaulted patients and attendants but less so latterly'.[148] Another patient, Mary L., 'pulled Maria's [the attendant's] hair and kicked her'.[149] Violent behaviour also extended to elderly patients. Thomas

Table 7.1 Proportion of patients described as 'Dangerous to Others' in case notes on Bloomfield, Stewarts, St John of God's, Hampstead and Highfield patients, c. 1890s

	Yes	Yes (%)	No	No (%)
Stewarts	4	10.3	35	89.7
Bloomfield	9	16.1	47	83.9
St John of God's	17	22.4	59	77.6
Hampstead	14	50.0	14	50.0
Highfield	4	66.7	2	33.3

Compiled from Bloomfield, Stewarts, St John of God's, Hampstead and Highfield casebooks

J.G., a seventy-eight-year-old retired bookkeeper, was believed to have attacked his wife and in consequence was sent to Bloomfield. While there, he struck another patient 'with a stick, cutting his head'. Although there was no record of him being punished or restrained for his actions, it was noted that 'since then we have not given him any stick'. Thomas was clearly of a violent temperament. He later became 'vexed because his room was being cleaned and struck the attendants and cursed violently'.[150]

Patients of all ages, both male and female, regularly attacked attendants and other patients.[151] Patient injuries included bruising, flesh wounds, scalp wounds and suspected fractures. Black eyes were particularly prominent among patients sent to Stewart's during the 1890s.[152] This is in stark contrast to a statement from the managing committee in 1894, which insisted:

> As far as possible, the admission of patients likely to be unsuitable and cause inconvenience to other patients is discouraged, and if any, after admission, are found objectionable, due notification is given to their friends in order that other arrangements may be made.[153]

Despite their reassurances, the managing committee did not discharge patients who were violent or disruptive and many 'harmless' patients were subjected to abuse.[154] Private asylum patients could also be violent. Highfield patient, Christina McF S., reportedly screamed, cursed and sometimes attacked the attendants.[155] At St John of God's, Joseph B. one night 'got up and beat a fellow patient sleeping in the same

Table 7.2 Recorded diagnoses of first admissions to the case studies, 1868–1900

Diagnosis	Belfast	(%)	Ennis	(%)	Enniscorthy	(%)	Richmond	(%)	Stewarts	(%)	Bloomfield	(%)	St John of God's	(%)
Mania	41	48.2	104	65.8	79	73.1	141	42.9	152	36.4	23	36.5	180	46.4
Melancholia	27	31.8	28	17.7	18	16.7	80	24.3	146	34.9	8	12.7	62	16.0
Dementia	11	12.9	20	12.7	6	5.6	60	18.2	58	13.9	2	3.2	70	18.0
Other	3	3.5	4	2.5	3	2.8	28	8.5	58	13.9	28	44.4	65	16.8
General paralysis	2	2.4	0	0.0	0	0.0	16	4.9	1	0.2	1	1.6	11	2.8
Epilepsy	1	1.2	2	1.3	2	1.9	4	1.2	3	0.7	1	1.6	0	0.0
Total	85	100.0	158	100.0	108	100.0	329	100.0	418	100.0	63	100.0	388	100.0

Compiled from Belfast, Ennis, Enniscorthy, Richmond, Stewarts, Bloomfield and St John of God's admissions registers dormitory with him. When I asked why he did it, he said so and so was laughing at him. Since then he sleeps in a locked room off the dormitory'.[156] Although this was apparently an isolated incident, other patients had a track record of violence. Patrick F., a medical student:

suddenly and without any provocation, came up behind Father P who was kneeling, pulled back his head and gave him a blow in the right eye. On August 8 in chapel, he got up and went over where Dr C was kneeling and struck him. Both acts were impulsive ... he had a fight with Father P and received a few blows on the right cheek [?] of the nose.

O'Connell noted, 'I am not sure that he was the aggressor. At any rate this is the second time within a year he struck Father P. against whom he seems to entertain a grudge'.[157]

Injuries were usually attributed to the violence of another patient. However, in some instances patients received injuries from attendants and doctors. The case of Frederick Healy W., a judge's son, reveals the extent to which violence had permeated the atmosphere at Stewarts in the 1890s. Frederick, who was very 'bad tempered' and had previously struck a fellow patient 'on [the] forehead with a poker', began to complain of a pain in his side where he said 'he was kicked by [another] patient'. Rainsford later noted that Frederick was 'very quarrelsome. Has both eyes blknd [sic] one by Dr. Hunt in a quarrel, the other by falling off a chair when quarrelling with the carpenter'.[158] Henrietta C.K., a 'lady', also received a black eye 'from struggling when being forcibly fed', while Margaret Anne C. 'got a push from a ward maid whilst interfering with bedmaking and falling cut her forehead against a rail'.[159] Although violence and bodily harm among patients and staff in public asylums is well documented, this high level of injury among voluntary asylum patients reveals that the often large sums of money paid to institutions such as Bloomfield and Stewarts did not guarantee patients' protection.

Importantly, tensions between patients and staff in voluntary asylums may have been amplified in the casebooks because asylum interactions were recorded selectively. While asylum doctors were compelled to account for patient injuries and violent incidents, they were not obliged to record amicable staff–patient interactions.[160] In this study, the degree to which staff mixed with patients is difficult to assess, given the relative absence of documentary evidence. Bloomfield's 'Notice of Particulars', kept by house stewards Hyde and later Stanley in the 1860s, is thus instructive in its more nuanced rendering of asylum life. It suggests that, at least in small asylums like Bloomfield, where low patient numbers still facilitated moral therapy, patients and staff could enjoy one another's company. Stanley, who ran errands on behalf of Bloomfield almost daily, often brought one or more patients along with him for the outing. Early on in his career as house steward, he apparently became attached to one patient, a William R.:

> Mr R[-] being so very steady today Mrs Pryor kindly gave me permission to bring him with me to Dublin where I had some business to transact. Being anxious to try the power of his memory, I asked him in the Roy. Bank ... the day of the month and he replied immediately the 28th without taking a moment's consideration. We then went to the North Wall to ascertain if the Steam Boats were plying to Kingstown as he is anxious to have a trip there, either by rail or boat ... It is, I believe, Mrs Pryor's intention to send him there as soon as it shall be found convenient.[161]

Stanley continued to bring William with him on errands for a number of days, on one occasion even buying him 'a pair of gloves which he wanted very badly'.[162] Sadly, when William relapsed a few days later, Stanley, who had commenced his position as house steward just two months earlier, was clearly unprepared:

> My poor friend Mr. R[-] I am sorry to say took a change last night although when I was leaving Bloomfield yesterday for home appeared to me to be as steady as he has been all the week ... One can scarcely imagine him to be the same person who accompanied me so often to Town and who reminded me of the different places to which we had to call. Here he is today crying and laughing at intervals – One time walking along the corridor as fast as he can, and another time tumbling head-over-heels from one side of it to the other. He will then come into the sitting room – take down the Testament, and read aloud five or six verses, crying and laughing over them alternately. Such is the state he would be seen in today after a week of steadiness spent in a way which he enjoyed so very much.[163]

Stanley's experience with William evidently did not deter him from socialising with the other patients. During his time as house steward, Stanley introduced 'football recreation' and actively joined in. He also played musical instruments for the patients in the evening, and he and his wife (who was the head attendant on the female side of Bloomfield) often brought groups of patients on trips together. While this portrayal of Stanley's relationship with his patients is rather positive, it offers an important counterpoint to the usual records of violence and tensions between patients and asylum staff.

The management techniques for violent patients in voluntary asylums were often similar to district asylums. However, patients maintained at high fees or whose relatives could afford to pay extra were sometimes given a personal attendant in place of the more usual method of restraint. By the late nineteenth century, the employment of special attendants for St Patrick's patients was less common and straitjackets became the preferred means of control.[164] Although Bloomfield remained a small institution and Stewarts was sometimes underfilled, several patients there were subject to restraint, seclusion or sedation, implying that these asylums had fewer disposable funds to supply special attendants. For example, in 1893, when Mary Elizabeth A. attacked a female attendant and tore her bedclothes, a 'restraining jacket' was applied for two hours and she was later given sulphonal. When the same patient attempted to 'throw herself downstairs' she was again restrained. Following another incident, the doctor noted that the jacket 'always quiets her and seems to do her good'. She later began to break windows in the asylum for which she was restrained and then given potassium bromide and cannabis. It is clear the straitjacket was being applied in a punitive manner. On one occasion, the reporting physician noted that 'the screaming was so bad that to try and stop it the straitjacket was put on about a month ago for a few hours at a time by way of punishment'.[165]

In keeping with moral therapy's emphasis on maintaining harmonious surroundings, staff in voluntary asylums seemed vigilant in their attempts to protect 'harmless' patients from those posing a threat to social order. Accordingly, reporting physicians judged patients' behaviour against that considered appropriate for the wealthier classes, frequently noting, for example, if a patient looked 'ladylike'.[166] Both the doctors and relatives of voluntary asylum patients assessed appropriate forms of female behaviour.[167] This included appraisal of their actions, language, clothing and appearance. Any form of embarrassing behaviour or deviation from social norms was considered evidence of mental illness. Thus, when Caroline J., a forty-seven-year-old governess was admitted to Stewarts in 1900, the asylum doctor reported that she had 'all her life strange views of men imagining they were in love with her and lately has imagined attempts were made to rob her of her virtue. Was inclined to be fond of alcohol and drank stout'. To his evident surprise, on admission she was 'quiet and ladylike. Took her meals and gave no trouble'.[168] The extent to which one was 'ladylike' was apparently a measure of sanity for female patients at Stewarts. When Charlotte Maria D. began to recover, it was noted that she was 'mentally much improved. Very quiet and ladylike'.[169]

Asylum doctors at both Stewarts and Bloomfield disapproved of patients using bad language or other 'indecorous behaviour' and frequently recorded incidents where the social decorum of the asylum had been breached.[170] In 1896, Charles Henry B. had reportedly been 'speaking so constantly ... to the gentlemen in the billiard room' at Bloomfield, that it was found 'necessary to keep him in his room upstairs'.[171] Charles Henry allegedly spoke 'in a most objectionable way' when the physician entered his room and accused the attendants of 'gross immorality'. The doctor, fearing other patients would hear him, placed Charles in solitary confinement:

> Every five days he goes out for two hours. I much regret his confinement in his room but I cannot see how it is to be avoided. He would greatly injure the other gentlemen if he talked to them in this manner.[172]

Likewise, at Hampstead, William Henry D. was removed from the main dining room to the 'second where the No 1 patients are' because:

> he continually annoyed a quiet harmless old patient. It is a relief to everyone that he has been removed as his conversation was continually turning on suicides, post mortems, abduction & similar cases. Another favourite topic was asylums & lunatics.[173]

One motivation to maintain a sense of social decorum in the asylum was to prepare patients for their return to the social circles they had previously inhabited. Richard P.F., a twenty-eight-year-old solicitor, was sent to Bloomfield by his father after failing to behave appropriately in the family home: 'when there he sat in the hall, said he was too bad to go upstairs, would not shake hands with anyone'.[174] Similarly, a Hampstead patient, Henry O.B., was described as having been 'formerly painfully polite now he will not raise his hat to a lady'.[175] Any breaches of the code of behaviour in public spaces posed serious problems and embarrassment for the relatives of the mentally ill.[176] This was certainly the case for the relatives of Annie Elizabeth W., a single, twenty-eight-year-old 'ladylike little woman', whom the physician at Bloomfield found 'quiet and pleasant to talk to'. He noted:

> I believe she thought she was married to some man in her neighbourhood – a preacher, and used to follow him about and went to him in a meeting and put arms around him, causing scandal.

Annie reportedly believed that 'her only prospect is of marrying this man'. She was sent away from home 'for a change' but was eventually committed to Bloomfield by her father.[177] The relatives of another Bloomfield patient, Cecil W.W., were also troubled by his behaviour, stating that 'before coming here he had been inclined to talk very indecently in the presence of ladies'. While a patient, he escaped and returned to a house where he used to lodge and 'frightened the woman in it by laughing and strange behaviour'.[178] Cecil's committal to Bloomfield, following this 'indecorous' behaviour, contradicts McCarthy's assumption, in her study of gender ideology and committal to the Enniscorthy asylum, that men's sexual urges were viewed as the fault of women.[179]

Inextricably linked to social decorum was patients' clothing and appearance. Patients and especially women were expected to be neat and tidy in dress and personal habits.[180] As discussed in Chap. 3, in the 1870s one Richmond paying patient was refused permission to wear his own clothes in the asylum, although presumably this changed under Norman's reign. By the 1890s, Richmond paying patients were photographed wearing their own outfits. Figure 7.2 shows one such patient, Rebecca B. While it is possible that Rebecca was allowed to dress in her own clothes only for this photograph,[181] her depiction in the case notes as being 'fantastically dressed. Wears white shoes with black tape rosettes' suggests otherwise.[182]

Wynter has argued that at the Staffordshire county asylum, which catered for patients from various social classes, 'clothing was woven into virtually every aspect of "life inside" during the first half of the nineteenth century', including dress, restraint, laundry and yarn.[183] At Staffordshire, clothing was the primary purchase of the wealthy and Wynter contends that 'for the rich, dress enabled participation in societal norms and the wider world'.[184] Patients in Bloomfield and Stewarts also purchased new clothing: Stanley accompanied Thomas S.W. into town

Fig. 7.2 Photograph of Rebecca B., female paying patient, Richmond district asylum, undated. Appended to 'Female Case Book, 1897–1898', (GM, Richmond District Lunatic Asylum, attached to pp. 337–338)

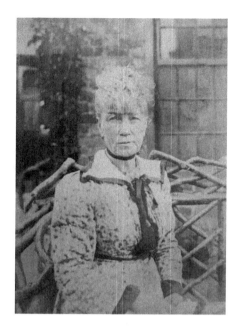

to order a new suit of clothes, while Stewarts patient, George J., was also allowed into town to purchase clothing.[185] Nineteenth-century asylum doctors often measured mental stability against patient's attire or general appearance. For instance, Andrews has demonstrated the relationship doctors perceived between nakedness and insanity, while patients who did not take care over their appearance were considered irrational and neglectful of the self.[186] Patients who stripped their clothes were deemed completely unacceptable at Bloomfield. When David S. became excited and 'gave liberty to his unruly member in the most disgraceful manner', Stanley proposed to have him sent directly to the padded-room but could not as it was already occupied by a female patient. Instead, he was sent to his room.[187] At Stewarts, Anna D.S. was reported to need a special attendant because she frequently took off her clothes.[188]

As part of his programme of reform at Richmond, Norman encouraged patients to make stylish individual clothes for themselves to promote their self-esteem.[189] This freedom was also apparent in voluntary asylums. When, in 1864, Bloomfield patient David S. decided he no longer required the services of the visiting barber and 'most strongly declared he would have his hair to grow both on the upper and lower part of his face', Stanley simply decided to observe whether the patient would continue 'firm in his word'.[190] When the barber arrived the following day, David went out for a walk and would not allow himself to be shaved.[191] On another occasion, the same patient decided to adopt a far more outlandish appearance:

> Took a strange notion to have his whiskers shaved off and also pierced his ears for earrings to make himself a female. He has written orders for a crinoline and for several changes of silk dresses.[192]

This 'wild notion' was entertained until one of his ears became swollen and inflamed and Duke's attention had to be called to it. Despite David's protests, the threads he had used to keep the puncture open were eventually removed and the ear healed. The extent to which asylum authorities did not wish to interfere in the patient's appearance or behaviour, even in cases where it breached conventional norms, is clear and Stanley was evidently relieved to report that 'the patient seems to have engendered no bad feeling towards any of us for having interfered in the matter'.[193]

At St John of God's, O'Connell often commented on the clothing and general appearance of the male patients.[194] He described James McL 'as slovenly and unkempt as ever ... never wears a coat—only a thin shirt and a "sweater" woollen jacket over it, and these he does not keep buttoned and tidy ... wears no hat, and often his shirt is hanging out over his trousers'.[195] Neat and tidy dress was considered essential and patients who removed their clothes were sometimes put in a lock suit.[196] Similarly, John Eustace Neilson described Hampstead patient Henry O'B. as being 'foolish in dress'.[197] At Stewarts, patients were encouraged to dress well. When Alice Julia B.'s mother sent her a new skirt, she was 'told she should wear it', although unfortunately she tore it up.[198] Physicians judged patients in accordance with contemporary fashions and what they considered normal.[199] For example, Elizabeth A. was reported as being 'rather fantastic in her dress, fond of decorations which are outré. Is silly in appearance and conversation'.[200] Robert Charles A. was described as being 'careless in dress', while Jane Thomasina J's progress was apparently mapped against her appearance: 'Seems gayer ... Tends to more personal decoration ... Is most demented. Has cut her hair does not know why'.[201] Joshua S.B., meanwhile, threw away his 'collar and tie frequently, believing he is not allowed to wear them'. He was described as being 'eccentric doing queer things' such as wearing 'his shirt back to front' and not 'wearing a tie and so on acting under high orders from a distance'.[202] Charles L. 'thinks he is a King. Walks around the grounds with a regal stride. His cap turned inside out to imitate a crown. His umbrella over his shoulders and his rug draped artistically from his shoulders'.[203]

CONCLUSION

This chapter has expanded on the work of Beveridge and Cox on experiences of asylum life. While both scholars have emphasised the influence of social class and status on patient experiences, this study has shown that these factors were especially significant among paying patients in Ireland's district asylums.[204] We have also seen how class identity influenced patients' expectations of their care and treatment, while simultaneously colouring their carers' expectations of their behaviour. In particular, accommodating new social classes in district asylums spawned changes in the social environment. The influx of paying patients who anticipated privileges beyond those permitted presented managerial challenges for their carers. This group was mindful of maintaining their class identity while housed in institutions intended for and accommodating primarily pauper patients. As Chaps. 3 and 4 have shown, this cohort was also more precariously positioned socially, a factor that only served to fuel their social apprehensions. Some paying patients therefore had expectations of better standards of treatment and criticised asylum conditions, particularly the food they were given.

Paying patients in district asylums were also troubled by mixing with pauper patients. This led to class tensions, which at times culminated in violence towards other patients and staff members. In an era when religious devotion was inextricably bound up with class identity and respectability, these patients were anxious to safeguard their religious identity. Some complained about having to interact with staff and patients of other denominations, expressed concern if told that their mental condition might prevent them from attending mass or church and feared exposure to proselytism. As Walsh has demonstrated, political affiliation was an equally important element of patient identity, evidenced by frequent discussions of key political figures and events.[205] While there is no record of political tensions between paying patients in the district asylums, the political unrest that characterised nineteenth-century Ireland clearly preoccupied some paying patients.

In voluntary and private asylums, conditions were apparently more in line with patients' expectations and relatively few had grievances. Likewise, there is little evidence of class or religious tensions among this cohort. Yet asylum doctors' expectations of respectable and class-appropriate behaviour from their wealthier patients were often frustrated by their regular violent outbursts. In fact, paying patients in the asylums studied evinced higher levels of violence than their pauper counterparts. This reveals that even when families invested large sums of money in asylum care, this did little to protect their relatives from violence. Patients' ill manners and strange dress and appearance also frustrated attempts to maintain harmonious surroundings in the asylum. Although moral therapy remained a dominant ideological framework for late nineteenth-century asylums and, in many respects, was still viable in the smaller, less crowded voluntary and private asylums, it was often the patients themselves who ultimately disrupted social codes and expectations of respectability.

Notes

1. Digby (1985, pp. 49–56). See also Scull (1982, pp. 186–253).
2. Finnane (1981, p. 175), Cox (2012, p. 229).
3. Ibid.
4. Cox (2012, p. 218).
5. Beveridge (1998).
6. Beveridge has found similar in Scotland: Ibid.
7. See, for example, Ibid., pp. 443–445.
8. Finnane (1981, pp. 39–40, 201–208), Cox (2012, pp. 207–212).
9. Cherry (1992).
10. Ibid.
11. Finnane (1981, p. 39).
12. Ibid.; Reynolds (1992, pp. 184–185). For more on Norman's reforms see Kelly (2016, pp. 111–114).
13. Reynolds (1992, p. 186).
14. *Annual Report of the State of the Retreat* (Dublin 1862), p. 8.
15. *The Stewart Institution and Asylum Report* (Dublin 1881), p. 14.
16. *Annual Report of the State of the Retreat* (Dublin 1865), p. 12.

17. Edward Hyde, Notice of Particulars (FHL, Bloomfield Records, 17 & 18 Dec. 1863).
18. Ibid., 19 Dec. 1863.
19. For example, Edward Hyde, Notice of Particulars (FHL, Bloomfield Records, 16 Jan. 1866).
20. Ibid., 30 Jan. 1866.
21. *Annual Report of the State of the Retreat* (Dublin 1867), p. 8.
22. For example, see Finnane's discussion of the contrasting therapeutic regimes in the Maryborough and Carlow asylums in the 1830s: Finnane (1981, p. 40).
23. For more on moral treatment and moral management, see Digby (1985, pp. 33–87).
24. Case Book 1889–1900 (Stewarts, Patient Records, pp. 108, 67).
25. Ibid., p. 46.
26. Ibid., p. 127.
27. Case Book (FHL, Bloomfield Records, p. 10).
28. Male Case Book, 1891–1892 (GM, Richmond District Lunatic Asylum, pp. 37–39).
29. Minute Book No. 12, 1867–1872 (NAI, Richmond District Lunatic Asylum, p. 285).
30. Male Case Book, 1887–1888 (GM, Richmond District Lunatic Asylum, p. 202; letter appended p. 203).
31. Office of Lunatic Asylums to Ennis District Lunatic Asylum, 4 Jun. 1891 (CCA, Our Lady's Hospital, OL1/7 Letter 1727).
32. Office of Lunatic Asylums to R.P. Gelston, 8 June 1891 (CCA, Our Lady's Hospital, OL1/7 Letter 1727a).
33. Cox (2012, pp. 210, 218).
34. Finnane (1981, p. 204).
35. Beveridge (1998, p. 432).
36. Cox (2012, p. 211).
37. Clinical Record Volume No. 4 (WCC, St Senan's Hospital, Enniscorthy, p. 360).
38. Clinical Record Volume No. 5 (WCC, St Senan's Hospital, Enniscorthy, p. 186).
39. Female Case Book, 1857–1887 (GM, Richmond District Lunatic Asylum, p. 528).
40. Beveridge (1998, p. 440).
41. Female Case Book 1897–1888 (GM, Richmond District Lunatic Asylum, pp. 533, 536).
42. Female Case Book, 1889–1890 (GM, Richmond District Lunatic Asylum, p. 607).

43. Male Case Book, 1894–1895 (GM, Richmond District Lunatic Asylum, p. 235).
44. Clinical Records Volume No. 4 (WCC, St Senan's Hospital, Enniscorthy, pp. 391–392).
45. Female Case Book, 1890–1891 (GM, Richmond District Lunatic Asylum, pp. 279, 294).
46. Female Case Book, 1892–1893 (GM, Richmond District Lunatic Asylum, pp. 530–532, 539).
47. Male Case Book, 1888–1889 (GM, Richmond District Lunatic Asylum, p. 777).
48. 'Female Case Book, 1900–1901' (GM, Richmond District Lunatic Asylum, pp. 773, 775).
49. Clarkson and Crawford (2001, pp. 105–107).
50. Clinical Record Volume No. 3 (WCC, St Senan's Hospital, Enniscorthy, p. 318).
51. Clinical Record Volume No. 6 (WCC, St Senan's Hospital, Enniscorthy, p. 30).
52. Ibid., p. 216.
53. Medical Superintendent's Memorandum Books, 1868–1889 (WCC, St Senan's Hospital, Enniscorthy, p. 138).
54. Female Case Book, 1893–1894 (GM, Richmond District Lunatic Asylum, pp. 261, 320, 323).
55. Male Case Book, 1892–1893 (GM, Richmond District Lunatic Asylum, p. 483).
56. Male Case Book, 1898 (GM, Richmond District Lunatic Asylum, appended to p. 761).
57. Female Case Book, 1891–1892 (GM, Richmond District Lunatic Asylum, p. 460).
58. Clinical Record Volume No. 3 (WCC, St Senan's Hospital, Enniscorthy, p. 336).
59. Andrews (1998, p. 266).
60. Male Case Book, 1892–1893 (GM, Richmond District Lunatic Asylum, pp. 338–339).
61. Cox (2012, pp. 211–212).
62. The Thirty-Ninth Report on the District, Criminal, and Private Lunatic Asylums in Ireland, H.C. 1890, p. 92.
63. Ibid., p. 93.
64. Malcolm (1989, p. 134).
65. *The Stewart Institution and Asylum Report* (Dublin 1890), p. 21.
66. *The Stewart Institution and Asylum Report* (Dublin 1892), p. 24.
67. *Annual Reports of the State of the Retreat.*
68. *The Stewart Institution and Asylum Report* (Dublin 1871), p. 13.

69. *The Stewart Institution and Asylum Report* (Dublin 1898), p. 24.
70. *Annual Report of the State of the Retreat* (Dublin 1855), p. 8.
71. Edward Hyde, Notice of Particulars (FHL, Bloomfield Records, 3 June 1864).
72. Ibid., 28 Jan. 1864.
73. Case Book (FHL, Bloomfield Records, p. 37).
74. Ibid., p. 59.
75. For example, Case Book 1889–1900 (Stewarts, Patient Records, pp. 73, 174).
76. Case Book (FHL, Bloomfield Records, pp. 39, 72).
77. Casebook Two (SJOGH, Patient Records, p. 54).
78. Ibid., p. 29.
79. Ibid.
80. Beveridge had found similar issues among patients in the Morningside asylum in Edinburgh. Beveridge (1998, p. 50).
81. Clinical Record Volume No. 7 (WCC, St Senan's Hospital, Enniscorthy, p. 44); Clinical Record Volume No. 4 (WCC, St Senan's Hospital, Enniscorthy, p. 386).
82. Female Case Book, 1899–1900 (GM, Richmond District Lunatic Asylum, p. 636).
83. Clinical Record Volume No. 6 (WCC, St Senan's Hospital, Enniscorthy, p. 120).
84. Female Case Book, 1889–1890 (GM, Richmond District Lunatic Asylum, p. 460).
85. Beveridge (1998, p. 442).
86. Finnane (1981, pp. 179–180).
87. Cox (2012, p. 203). For the English context, see Melling and Forsythe (2006, p. 57).
88. Female Case Book, 1889–1890 (GM, Richmond District Lunatic Asylum, p. 430).
89. Female Case Book, 1897–1898 (GM, Richmond District Lunatic Asylum, p. 340); Female Case Book, 1898–1899 (GM, Richmond District Lunatic Asylum, pp. 852, 868).
90. Female Case Book, 1895–1897 (GM, Richmond District Lunatic Asylum, p. 26).
91. Female Case Book, 1892–1893 (GM, Richmond District Lunatic Asylum, p. 848).
92. Clinical Record Volume No. 7 (WCC, St Senan's Hospital, Enniscorthy, p. 43).
93. Ibid., p. 44.
94. Ibid., p. 57.
95. Reynolds (1992, p. 88), Cox (2012, p. 206).

96. Hampstead Casebook 1890s (Highfield Hospital Group, Hampstead and Highfield Records, p. 24).
97. Casebook Two (SJOGH, Patient Records, p. 6).
98. Ibid., p. 26.
99. Ibid., p. 30.
100. Ibid., p. 45.
101. Early Hampstead Casebook 1840s (Highfield Hospital Group, Hampstead and Highfield Records, p. 14).
102. Hampstead Casebook 1890s (Highfield Hospital Group, Hampstead and Highfield Records, p. 46).
103. Digby (1985, p. 54).
104. Case Book (FHL, Bloomfield Records, p. 64).
105. Case Book 1889–1900 (Stewarts, Patient Records, p. 175).
106. Ibid., p. 137.
107. Ibid., pp. 27, 137.
108. Davidoff and Hall (1987, p. 76).
109. Ibid.
110. Comerford (1989).
111. Cox (2012, pp. 214–215).
112. Ibid.
113. Prior and Griffiths (2012).
114. Ibid., pp. 169, 182.
115. Walsh (1999, pp. 228–233).
116. Clinical Record Volume No. 7 (WCC, St Senan's Hospital, Enniscorthy, p. 465). Drapes was on the Synod of his diocese and secretary of the local choir union for 30 years. Kelly (2016, p. 95).
117. Clinical Record Volume No. 5 (WCC, St Senan's Hospital, Enniscorthy, pp. 410–411).
118. Female Case Book, 1892–1893 (GM, Richmond District Lunatic Asylum, pp. 769, 772).
119. Male Case Book, 1882–1883 (GM, Richmond District Lunatic Asylum, p. 50).
120. Female Case Book, 1898–1899 (GM, Richmond District Lunatic Asylum, pp. 489, 491).
121. *Annual Report of the State of the Retreat* (Dublin 1863), p. 12.
122. Report into the State of Lunatic Asylums, Part II, p. 161.
123. Forty-Fourth Report of the Inspectors of Lunatics (Ireland), H.C. 1895, p. 170.
124. *The Stewart Institution and Asylum Report* (Dublin 1883), p. 21.
125. *The Stewart Institution and Asylum Report* (Dublin 1896), p. 24.
126. Case Book 1889–1900 (Stewarts, Patient Records, pp. 87, 161).
127. Ibid., p. 150.

128. Edward Hyde, Notice of Particulars (FHL, Bloomfield Records, 6 Jan. 1868).
129. Daly (1984, p. 124).
130. Walsh (1999, p. 223).
131. Drapes (1894).
132. As Cox has observed, 'when Drapes was writing in 1894, the country had gone through two decades of turbulent and disruptive events', including political agitation over land ownership and tenant's rights and the Home Rule movement. Cox (2012, pp. 63–64).
133. Female Case Book, 1888–1889 (GM, Richmond District Lunatic Asylum, pp. 530–531).
134. Male Case Book, 1890–1891 (GM, Richmond District Lunatic Asylum, p. 921); Katharine O'Shea was best known for her love affair with Parnell during her marriage to Captain William O'Shea, a Catholic Nationalist MP for Galway borough. This affair, and Katharine's subsequent divorce, created a very public scandal and had negative implications for Parnell's political career. Katharine and Parnell were married in 1891.
135. Female Case Book, 1890–1891 (GM, Richmond District Lunatic Asylum, pp. 445, 450).
136. Female Case Book, 1891–1892 (GM, Richmond District Lunatic Asylum, p. 83); Female Case Book, 1898–1899 (GM, Richmond District Lunatic Asylum, p. 247).
137. Female Case Book, 1897–1898 (GM, Richmond District Lunatic Asylum, p. 535).
138. Malcolm (1989, pp. viii–x, 243–245).
139. Ibid., pp. x, 243. William Saunders Hallaran established the Cittadella private asylum in Cork. For more, see Kelly (2008, pp. 79–84).
140. Case Book (FHL, Bloomfield Records, p. 22).
141. For example, Cox (2012), Finnane (1981), Walsh (2001).
142. Cox (2012).
143. See Cox (2012), Finnane (1981, 1985), Malcolm (1999, 2003), Walsh (2001, 2004).
144. Lunacy (Ireland) Act, 1867, 30 & 31 Vic., c. 117, s. 10. For further explanation of district asylum admission procedures see Cox (2012, pp. 73–96).
145. Finnane (1981, p. 161).
146. Cox (2012, p. 220).
147. Ibid.
148. Case Book (FHL, Bloomfield Records, p. 11).
149. Ibid., p. 57.
150. Ibid., p. 63.

151. See, for example, Ibid., pp. 45, 58; Case Book 1889–1900 (Stewarts, Patient Records, pp. 5, 46, 49, 56, 77, 84, 95, 99, 115, 119, 135, 142, 144, 161, 175).

152. For example, Case Book 1889–1900 (Stewarts, Patient Records, pp. 11, 82, 77, 94, 49, 113, 144).

153. *The Stewart Institution and Asylum Report* (Dublin 1894), p. 20.

154. For example, Case Book 1889–1900 (Stewarts, Patient Records, pp. 141, 142, 143, 175).

155. Highfield Casebook (Highfield Hospital Group, Hampstead and Highfield Records, p. 21).

156. Casebook Two (SJOGH, Patient Records, p. 19).

157. Ibid., p. 40.

158. Case Book 1889–1900 (Stewarts, Patient Records, p. 100).

159. Ibid., pp. 94, 75.

160. Cox (2012, p. 206).

161. Edward Hyde, Notice of Particulars (FHL, Bloomfield Records, 28 Dec. 1863).

162. Ibid., 30 Dec. 1863.

163. Ibid., 1 Jan. 1864.

164. Malcolm (1989, p. 209).

165. Case Book (FHL, Bloomfield Records, pp. 38, 45, 71).

166. For example, Ibid., p. 27.

167. Elaine Showalter has also found this in nineteenth-century Britain: see Showalter (1986).

168. Case Book 1889–1900 (Stewarts, Patient Records, p. 167).

169. Ibid., p. 118. For other examples see Ibid., pp. 32, 44.

170. For example, Ibid., p. 44.

171. Case Book (FHL, Bloomfield Records, p. 70).

172. Ibid.

173. Hampstead Casebook 1890s (Highfield Hospital Group, Hampstead and Highfield Records, p. 12).

174. Case Book (FHL, Bloomfield Records, p. 80).

175. Hampstead Casebook 1890s (Highfield Hospital Group, Hampstead and Highfield Records, p. 16).

176. Suzuki (2001, pp. 121–122).

177. Case Book (FHL, Bloomfield Records, p. 62).

178. Ibid., pp. 73, 75.

179. McCarthy (2004, p. 122).

180. Ibid., p. 131.

181. See Gilman (1996).

182. Female Case Book, 1897–1898 (GM, Richmond District Lunatic Asylum, p. 340).

183. Wynter (2010, p. 41).
184. Ibid., pp. 41–42.
185. Edward Hyde, Notice of Particulars (FHL, Bloomfield Records, 8 Apr. 1864); Case Book 1889–1900 (Stewarts, Patient Records, p. 72).
186. Andrews (2007).
187. Edward Hyde, Notice of Particulars (FHL, Bloomfield Records, 18 Jan. 1864).
188. Case Book 1889–1900 (Stewarts, Patient Records, p. 88).
189. Reynolds (1992, pp. 183–184).
190. Edward Hyde, Notice of Particulars (FHL, Bloomfield Records, 12 Feb. 1864).
191. Ibid., 13 Feb. 1864.
192. Ibid., 6 Dec. 1865.
193. Ibid., 13 Dec. 1865.
194. For example, Casebook Two (SJOGH, Patient Records, pp. 39, 53, 22).
195. Ibid., p. 15.
196. For example, Ibid., pp. 15, 24.
197. Hampstead Casebook 1890s (Highfield Hospital Group, Hampstead and Highfield Records, p. 32).
198. Case Book 1889–1900 (Stewarts, Patient Records, p. 29).
199. This was not exclusive to Stewart's. See Showalter (1982, p. 84). Malcolm has noted similar concerns regarding patients' appearance in St Patrick's Hospital. See Malcolm (1989, p. 169).
200. Case Book 1889–1900 (Stewarts, Patient Records, p. 157).
201. Ibid., pp. 122, 35, 44.
202. Ibid., pp. 59, 25.
203. Ibid., p. 26.
204. Cox (2012, p. 218); Beveridge (1998, pp. 442–453).
205. Walsh (1999, p. 223).

References

Andrews, Jonathan. 'Case Notes, Case Histories and the Patient's Experience of Insanity at Gartnaval Royal Asylum, Glasgow, in the Nineteenth Century.' *Social History of Medicine* 11, no. 2 (1998): 255–281.

Andrews, Jonathan. 'The (Un)dress of the Mad Poor in England, c. 1650–1850.' Parts I and II. *History of Psychiatry* 18, no. 1 (2007): 5–24; 18, no. 2 (2007): 131–156.

Beveridge, Allan. 'Life in the Asylum: Patient's Letters from Morningside, 1873–1908.' *History of Psychiatry* 9 (1998): 431–469.

Cherry, Charles L. 'An Anglo-Irish Connection: York Retreat and Bloomfield Hospital.' Paper presented at the conference of Quaker Historians and Archivists, Willmington College, Ohio, USA, June 1992.

Clarkson, L. A. and E. Margaret Crawford. *Feast and Famine: A History of Food and Nutrition in Ireland, 1500–1920*. Oxford and New York: Oxford University Press, 2001.

Comerford, R. V. 'Ireland 1850–1870: Post-Famine and Mid-Victorian.' In *A New History of Ireland V: Ireland under the Union, I, 1801–1870*, edited by W. E. Vaughan, 371–385. Oxford: Oxford University Press, 1989.

Cox, Catherine. *Negotiating Insanity in the Southeast of Ireland 1830–1900*. Manchester: Manchester University Press, 2012.

Daly, Mary E. *Dublin, The Deposed Capital: A Social and Economic History, 1860–1914*. Cork: Cork University Press, 1984.

Davidoff, Leonore and Catherine Hall. *Family Fortunes: Men and Women of the English Middle Class 1780–1850*. Chicago: University of Chicago Press, 1987.

Digby, Anne. *Madness, Morality and Medicine: A Study of the York Retreat, 1796–1914*. Cambridge: Cambridge University Press, 1985.

Drapes, Thomas. 'On the Alleged Increase of Insanity in Ireland.' *Journal of Mental Science* 40 (1894): 519–543.

Finnane, Mark. *Insanity and the Insane in Post-Famine Ireland*. London: Croom Helm, 1981.

Finnane, Mark. 'Asylums, Families and the State.' *History Workshop Journal* 20, no. 1 (1985): 134–148.

Gilman, Sander. *Seeing the Insane*. Lincoln: University of Nebraska Press, 1996.

Kelly, Brendan D. 'Dr. William Saunders Hallaran and Psychiatric Practice in Nineteenth-Century Ireland.' *Irish Journal of Medical Science*, 117, no. 1 (2008): 79–84.

Kelly, Brendan. *Hearing Voices: The History of Psychiatry in Ireland*. Newbridge: Irish Academic Press, 2016.

Malcolm, Elizabeth. *Swift's Hospital: A History of St. Patrick's Hospital, Dublin, 1746–1989*. Dublin: Gill and Macmillan, 1989.

Malcolm, Elizabeth. 'The House of Strident Shadows: The Asylum, the Family and Emigration in Post-Famine Rural Ireland.' In *Medicine, Disease and the State in Ireland 1650–1940*, edited by Elizabeth Malcolm and Greta Jones, 177–195. Cork: Cork University Press, 1999.

Malcolm, Elizabeth. '"Ireland's Crowded Madhouses": The Institutional Confinement of the Insane in Nineteenth- and Twentieth-Century Ireland.' In *The Confinement of the Insane: International Perspectives, 1800–1965*, edited by Roy Porter and David Wright, 315–333. Cambridge: Cambridge University Press, 2003.

McCarthy, Áine. 'Hearths, Bodies and Minds: Gender Ideology and Women's Committal to Enniscorthy Lunatic Asylum, 1916–1925.' In *Irish Women's*

History, edited by Alan Hayes and Diane Urquhart, 115–136. Dublin: Irish Academic Press, 2004.

Melling, Joseph and Bill Forsythe. *The Politics of Madness: The State, Insanity and Society in England, 1845–1814.* London and New York: Routledge, 2006.

Prior, Pauline M. and David V. Griffiths. 'The "Chaplaincy Question" at Belfast District Asylum, 1834–1870.' In *Asylums, Mental Health Care and the Irish: Historical Studies, 1800–2010*, edited by Pauline M. Prior, 167–184. Dublin and Portland: Irish Academic Press, 2012.

Reynolds, Joseph. *Grangegorman: Psychiatric Care in Dublin Since 1815.* Dublin: Institute of Public Administration, 1992.

Scull, Andrew. *Museums of Madness: The Social Organisation of Insanity in Nineteenth-Century England.* Harmondsworth: Penguin, 1982.

Showalter, Elaine. *The Female Malady: Women Madness and Culture in England, 1830–1980.* New York: Pantheon Book, 1986.

Suzuki, Akihito. 'Enclosing and Disclosing Lunatics within the Family Walls: Domestic Psychiatric Regime and the Public Sphere in Early Nineteenth-Century England.' In *Outside the Walls of the Asylum: The History of Care in the Community, 1750–2000*, edited by Peter Bartlett and David Wright, 115–132. London: Athlone Press, 2001.

Walsh, Oonagh. '"The Designs of Providence": Race, Religion and Irish Insanity.' In *Insanity, Institutions and Society, 1800–1914: A Social History of Madness in Comparative Perspective*, edited by Joseph Melling and Bill Forsythe, 223–242. London and New York: Routledge, 1999.

Walsh, Oonagh. 'Lunatic and Criminal Alliances in Nineteenth-Century Ireland.' In *Outside the Walls of the Asylum: The History of Care in the Community 1750–2000*, edited by Peter Bartlett and David Wright, 132–152. London: Athlone Press, 2001.

Walsh, Oonagh. 'Gender and Insanity in Nineteenth-Century Ireland.' In *Sex and Seclusion, Class and Custody: Perspectives on Gender and Class in the History of British Psychiatry*, edited by Jonathan Andrews and Anne Digby, 69–93. Amsterdam and New York: Rodopi, 2004.

Wynter, Rebecca. 'Good in all Respects: Appearance and Dress at Staffordshire County Lunatic Asylum, 1818–1854.' *History of Psychiatry* 22, no. 1 (2010): 40–57.

CONCLUSION

The state occupied an uncomfortable position within debates on how to provide for paying patients. Contrary to prompt and substantial state involvement in pauper lunacy provision in the form of the ever-growing district asylum system, other social groups were not subject to any state-sponsored strategy until 1870. In the interim, the public demanded recognition of the needs of the common man or 'the great class which lies between'. The state's eventual response was to sanction the admission of paying patients in the district asylum system. The Privy Council rules for asylums regulated this practice but placed crippling limitations upon how many would be eligible and how they were to be treated.[1] Those whose relatives paid for their care in district asylums suffered the ultimate indignity of being subject to the same treatment, care and accommodation as the resident pauper patients. This accommodation therefore remained an unfavourable solution for many. Voluntary and private asylums tailored care to cost and those who could afford to were likely to pay for this alternative.

No single initiative proved effective or popular enough to monopolise provision for fee-paying patients. Instead, what resulted was a patchwork of public, voluntary and private care, intended for distinctive social groups and providing very different kinds of accommodation. At local level, the blurring of the lines between those groups eligible for and able to afford district, voluntary or private asylum care gave rise to an institutional marketplace for the non-pauper insane. Its currency was

© The Editor(s) (if applicable) and The Author(s) 2018   253
A. Mauger, *The Cost of Insanity in Nineteenth-Century Ireland*,
Mental Health in Historical Perspective,
https://doi.org/10.1007/978-3-319-65244-3

the financial means of the insane or their relatives and friends. In keeping with Cox's emphasis on the central role of the family in negotiations with asylum authorities, patients' relatives were usually responsible not only for determining when it was time to commit someone, but also where to commit them and how much should be paid for their care.[2] Factors such as cost, spending power, standard of accommodation, an institution's religious ethos and the sort of people confined there all coloured these decisions. Accordingly, and broadly speaking, certain social groups tended to utilise certain asylums.

It was within this institutional marketplace that private and voluntary asylums were eventually compelled to compete. Private asylum proprietors were popularly perceived as being intent on obtaining profits at the expense of their professional integrity and their patients' wellbeing. Yet, the lunacy inspectors paradoxically castigated these proprietors for their attempts to provide less expensive accommodation, arguing that these low rates were insufficient to finance even the most basic accommodation and care, let alone generate profits. The motivations of proprietors who continued to offer lower rates remain remote. In the English context, Parry-Jones has suggested that some proprietors felt a benevolent duty to retain patients who in reality could no longer afford expensive private accommodation.[3] However, this book has shown that proprietors who kept patients at low rates or free of charge also did so as an alternative to expelling them in order to maintain the reputation of their establishments.

Those involved in the establishment and management of the voluntary asylums met with a comparatively warm response both from the national press and the lunacy inspectors. These managing bodies flaunted the charitable nature of their initiatives—the ultimate symbol of their benevolence resting in their professed disregard for profit. As with private asylums, however, good reputation was an essential prerequisite for voluntary asylums hoping to attract a high-spending clientele. The high fees charged for many patients produced profits but these were used to house the 'respectable' or the 'fallen'—those who could no longer afford the luxuries they were accustomed to but were deemed 'deserving' nonetheless. The lunacy inspectors championed these voluntary institutions, along with St John of God's and Belmont private asylums, because they conveniently alleviated the pressure on the state and/or local rates to provide for that 'middling' sector of society not hitherto catered for.

These asylums were also considered a more acceptable alternative to the expensive private establishments.

This book has provided the first comparative study of the social profile of fee-paying patients in Irish asylums. In doing so, it complements and expands on existing analyses of patient populations in Ireland and Britain. Gender presents an interesting conundrum. Historians including MacKenzie, in the English context, and Walsh, in the Irish, have presented families as being less than willing to invest in asylum care for their female relatives.[4] Yet women were committed to even the most expensive asylums in Ireland. Further proof of the existence of a market for expensive female asylum care lies in the fact that some voluntary and private asylums limited their provision to women only. Inside the asylum, gender trumped class, as women and men were segregated by sex before social status. Patients' gender also informed asylum doctors' depictions of what had caused their illness. Women were defined by their performance in the domestic sphere, while men were measured against their roles in the public sphere—often the workplace.

A key area of difference between paying patients and their pauper counterparts was occupational profile. In contrast to district asylum patients, who were usually labourers, or from a labouring or small farming family,[5] voluntary and private asylums largely catered for merchants, white-collar workers, professionals, wealthy farmers and 'respectable' women who were not economically compelled to work. By comparison, paying patients in district asylums were more precariously positioned. Many occupied the socio-economic stratum just above the level of the pauper patients, while others were slightly better off, such as clerks, policemen and shop owners. Building on the findings of Suzuki and Levine-Clark concerning working-class asylum patients in England,[6] this book has argued that work-related causes were often ascribed to patients' illness, both in lay and medical narratives. It has also identified that paying patients entertained similar apprehensions concerning their economic condition to those expressed by patients in Cox's study of Enniscorthy and Carlow district asylums.[7]

Patients' religious denomination often determined to which asylums they were committed. While there is evidence that the emerging Catholic middle classes utilised district asylums and Catholic asylums such as St Vincent's and St John of God's, Protestants, and particularly members of the Church of Ireland, were more likely to seek accommodation in asylums that shared their religious ethos. This confirms Malcolm's contention that Protestants were probably over-represented in private asylums and hints at the superior spending power of many Protestant families in nineteenth-century Ireland.[8]

Expanding on the work of Beveridge, Cox and Walsh,[9] this book has argued that social class, status and religious affiliation informed paying patients' experiences and expectations of asylum care. Patients in this study were quick to complain if they felt that they had been treated without a due degree of 'respect', a particular concern for those in the district asylums, who were eager to distance themselves from the pauper patients they were forced to cohabit with. This informs on the fragility of paying patients' class identity as members of the Catholic and Protestant rising middle classes fiercely asserted their 'respectability' and social values. Religious tensions were also more liable to surface in district asylums than in voluntary or private ones, as the Protestant minority struggled to coexist with the Catholic majority.

Meanwhile, the families of paying patients placed high value on privacy and many invested large sums of money to secure 'appropriate' standards of accommodation and treatment. Paying for accommodation also allowed families to avoid the public scandal of dangerous lunatic certification.[10] However, the influence of the family over patients' care was limited. District asylums often prohibited relatives from supplying paying patients with clothing and food. Moreover, paying for asylum care did not guarantee patients protection from violence and injury once accommodated. This study has revealed high levels of violence among paying patients and staff in even the most expensive asylums under analysis. Private asylum patients, however, had relatively greater influence over their conditions of care than those in district asylums, as evidenced by the dismissal of staff members following patients' complaints.

Finally, asylum doctors' expectations of paying patients were often frustrated when even the wealthiest 'lady' or 'gentleman' persisted in subverting the accepted codes of behaviour for a person of their standing. In addition to violence, peculiar dress sense and general breaches of social decorum shattered the illusion of a 'domestic milieu' so central to the operation of moral therapy or management. Insanity, after all, was neither rational nor courteous and those who suffered from it were often hard pressed to behave 'appropriately'. Ultimately, providing satisfactory and effective accommodation for the non-pauper insane remained a challenging and intricate process.

NOTES

1. Cox (2012, p. 23).
2. Ibid., pp. 97–132, 148, 154–159.
3. Parry-Jones (1972), p. 86.
4. MacKenzie (1992), pp. 129, 135–136; Walsh (2004), pp. 73–74.
5. Malcolm (1999), p. 182.
6. Suzuki (2007); Levine-Clark (2004).
7. Cox (2012), p. 59, 121.
8. Malcolm (1999), p. 179.
9. Cox (2012), p. 218; Beveridge (1998), pp. 442–453; Walsh (1999), pp. 223–242.
10. Cox (2012), pp. 97–132.

REFERENCES

Beveridge, Allan. 'Life in the Asylum: Patient's Letters from Morningside, 1873–1908.' *History of Psychiatry* 9 (1998): 431–469.

Cox, Catherine. *Negotiating Insanity in the Southeast of Ireland 1830–1900.* Manchester: Manchester University Press, 2012.

Levine-Clark, Marjorie. '"Embarrassed Circumstances": Gender, Poverty and Insanity in the West Riding of England in the Early Victorian Years.' In *Sex and Seclusion, Class and Custody: Perspectives on Gender and Class in the History of British and Irish Psychiatry*, edited by Jonathan Andrews and Anne Digby, 123–148. Amsterdam and New York: Rodopi, 2004.

MacKenzie, Charlotte. *Psychiatry for the Rich: A History of the Private Madhouse at Ticehurst in Sussex, 1792–1917.* London: Routledge, 1992.

Malcolm, Elizabeth. 'The House of Strident Shadows: The Asylum, the Family and Emigration in Post-Famine Rural Ireland.' In *Medicine, Disease and the State in Ireland 1650–1940*, edited by Elizabeth Malcolm and Greta Jones, 177–195, Cork: Cork University Press, 1999.

Parry-Jones, William Ll. *The Trade in Lunacy: A Study of Private Madhouses in England in the Eighteenth and Nineteenth Centuries.* London: Routledge & Kegan Paul, 1972.

Suzuki, Akihito. 'Lunacy and Labouring Men: Narratives of Male Vulnerability in Mid-Victorian London.' In *Medicine, Madness and Social History: Essays in Honour of Roy Porter*, edited by Roberta Bivins and John V. Pickstone, 118–128. Basingstoke: Palgrave Macmillan, 2007.

Walsh, Oonagh. '"The Designs of Providence": Race, Religion and Irish Insanity.' In *Insanity, Institutions and Society, 1800–1914: A Social History of Madness in Comparative Perspective*, edited by Joseph Melling and Bill Forsythe, 223–242. London and New York: Routledge, 1999.

Walsh, Oonagh. 'Gender and Insanity in Nineteenth-Century Ireland.' In *Sex and Seclusion, Class and Custody: Perspectives on Gender and Class in the History of British Psychiatry*, edited by Jonathan Andrews and Anne Digby, 69–93. Amsterdam and New York: Rodopi, 2004.

APPENDIX: A METHODOLOGY AND SOURCES FOR CHAPTER 4

The socio-economic profile of fee-paying patients was assessed through analysis of the records of the nine selected asylums: Belfast, Ennis, Enniscorthy and Richmond district asylums, Stewarts and Bloomfield voluntary asylums, and St John of God's, Hampstead and Highfield private asylums. Admissions registers provided data on patients' gender, age, marital status, occupational background, religious persuasion, date of admission, date of discharge and length of stay. Nine separate datasets were constructed with fields containing this information. Following completion, these datasets were merged to form two separate 'master' datasets: 'pre-1868' and 'post-1868'.

The 'post-1868' dataset forms the basis for most of the analysis in Chap. 4. While Richmond opened in 1815 and received some paying patients prior to the Privy Council's sanction in 1870, paying patients were neither clearly nor systematically identifiable in the hospital's records before this date. Belfast, which opened in 1829, refused to admit paying patients until 1870 and Enniscorthy and Ennis, both founded in 1868, each received a handful of paying patients prior to 1870. For these reasons, analysis of the social profile of paying patients in the district asylums is for the period 1868–1900. The voluntary asylums, Bloomfield and Stewarts, were both accepting fee-paying patients prior to this period: Bloomfield from 1812 and Stewarts from 1857. In relation to

© The Editor(s) (if applicable) and The Author(s) 2018   259
A. Mauger, *The Cost of Insanity in Nineteenth-Century Ireland*,
Mental Health in Historical Perspective,
https://doi.org/10.1007/978-3-319-65244-3

private asylums, Hampstead admitted its first patient in 1826, Highfield in 1862 and St John of God's in 1885. Because Stewarts and Highfield had admitted only thirty and twenty-nine patients by 1867 respectively (compared with 492 and 124 after this year), analysis of admissions to these asylums is also confined to the period 1868–1900. Examination of admissions to Bloomfield and Hampstead is split between two time periods: the first, 1826–1867, and the second, 1868–1900. The latter period enables comparison between all nine asylums.

Analysis of patients is confined to first admissions. Between 1826 and 1867, 730 fee-paying patients were admitted to Bloomfield and Hampstead, ninety-nine of which were readmissions (13.6%). Between 1868 and 1900, 2411 fee-paying patients were admitted to the nine case study institutions and 288 of these were readmissions (11.9%). The district asylum datasets were constructed from a range of asylum records. Firstly, paying patients were identified in the admissions registers of the four district asylums. In the registers for Enniscorthy, Belfast and Richmond, paying patients were clearly marked. In the Ennis registers, paying patients were not readily identifiable in the admissions registers. Their names were instead found in the minute books and nominally linked to the corresponding entries in the admissions registers. Casebooks exist for Richmond (beginning in 1881) and Enniscorthy (beginning in 1891), and through nominal linkage with the datasets, paying patients' case notes were identified. Following this, five additional databases were constructed from the admissions registers of the voluntary and private asylums. With the exception of Bloomfield, these registers contained fee-paying patients only. Fee-paying patients were not distinguished from free patients in the Bloomfield registers and, accordingly, could not be identified. However, through nominal linkage with the accounts, a number of these free patients were identified. Drawing from the asylums' financial records and minute books, an additional field was created in the datasets under the heading of maintenance fees to compare rates of payment with social characteristics such as gender, religion and former occupation. These final datasets have enabled a thorough investigation of the social profile of fee-paying patients.

SELECT BIBLIOGRAPHY

Archives and Manuscripts

Clare County Archives
Records of Ennis District Lunatic Asylum:
OL1/1/1 Minute Book, 1874–1880.
OL1/1/3 Minute Book, 1880–1885.
OL1/1/5 Minute Book, 1888–1891.
OL1/1/6 Minute Book, 1891–1894.
OL1/1/7 Minute Book, 1894–1898.
OL1/1/8 Minute Book, 1898–1902.
OL1/2 Rough Minute Book, 1867–1871.
OL1/7 Correspondence, 1867–1900.
OL3/1.3 Admissions-Refusals, 1868–1900.

Friends Historical Library, Rathfarnham, Dublin
Records of Bloomfield Retreat:
Admissions Registers, 1812–1900.
Bloomfield Case Book, 1891–1898.
Edward Hyde, Notice of Particulars, 1862–1868.

Grangegorman Museum
Records of Richmond District Lunatic Asylum:
Admissions Registers, 1870–1900.
Female Case Book, 1857–1887.
Female Case Book, 1888–1889.
Female Case Book, 1889–1890.
Female Case Book, 1890–1891

© The Editor(s) (if applicable) and The Author(s) 2018
A. Mauger, *The Cost of Insanity in Nineteenth-Century Ireland*,
Mental Health in Historical Perspective,
https://doi.org/10.1007/978-3-319-65244-3

Female Case Book, 1891–1892.
Female Case Book, 1892–1893.
Female Case Book, 1893–1894.
Female Case Book, 1895–1897.
Female Case Book, 1897–1898.
Female Case Book, 1898–1899.
Female Case Book, 1899–1900.
Female Case Book, 1900–1901.
Male Case Book, 1887–1888.
Male Case Book, 1888–1889.
Male Case Book, 1890–1891.
Male Case Book, 1891–1892.
Male Case Book, 1892–1893.
Male Case Book, 1893–1894.
Male Case Book, 1894–1895.
Male Case Book, 1898.
Male Case Book, 1899–1900.
Male Case Book, 1900–1901.

Highfield Hospital Group
Records of Hampstead House and Highfield House:
Admissions Registers, 1826–1900.
Eustace Family Tree.
Hampstead Casebook 1845–1856.
Hampstead Casebook, 1891–1900.
Hampstead Proceedings, 1825–1831.
Highfield Casebook, 1891–1900.
Patient Accounts, 1896–1900.

National Archives of Ireland
Chief Secretary Office, Registered Papers.
Records of Richmond District Lunatic Asylum:
Minute Book No. 12, 1867–1872.
Minute Book No. 13, 1872–1877.
Minute Book No. 14, 1877–1881.

Public Records Office of Northern Ireland
Records of Belfast District Lunatic Asylum:
HOS/28/1/1/4 Minute Book, 1870–1882.
HOS/28/1/1/5 Minute Book, 1882–1893.
HOS/28/1/3 Admissions and Reception Registers, 1841–1900.

St. John of God's Hospital
Records of the Hospital of St. John of God:
Admissions Registers, 1885–1900.

Casebook Two, 1901–1911.
Prospectus of St. John of God Hospital, 1884.

Stewarts
Records of Stewart's Institution:
Admissions Registers, 1858–1900.
Case Book, 1889–1900.
Patient Accounts, 1858–1900.

Wexford County Council
Records of Enniscorthy District Lunatic Asylum:
Admissions Registers, 1868–1900.
Clinical Record Volume No. 3.
Clinical Record Volume No. 4.
Clinical Record Volume No. 5.
Clinical Record Volume No. 6.
Clinical Record Volume No. 7.
Medical Superintendent Memorandum Books, 1868–1889.
Minutes of the Governors of Enniscorthy District Lunatic Asylum, 1867–1882;
    1883–1898; 1898–1915.

Newspapers and Journals

Clonmel Chronicle
Dublin Journal of Medical Science
Freeman's Journal
Irish Times
Journal of Mental Science
Nenagh Guardian
The Nation

Parliamentary Papers

Annual Reports of the Inspectors General of the Prisons of Ireland, 1823–1843.
Annual Reports of the Inspectors of Criminal, District and Private Lunatic Asylums in Ireland, 1844–1919.
First and Second Report of the Committee appointed by the Lord Lieutenant of Ireland on Lunacy Administration (Ireland), 1890–1891.
Report of the Royal Commissioners of Inquiry into the State of Lunatic Asylums and other Institutions for the Custody and Treatment of the Insane in Ireland, 1857–1858.
Report and Minutes of Evidence of the Select Committee on Poor Law Union and Lunacy Inquiry (Ireland), 1878–1879.

Contemporary Printed Material

Annual Reports of the State of the Retreat (Dublin, 1811); (Dublin, 1814); (Dublin, 1836); (Dublin, 1839); (Dublin, 1849); (Dublin, 1850); (Dublin, 1852); (Dublin, 1855); (Dublin, 1856); (Dublin, 1860); (Dublin, 1862); (Dublin, 1863); (Dublin, 1864); (Dublin, 1865); (Dublin, 1866); (Dublin, 1867); (Dublin, 1901).

Drapes, Thomas. 'On the Alleged Increase of Insanity in Ireland.' *Journal of Mental Science* 40 (1894): 519–543.

Duncan, James Foulis. *Popular Errors on the Subject of Insanity Examined and Exposed* (Dublin, 1853).

MacCabe, Frederick. 'On Mental Strain and Overwork.' *Journal of Mental Science* 21 (Oct., 1875): 388–402.

Stewart Institution and Asylum Report (Dublin, 1871); (Dublin, 1872); (Dublin, 1873); (Dublin, 1874); (Dublin, 1878); (Dublin, 1879); (Dublin, 1881); (Dublin, 1883); (Dublin, 1884); (Dublin, 1885); (Dublin,1886); (Dublin, 1887); (Dublin, 1888); (Dublin, 1889); (Dublin, 1890); (Dublin, 1891); (Dublin, 1892); (Dublin, 1893); (Dublin, 1894); (Dublin, 1895); (Dublin, 1896); (Dublin, 1897); (Dublin, 1898); (Dublin, 1899); (Dublin, 1900).

Tuke, Samuel. *Description of the Retreat: An Institution near York for Insane Persons of the Society of Friends.* York: W. Alexander, 1813.

Articles and Book Chapters

Andrews, Jonathan. 'Case Notes, Case Histories and the Patient's Experience of Insanity at Gartnaval Royal Asylum, Glasgow, in the Nineteenth Century.' *Social History of Medicine* 11, no. 2 (1998): 255–281.

Andrews, Jonathan. 'Hardly a Hospital, But Charity for Pauper Lunatics?' In *Medicine and Charity before the Welfare State*, edited by Jonathan Barry and Colin Jones, 63–81. London: Routledge, 1991.

Andrews, Jonathan. 'The (Un)dress of the Mad Poor in England, c. 1650–1850.' Parts I and II. *History of Psychiatry* 18, no. 1 (2007): 5–24; 18, no. 2 (2007): 131–156.

Bartlett, Peter. 'The Asylum and the Poor Law: The Productive Alliance.' In *Insanity, Institutions and Society, 1800–1914*, edited by Joseph Melling and Bill Forsythe, 48–67. London and New York: Routledge, 1999.

Beveridge, Allan. 'Life in the Asylum: Patient's Letters from Morningside, 1873–1908.' *History of Psychiatry* 9 (1998): 431–469.

Breathnach, C.S. 'Henry Hutchinson Stewart (1798–1879): From Page to Philanthropist.' *History of Psychiatry* 9 (1998): 27–33.

Busfield, Joan. 'The Female Malady? Men, Women and Madness in Nineteenth-Century Britain.' *Sociology* 27, no. 1 (1994): 259–277.

Cherry, Steven and Munting, Roger. '"Exercise is the Thing"? Sport and the Asylum c. 1850–1950.' *The International Journal of the History of Sport* 22, no. 1 (2005): 42–58.

Comerford, R. V. 'Ireland 1850–1870: Post-Famine and Mid-Victorian.' In *A New History of Ireland V: Ireland under the Union, I, 1801–1870*, edited by W. E. Vaughan, 371–385. Oxford: Oxford University Press, 1989.

Condrau, Flurin. 'The Patient's View meets the Clinical Gaze.' *Social History of Medicine* 20, no. 3 (Dec 2007): 525–540.

Connell, K.H. 'Peasant Marriage in Ireland: Its Structure and Development since the Famine.' *Economic History Review* 14, no. 3 (1962): 502–523.

Cox, Catherine and Hilary Marland. '"A Burden on the County": Madness, Institutions of Confinement and the Irish Patient in Victorian Lancashire'. *Social History of Medicine* 28, no. 2 (2015): 263–287.

Cox, Catherine. 'Access and Engagement: The Medical Dispensary System in Post-Famine Ireland.' In *Cultures of Care in Irish Medical History, 1750–1970*, edited by Catherine Cox and Maria Luddy, 57–78. Basingstoke, 2010.

Cox, Catherine. 'Health and Welfare in Enniscorthy, 1850–1920.' In *Enniscorthy: A History*, edited by Colm Tóibín, 265–287. Wexford: Wexford County Council Public Library Service, 2010.

Cronin, Maura. '"You'd be Disgraced!": Middle-Class Women and Respectability in Post-Famine Ireland.' In *Politics, Society and Middle Class in Modern Ireland*, edited by Fintan Lane, 107–129. Basingstoke: Palgrave MacMillan, 2010.

Crossman, Virginia. 'Middle-Class Attitudes to Poverty and Welfare in Post-Famine Ireland.' In *Politics, Society and the Middle Class in Modern Ireland*, edited by Fintan Lane, 130–147. Basingstoke: Palgrave Macmillan, 2010.

Digby, Anne. 'Moral Treatment at the Retreat 1796–1846.' In *The Anatomy of Madness: Essays in The History of Psychiatry Vol. II: Institutions and Society*, edited by W.F. Bynum, Roy Porter and Michael Shepherd, 52–72. London and New York: Tavistock, 1983.

Digby, Anne. 'Women's Biological Straitjacket.' In *Sexuality and Subordination: Interdisciplinary Studies of Gender in the Nineteenth Century*, edited by Susan Mendes and Jane Rendall, 192–220. London and New York: Routledge, 1989.

Donnelly, James S. 'Landlords and Tenants.' In *A New History of Ireland V: Ireland Under the Union, I, 1801–1870*, edited by W.E. Vaughan, 332–349. Oxford: Oxford University Press, 1989.

Ellis, Rob. '"A Constant Irritation to the Townspeople"?: Local, Regional and National Politics and London's County Asylums at Epsom.' *Social History of Medicine* 26, no. 4 (2013): 653–667.

Ernst, Waltraud. 'European Madness and Gender in Nineteenth-Century British India.' *Social History of Medicine* 9 (1996): 357–382.

Finnane, Mark. 'Asylums, Families and the State.' *History Workshop Journal* 20, no. 1 (1985): 134–148.

Finnane, Mark. 'Law and the Social Uses of the Asylum in Nineteenth-Century Ireland.' In *Asylum in the Community*, edited by John Carrier and Dylan Tomlinson, 88–107. London, 1996.

Fitzpatrick, David. 'Irish Farming Families before the First World War.' *Comparative Studies in History and Society* 25 (1980): pp. 339–384.

Fitzpatrick, David. 'Marriage in Post-Famine Ireland.' In *Marriage in Ireland*, edited by Art Cosgrove, 116–131. Dublin: College Press, 1985.

Forsythe, Bill, Joseph Melling and Richard Adair. 'Politics of Lunacy: Central State Regulation and the Devon Pauper Lunatic Asylum, 1845–1914.' In *Insanity, Institutions and Society, 1800–1914*, edited by Joseph Melling and Bill Forsythe, 68–92. London and New York: Routledge, 1999.

Gribbon, H.D. 'Economic and Social History, 1850–1921.' In *A New History of Ireland VI: Ireland Under Union, 1870–1921*, edited by W.E. Vaughan, 260–356. Oxford: Oxford University Press, 1989.

Griffin, Brian. 'The Irish Police: Love Sex and Marriage in the Nineteenth and Early Twentieth Centuries.' In *Gender Perspectives in Nineteenth-Century Ireland: Public and Private Spheres*, edited by Margaret Kelleher and James H. Murphy, 168–178. Dublin: Irish Academic Press, 1997.

Healy, David. 'Irish Psychiatry. Part 2: Use of the Medico-Psychological Association by its Irish Members—Plus ça Change!' In *150 Years of British Psychiatry*, edited by Hugh Freeman and German E. Berrios, 314–320. London: Athlone Press, 1996.

Houston, Robert A. '"Not Simply Boarding": Care of the Mentally Incapacitated in Scotland during the long Eighteenth Century.' In *Outside the Walls of the Asylum: The History of Care in the Community, 1750–2000*, edited by Peter Bartlett and David Wright, 19–44. London: Athlone Press, 2001.

Houston, Robert A. 'Class, Gender and Madness in Eighteenth-Century Scotland.' In *Sex and Seclusion, Class and Custody: Perspectives on Gender and Class in the History of British and Irish Psychiatry*, edited by Jonathan Andrews and Anne Digby, 45–68. Amsterdam and New York: Rodopi, 2004.

Jones, Greta and Elizabeth Malcolm. 'Introduction: An Anatomy of Irish Medical History.' In *Medicine, Disease and the State in Ireland, 1650–1940*, edited by Elizabeth Malcolm and Greta Jones, 1–17. Cork: Cork University Press, 1999.

Lane, Joan. '"The Doctor Scolds Me": The Diaries and Correspondence of Patients in Eighteenth-Century England.' In *Patients and Practitioners: Lay Perceptions of Medicine in Pre-Industrial Society*, edited by Roy Porter, 205–248. Cambridge: Cambridge University Press, 2002.

Levine-Clark, Marjorie. '"Embarrassed Circumstances": Gender, Poverty and Insanity in the West Riding of England in the Early Victorian Years.' In *Sex and Seclusion, Class and Custody: Perspectives on Gender and Class in the History of British and Irish Psychiatry*, edited by Jonathan Andrews and Anne Digby, 123–148. Amsterdam and New York: Rodopi, 2004.

Luddy, Maria. 'Women and Work in Nineteenth- and Early Twentieth-Century Ireland: An Overview.' In *Women and Paid Work in Ireland, 1500–1930*, edited by Bernadette Whelan, 44–56. Dublin: Four Courts Press, 2000.

MacDonagh, Oliver. 'Ideas and Institutions, 1830–1845.' In *A New History of Ireland V: Ireland under the Union, I, 1801–1870*, edited by W.E. Vaughan, 193–217. Oxford: Oxford University Press, 1989.

Malcolm, Elizabeth. '"Ireland's Crowded Madhouses": The Institutional Confinement of the Insane in Nineteenth- and Twentieth-Century Ireland.' In *The Confinement of the Insane: International Perspectives, 1800–1965*, edited by Roy Porter and David Wright, 315–333. Cambridge: Cambridge University Press, 2003.

Malcolm, Elizabeth. 'The House of Strident Shadows: The Asylum, the Family and Emigration in Post-Famine Rural Ireland.' In *Medicine, Disease and the State in Ireland 1650–1940*, edited by Elizabeth Malcolm and Greta Jones, 177–195. Cork: Cork University Press, 1999.

Mauger, Alice. '"Confinement of the Higher Orders": The Social Role of Private Lunatic Asylums in Ireland, c. 1820–1860.' *Journal of the History of Medicine and Allied Sciences* 67, no. 2 (2012): 281–317.

McCarthy, Áine. 'Hearths, Bodies and Minds: Gender Ideology and Women's Committal to Enniscorthy Lunatic Asylum, 1916–25.' In *Irish Women's History*, edited by Alan Hayes and Diane Urquhart, 115–136. Dublin: Irish Academic Press, 2004.

Melling, Joseph, Bill Forsythe and Richard Adair. 'Families, Communities and the Legal Regulation of Lunacy in Victorian England: Assessments of Crime, Violence and Welfare in Admissions to the Devon Asylum, 1845–1914.' In *Outside the Walls of the Asylum: The History of Care in the Community, 1750–2000*, edited by Peter Bartlett and David Wright, 153–180. London: Athlone Press, 2001.

Melling, Joseph. 'Sex and Sensibility in Cultural History: The English Governess and the Lunatic Asylum, 1845–1914.' In *Sex and Seclusion, Class and Custody: Perspectives on Gender and Class in the History of British Psychiatry*, edited by Jonathan Andrews and Anne Digby, 177–221. Amsterdam and New York: Rodopi, 2004.

Michael, Pamela. 'Class, Gender and Insanity in Nineteenth-Century Wales.' In *Sex and Seclusion, Class and Custody: Perspective in Gender and Class in the History of British and Irish Psychiatry* edited by Jonathan Andrews and Anne Digby, 95–122. Amsterdam and New York: Rodopi, 2004.

Ó Gráda, Cormac. 'Industry and Communications, 1801–45.' In *A New History of Ireland V: Ireland under the Union, I, 1801–70*, edited by W. E. Vaughan, 137–157. Oxford: Oxford University Press, 1989a.

Ó Gráda, Cormac. 'Poverty, Population, and Agriculture, 1801–1845.' In *A New History of Ireland V: Ireland under the Union, I, 1801–70*, edited by W.E. Vaughan, 108–136. Oxford: Oxford University Press, 1989b.

Porter, Roy. 'The Patient's View: Doing Medical History from Below.' *History and Society*, 14 (1985): 175–198.

Prior, Pauline M. and David V. Griffiths. 'The "Chaplaincy Question" at Belfast District Asylum, 1834–1870.' In *Asylums, Mental Health Care and the Irish: Historical Studies, 1800–2010*, edited by Pauline M. Prior, 167–184. Dublin and Portland: Irish Academic Press, 2012.

Rosenberg, Charles E. 'Framing Disease: Illness, Society and History.' In *Framing Disease: Studies in Cultural History*, edited by Charles E. Rosenbery and Janet Golden, xiii–xxvi. New Brunswick and New Jersey: Rutgers University Press, 1992.

Showalter, Elaine. 'Victorian Women and Insanity.' In *Madhouses, Mad-Doctors and Madmen: The Social History of Psychiatry in the Victorian Era*, edited by Andrew Scull, 157–181. Philadelphia: University of Pennsylvania Press, 1981.

Smith, Leonard D. 'Close Confinement in a Mighty Prison: Thomas Bakewell and his Campaign against Public Asylums, 1810–1830.' *History of Psychiatry*, 5, no. 18 (1994): 191–214.

Smith, Leonard D. 'The County Asylum in the Mixed Economy of Care, 1808–1845.' In *Insanity, Institutions and Society, 1800–1914*, edited by Joseph Melling and Bill Forsythe, 33–47. London and New York: Routledge, 1999b.

Suzuki, Akihito. 'Enclosing and Disclosing Lunatics within the Family Walls: Domestic Psychiatric Regime and the Public Sphere in Early Nineteenth-Century England.' In *Outside the Walls of the Asylum: The History of Care in the Community, 1750–2000*, edited by Peter Bartlett and David Wright, 115–132. London: Athlone Press, 2001.

Suzuki, Akihito. 'Lunacy and Labouring Men: Narratives of Male Vulnerability in Mid-Victorian London.' In *Medicine, Madness and Social History: Essays in Honour of Roy Porter*, edited by Roberta Bivins and John V. Pickstone, 118–128. Basingstoke: Palgrave Macmillan, 2007.

Suzuki, Akihito. 'Lunacy in Seventeenth- and Eighteenth-Century England: Analysis of Quarter Sessions Records.' Parts I and II. *History of Psychiatry* 2 (1991): 437–456; 3 (1992): 29–44.

Theriot, Nancy M. 'Women's Voices in Nineteenth-Century Medical Discourse: A Step towards Deconstructing Science.' *Signs: Journal of Women in Culture and Society* 29 (1993): 1–31.

Walsh, Lorraine. 'A Class Apart? Admissions to the Dundee Royal Lunatic Asylum, 1890–1910.' In *Sex and Seclusion, Class and Custody: Perspectives* on *Gender and Class in the History of British and Irish Psychiatry*, edited by Jonathan Andrews and Anne Digby, 249–269. Amsterdam and New York: Rodopi, 2004.

Walsh, Oonagh. '"The Designs of Providence": Race, Religion and Irish Insanity.' In *Insanity, Institutions and Society, 1800–1914: A Social History of Madness in Comparative Perspective*, edited by Joseph Melling and Bill Forsythe, 223–242. London and New York: Routledge, 1999.

Walsh, Oonagh. 'Gender and Insanity in Nineteenth-Century Ireland.' In *Sex and Seclusion, Class and Custody: Perspectives on Gender and Class in the History of British Psychiatry*, edited by Jonathan Andrews and Anne Digby, 69–93. Amsterdam and New York: Rodopi, 2004.

Walsh, Oonagh. 'Lunatic and Criminal Alliances in Nineteenth-Century Ireland.' In *Outside the Walls of the Asylum: The History of Care in the Community 1750–2000*, edited by Peter Bartlett and David Wright, 132–152. London: Athlone Press, 2001.

Walton, John. 'Lunacy in the Industrial Revolution: A Study of Asylum Admission in Lancashire, 1848–1850.' *Journal of Social History* 13, no. 1 (1979–1980): 1–22.

Wright, David. 'Family Strategies and the Institutional Confinement of "Idiot" Children in Victorian England.' *Journal of Family History*, 23, no. 2 (April, 1998): 190–208.

Wright, David. 'Getting out of the Asylum: Understanding the Confinement of the Insane in the Nineteenth Century.' *Social History of Medicine* 10, no. 1 (1997): 137–155.

Wynter, Rebecca. 'Good in all Respects: Appearance and Dress at Staffordshire County Lunatic Asylum, 1818–1854.' *History of Psychiatry* 22, no. 1 (2010): 40–57.

Books

Andrews, Jonathan and Anne Digby (eds.). *Sex and Seclusion, Class and Custody: Perspectives on Gender and Class in the History of British Psychiatry.* Amsterdam and New York: Rodopi, 2004.

Bielenberg, Andy. *Ireland and the Industrial Revolution: The Impact of the Industrial Revolution on Irish Industry, 1809–1822.* London and New York: Routledge, 2009.

Bourke, Joanna. *Husbandry to Housewifery: Women, Economic Change and Housework in Ireland, 1890–1914.* Oxford: Clarendon Press, 1993.

Busfield, Joan. *Managing Madness: Changing Ideas and Practices.* London, 1986.

Cherry, Steven. *Mental Healthcare in Modern England: The Norfolk Lunatic Asylum/St Andrew's Hospital circa 1810–1998*. Suffolk: The Boydell Press, 2003.

Clarkson, L. A. and E. Margaret Crawford. *Feast and Famine: A History of Food and Nutrition in Ireland, 1500–1920*. Oxford and New York: Oxford University Press, 2001.

Cox, Catherine. *Negotiating Insanity in the Southeast of Ireland 1830–1900*. Manchester: Manchester University Press, 2012.

Daly, Mary E. *Dublin, The Deposed Capital: A Social and Economic History, 1860–1914*. Cork: Cork University Press, 1984.

Daly, Mary E. *The Famine in Ireland*. Dublin: Dundalgan Press, 1986.

Daly, Mary E. *Women and Work in Ireland*. Dundalk: Dundalgan Press, 1997.

Davidoff, Leonore and Catherine Hall. *Family Fortunes: Men and Women of the English Middle Class 1780–1850*. Chicago: University of Chicago Press, 1987.

Digby, Anne. *Madness, Morality and Medicine: A Study of the York Retreat, 1796–1914*. Cambridge: Cambridge University Press, 1985.

Earner-Byrne. Lindsey. *Mother and Child: Maternity and Child Welfare in Dublin, 1922–1960*. Manchester: Manchester University Press, 2007.

Finnane, Mark. *Insanity and the Insane in Post-Famine Ireland*. London: Croom Helm, 1981.

Garton, Stephen. *Medicine and Madness: A Social History of Insanity in New South Wales, 1880–1940*. Kensington, New South Wales, Australia: New South Wales University Press, 1988.

Gilman, Sander. *Seeing the Insane*. Lincoln: University of Nebraska Press, 1996.

Guinnane, Timothy. *The Vanishing Irish: Households, Migration, and the Rural Economy in Ireland, 1850–1914*. Princeton: Princeton University Press, 1997.

Harrison, Brian. *Drink and the Victorians: The Temperance Question in England, 1815–72*. London: Faber, 1971.

Hoppen, K. Theodore. *The Mid-Victorian Generation, 1846–1886*. Oxford: Oxford University Press, 1998.

Ingram, Allan. *Patterns of Madness in the Eighteenth Century: A Reader*. Liverpool: Liverpool University Press, 1998.

Jones, David Seth. *Graziers, Land Reform, and Political Conflict in Ireland*. Washington D.C.: Catholic University of America Press, 1995.

Kelly, Brendan. *Hearing Voices: The History of Psychiatry in Ireland*. Newbridge: Irish Academic Press, 2016.

Lane, Fintan (ed.). *Politics, Society and the Middle Class in Modern Ireland*. Basingstoke: Palgrave Macmillan, 2010b.

Luddy, Maria. *Women and Philanthropy in Nineteenth-Century Ireland*. Cambridge: Cambridge University Press, 1995.

MacDonagh, Oliver. *Ireland: The Union and Its Aftermath*. London: Allen and Unwin, 1977.

MacKenzie, Charlotte. *Psychiatry for the Rich: A History of the Private Madhouse at Ticehurst in Sussex, 1792–1917.* London: Routledge, 1992.

Malcolm, Elizabeth. *Ireland Sober, Ireland Free: Drink and Temperance in Nineteenth-Century Ireland.* Dublin: Gill and Macmillan, 1986.

Malcolm, Elizabeth. *Swift's Hospital: A History of St Patrick's Hospital, Dublin, 1746–1989.* Dublin: Gill and Macmillan, 1989.

Marland, Hilary. *Dangerous Motherhood: Insanity and Childbirth in Victorian Britain.* Basingstoke: Palgrave Macmillan, 2004.

Melling, Joseph and Bill Forsythe. *The Politics of Madness: The State, Insanity and Society in England, 1845–1914.* London and New York: Routledge, 2006.

Michael, Pamela. *Care and Treatment of the Mentally Ill in North Wales 1800–2000.* Cardiff: University of Wales Press, 2003.

Ó Gráda, Cormac. *Black '47 and Beyond: The Great Irish Famine in History, Economy, and Memory.* Princeton: Princeton University Press, 1999.

Ó Gráda, Cormac. *Ireland before and after the Famine: Exploration in Economic History, 1800–1925.* Manchester: Manchester University Press, 1993.

Ó Gráda, Cormac. *Ireland: A New Economic History, 1780–1939.* Oxford: Oxford University Press, 1994.

O'Hare, Pauline. *In the Care of Friends.* Dublin: Highfield Healthcare, 1998.

Oppenheim, Janet. *'Shattered Nerves': Doctors, Patients and Depression in Victorian England.* New York and Oxford: Oxford University Press, 1991.

Parry-Jones, William Ll. *The Trade in Lunacy: A Study of Private Madhouses in England in the Eighteenth and Nineteenth Centuries.* London: Routledge & Kegan Paul, 1972.

Pick, Daniel. *Faces of Degeneration: A European Disorder, c. 1848–1918.* Cambridge: Cambridge University Press, 1989.

Porter, Roy. *A Social History of Madness: Stories of the Insane.* London: Weidenfeld and Nicolson, 1987.

Preston, Margaret H. *Charitable Words: Women, Philanthropy and the Language of Charity in Nineteenth-Century Dublin.* Westport, Conn.: Praeger, 2004.

Prunty, Jacinta. *Dublin Slums, 1800–1925: A Study in Urban Geography, 1800–1925.* Dublin and Portland: Irish Academic Press, 1998.

Rains, Stephanie. *Commodity, Culture and Social Class in Dublin 1850–1916.* Dublin and Portland: Irish Academic Press, 2010.

Reynolds, Joseph. *Grangegorman: Psychiatric Care in Dublin Since 1815.* Dublin: Institute of Public Administration, 1992.

Robins, Joseph. *Fools and Mad: A History of the Insane in Ireland.* Dublin: Institute of Public Administration, 1986.

Scull, Andrew. *Museums of Madness: The Social Organisation of Insanity in Nineteenth-Century England.* Harmondsworth: Penguin, 1982.

Scull, Andrew. *The Most Solitary of Afflictions: Madness and Society in Britain, 1700–1900.* New Haven: Yale University Press, 1993.

Showalter, Elaine. *The Female Malady: Women Madness and Culture in England, 1830–1980*. New York, Pantheon Book, 1986.

Smith, Leonard D. *Cure, Comfort and Safe Custody: Public Lunatic Asylums in Early Nineteenth-Century England*. London and New York: Leicester University Press, 1999.

Suzuki, Akihito. *Madness at Home: The Psychiatrist, the Patient and the Family in England, 1820–1860*. Berkeley and Los Angeles: University of California Press, 2006.

Vaughan, W.E. *Landlords and Tenants in Mid-Victorian Ireland*. New York: Oxford University Press, 1994.

Walsh, Oonagh. *Anglican Women in Dublin: Philanthropy, Politics and Education in the Early Twentieth Century*. Dublin, 2005.

Theses

Byrne, Fiachra. 'Madness and Mental Illness in Ireland: Discourses, People and Practices, 1900 to c. 1960.' PhD diss., University College Dublin, 2011.

Cox, Catherine. 'Managing Insanity in Nineteenth-Century Ireland.' PhD diss., University College Dublin, 2003.

INDEX

© The Editor(s) (if applicable) and The Author(s) 2018   273
A. Mauger, *The Cost of Insanity in Nineteenth-Century Ireland*,
Mental Health in Historical Perspective,
https://doi.org/10.1007/978-3-319-65244-3

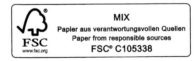